**Bethlem
Royal and
Maudsley
Hospital**

manual of

Clinical Psychiatric Nursing Principles and Procedures

Bethlem Royal and Maudsley Hospital

manual of
Clinical Psychiatric Nursing Principles and Procedures

by

Susan Ritter BA MA RGN RMN
Lecturer in Psychiatric Nursing, Institute of
Psychiatry, University of London, and Honorary
Clinical Nurse Specialist, Bethlem Royal and
Maudsley Hospital

Harper & Row, Publishers

Philadelphia
New York
St. Louis
Sydney

San Francisco
London
Singapore
Tokyo

Harper & Row Ltd.
Middlesex House
34–42 Cleveland Street
London
W1P 5FB

British Library Cataloguing in Publication Data

Ritter, Susan
    Manual of clinical psychiatric nursing.
    1. Psychiatric patients. Nursing
    I. Title
    610.73′68

    ISBN 0–06–318436–2

Typeset by Inforum Typesetting, Portsmouth
Printed and bound by The Alden Press, Oxford

Contents

Preface

I am honoured to write the preface to this significant publication, which will have a powerful impact on psychiatric nursing practice in the UK.

Following the success of the first edition of The Royal Marsden Hospital Manual of Clinical Nursing Procedures, Harper & Row approached the Bethlem Royal and Maudsley Hospital Special Health Authority to discuss the possibility of publishing a comparable book for psychiatric nurses. Thanks to the commitment of the Special Health Authority and the hard work of the author and the Editorial Board this innovative work has at last come to fruition. The Directors of Nursing Services, Mrs Pamela Tibbles and Mr David Russell, the Director of Nurse Education, Mr Robert Combes and a Senior Tutor, Mrs Joan Smith, took the lead in establishing the project with the Chief Nursing Officer, Miss Juliette Wiltshire and the General Manager, Mr Eric Byers. A multidisciplinary editorial board was set up, chaired by a Member of the Special Health Authority.

To ensure the success of the project, the Special Health Authority nominated a Senior Charge Nurse, Miss Susan Ritter, as author supported by Trust Funds, to work full-time on the project for two years. Miss Ritter reviewed the relevant literature and produced successive drafts for critical discussion with nurses and other colleagues.

Both this book and its companion volume have been produced in London postgraduate University hospitals. With their associated Institutes, these hospitals provide a suitable environment in which to promote clinical practice informed by nursing research and education. It is that combination of the academic and the practical which gives this book its value. Using these procedures nurses can be confident that patients will receive care in accordance with recent research findings and well established clinical principles.

Dr Julia Brooking
Senior Lecturer and Head of the Section of Psychiatric Nursing, Institute of Psychiatry
Chief Nursing Adviser to the Bethlem Royal and Maudsley Hospital

July 1989

Acknowledgements

John Barker, Professor Robert Cawley, Padmal De Silva, Bob Combes, Jo Brand, Alastair Williamson, Griselda Campbell and David Russell were the Editorial Board. Despite their already immensely busy schedules, they diligently read, criticised and discussed successive drafts of the manual, and attended many editorial meetings over more than two years.

My thanks are also due to Peter Pocock, Bob Chapman, Phil Barker and Bill Yule who reviewed the whole MS in detail. Their advice was carefully considered, if not always heeded. I think, and I hope they agree, that it led to improvements.

I acknowledge the generous permission by Reginald Pyne, on behalf of the United Kingdom Central Council for Nursing, Midwifery and Health Visiting to reprint copies of the UKCC leaflets setting out the various aspects of the Code of Professional Conduct.

A Macintosh Plus computer simplified the word processing immeasurably.

The people whose names follow represent the many who gave me help, contributions and encouragement in the preparation of the manual.

King Edward's Hospital Fund Librarians, Royal College of Nursing Librarians, Institute of Psychiatry Librarians, Normanby College Librarians, Eric Byers, David Woodward, Juliette Wiltshire, John Foskett, John Roscoe, Helen Costigan, Janine James, John Corbett, Philippa Geraghty, Tom Carrigan, Rob Burrows, Paul Williams, Beatrice Stevens, Rita Bourke, Mrs King, Murray Jackson, Barbara Pottle, Theresa Wilkinson, Buddah Singh, Pamela Tibbles, Geoff Haines, Jamie Gillespie, Fay Hall, Susan Smith, Breda O'Neill, Maureen Cunningham, Gillian Cormack, Vi Cain, Michael Wilding, David Morrison, Conor Duggan, Peter May, Lee Frisby, Chris Rance, Sue Davison, Robin Jacobson, Ivan Clout, Joe Connolly, Julia Brooking, Gerald Russell, Stuart Checkley, Gunna Dietrich, Sally Jacobson, Mary Watkins, Robin Murray, Ben Thomas, Debbie Heavey, and Ulla Arnel.

Introduction

The aims of this manual are, first, to set out general principles and procedures for the practice of psychiatric nursing; second, to provide guidelines for consideration by psychiatric nurses of the most common issues which arise in the course of the nurse–inpatient relationship in mental illness hospitals in the UK; third, to encourage creativity and initiative by psychiatric nurses who are interested in operationalizing psychiatric nursing practice.

The procedures documented in the manual derive from the policies and practice of the Bethlem Royal and Maudsley Hospital, but the book is intended to review general aspects of the issues involved. In so doing it is intended to be relevant to all adult inpatient units in the National Health Service in the UK.

This procedure manual is designed to be a step in the process of identifying the components of psychiatric nursing as a discipline, and of enhancing traditional nursing activities with research-based ones. It is recognized that considerable progress has been made in specialist areas such as behaviour therapy, liaison psychiatry and community psychiatric nursing, but the manual was deliberately planned within the specific limits of adult, inpatient general psychiatric nursing. Users' criticisms will be warmly welcomed.

The succession of scandals of ill-treatment of patients in hospitals in the UK in the 1960s and 1970s was accompanied by a polarization of psychiatry and anti-psychiatry within hospitals as well as outside them. Task-based nursing has become associated with practices which dehumanize both nurses and patients, but in order that audit and other evaluation can be routinely carried out, the elements of psychiatric nursing practice must be identified.

Each chapter begins with an introductory discussion which refers to selected material from the relevant literature. The procedures themselves are more or less detailed depending on the degree to which it is thought that nurses are free to interpret the principles behind each nursing activity. For example, in procedures where nurses have specific statutory obligations the tasks are analysed more specifically and allow less flexibility than where nurses have more general professional obligations.

As well as specific reference material for each section of the manual a selection has been compiled which is recommended for further reading. The literature is biased towards practice in the UK, although it is acknowledged that the bulk of relevant nursing research originates in the USA.

The focus of this book is the person who has been admitted to a mental illness hospital. For this reason, the terminology of the manual follows the currently accepted practice in the UK of referring to such people as 'patients', and to diagnoses as defined in the International Classification of Diseases (ICD-9). It is emphasized that the word 'patient' describes a person who one minute has needs, the next rights, and the next represents the object of that other, far from unitary phenomenon: nursing care.

As has been said, the psychiatric nursing practice that is recommended in the manual is based on a multiplicity of sources. It is hoped that in order to provide the most effective, most humane care possible, psychiatric nurses will be encouraged to use the wealth of material available from clinical science, the social and natural sciences and from the humanities in order to define their personal philosophies for their nursing practice.

In procedures where pronouns are used and the gender of a person could be understood to be that of either a woman or a man, both sexes are referred to. It is acknowledged that the practice may appear cumbersome. The aim was to conform with accepted English usage.

Susan Ritter

July 1989

Part One

Nursing Process

1

Nursing Assessment

DEFINITION

Assessment is defined as the collection and documentation of primary and secondary information about a patient (Whyte and Youill, 1984), and the re-examination of this information in the light of outcomes of nursing plans and interventions.

Assessment is a dynamic activity. That is, it changes constantly in response to changes in the patient as well as in the nurses performing the assessment. Recordings of assessments occur in at least five forms: on admission, in objective measurements, in interaction process recordings, in progress notes and in the evaluation of plans. For this reason portions of records of assessment activities are found throughout the nursing process documentation.

DISCUSSION
Aims of assessment

The purpose of psychiatric nursing assessment has often been seen as being to facilitate a psychiatric diagnosis. While the psychiatric nurse's assessment may contribute to the diagnostic process employed by the psychiatrist, the patient's expression of symptoms may differ with each person with whom he or she comes into contact, depending on the quality of the relationship and other contextual variables. Although patients who experience hallucinations may be described as 'hallucinated' as though one hallucinated patient is like another, the nature of the symptom may well be different for each patient. Moreover, there is no objective way to determine if hallucinations or complaints of pain are 'real' whereas some other forms of behaviour can be measured and confirmed experimentally if necessary (Ludwig, 1980).

Walton (1986) suggests that the nursing process has been interpreted at four levels: as a system of recording; a system for organizing work; a tool for education and practice; and as an ideology. As a system of recording, it is relatively easy to operationalize, but the other levels are much more difficult. To employ the nursing process at these levels requires the user to identify the models and beliefs by which he or she intends to work.

The account of the stages of the nursing process in this manual is weighted towards their role in systematizing record-keeping. Nursing models, the organizational methods for delivering nursing care and the means by which they are learned and taught are only briefly discussed or represented in the actual procedures.

If the nursing process is viewed at the level of recording nursing care, the problem-solving method provides an economical way of identifying its components. The nursing process is thus agreed to be a 'deliberate organised problem-solving approach incorporating the principles of scientific method' (Ashworth et al., 1987, p. 36). According to this view the nurse who uses a scientific approach makes nursing observations, which lead to the formation of hypotheses or assessments, which in turn lead to predictions or plans. Verification of predictions or plans comes about by observation of their outcomes. Testing predictions leads to verification or to new hypotheses. Implementation of plans leads to reassessment. Just as testing predictions leads to knowledge and understanding of natural phenomena, so implementing plans, it is said, leads to knowledge and understanding of the individual patient.

Decision-making

Problem-solving is one type of aid to decision-making. De la Cuesta (1983) notes that in the UK, nursing assessments have not been generally used as the preliminary step to planning, but as ends in themselves. That is, they have not been used to help nurses make decisions. Ashworth (Ashworth et al., 1987) implies that this was the case when she was selecting centres to participate in the World Health Organization's study of nursing care. De la Cuesta also noted that in the UK, use of the nursing process involves patients' co-operation in nursing care, rather than their participation, so that patients may not be required to make decisions either.

Another main approach to decision-making is that of systems analysis. Leaving aside the question of the extent to which problem-solving is actually practised, a tension exists between it and the systems approach, particularly for psychiatric nurses (Altschul, 1978). The notion that a complex system like human service delivery represents a cause and effect process moving through time in straight lines was criticized by Levin *et al.* (1976), working from a systems perspective. The approach in this procedure attempts to combine elements from problem-solving and systems methods.

The problem-solving view assumes that the knowledge and understanding derived from assessment and planning enable nurses to help patients to meet needs and to solve their problems. However, as Cronenwett (1983) points out, different assumptions about the nature of helping will lead to different interventions by the helper. She recommends that when applying the nursing process the nurse should focus on the problem-solving approach as it applies to both client and nurse. The nurse who involves the patient in the assessment process is, according to Cronenwett, more likely to be able to select a model of helping or nursing care appropriate to that person.

Holism and reductionism
Systems approaches have been identified with holism (Riehl and Roy, 1980). Both holistic and reductionist approaches attempt to understand complex situations. In recent years a holistic approach to nursing has been esteemed at the expense of a reductionist approach, although as Cronenwett (1983) indicates, a reductionist or 'medical-model approach' allows nurses and patients to ignore the difficult-to-control psychological and physical aspects of disease processes and crises. Reductionism, the breaking down of complex situations into simple components, has the merit of making complexity manageable.

Assessment
The nurse may use many models of assessment, including family systems, adaptation and crisis intervention. Two main models are discussed in this procedure: the medical model and the behavioural assessment.

Medical model
The medical model relies on precision of diagnosis to organize treatment. That is, the clinician is required to collect data in order to make inferences from them and to construct the treatment plan on the basis of a diagnosis.

Behavioural assessment
The need to make inferences is reduced in a behavioural assessment because, unlike the medical model, the focus is on observable behaviours.

A behavioural assessment is based on the view that there are three main categories of behaviour or responses, and that all activity by an organism can be termed behaviour. Weick's (1985) classification is of 'three major response systems – verbal, overt, physiological' (p. 601). Nelson and Hayes (1981) describe the categories of 'overt motor behaviour, physiological-emotional behaviour, and cognitive-verbal behaviour' (p. 17). They cite Lang (1968) in noting that 'these three systems do not necessarily covary' (p. 17). However, systematic covariation is found in the major disorders such as depression, schizophrenia and organic brain reactions. The diagnosis of depression or schizophrenia is made as an inference from observations of the variations in behaviour within the three systems and of the ways in which they do or do not covary.

In contrast to the psychiatric nurse, other members of the multidisciplinary team, such as psychologists and doctors, have well-defined categories of assessment. The heterogeneous data that form the basis of a psychiatric nursing assessment need to be organized in such a way that they make sense to people other than the individual nurse and patient. Observations, interactions, negotiations between the patient and the nursing and multidisciplinary teams, definitions of problems, plans, evaluations and assessments are activities which cause complex records to be accumulated. These records are tools for organizing nursing care, means of communication within and between disciplines, and evidence of the nurse's fulfilment of his or her duty of care to the patient.

TECHNIQUES OF ASSESSMENT
Since 1978 a good deal of work has been done by nurses trained as behavioural therapists, in whose discipline the accurate measurement and classification of behaviour are essential for targeting desired change. Much of this work is summarized by Barker (1985).

Nursing history
The idea of a nursing history derives from the medical model, which hypothesizes that careful analysis of events and symptoms preceding the current episode will lead eventually by inductive steps to a diagnosis and therefore to a specific treatment. Because of the difficulty in psychiatry of formulating a diagnosis and treatment plan, the significance of a patient's history depends on other kinds of information.

The decision to take a nursing history will be made by the nursing team and, possibly, the multidisciplinary clinical team for the individual patient. A standardized nursing history form is generally not found particularly useful, although it is helpful in three sets of circumstances:

1 admission of any patient likely to cause hazards;
2 admission of a violent or potentially violent patient;
3 when a patient is transferred from another hospital.

Diagnosis

Nelson and Hayes (1981, p. 10) recommend that 'an idiosyncratic behavioural classification schema' is not used when assessing patients. They recommend the use of DSM–III (revised 1987) in order to communicate with the scientific community generally, and to take advantage of its reliability, and the number of aids to diagnosis which have been devised to make use of DSM–III. The International Classification of Diseases (ICD–9) provides similar advantages to those of DSM–III (Revised).

DOCUMENTATION

The content of assessment documentation varies according to the organizational system and the model of nursing used in the individual ward or department. However, the documents themselves will include the following:

1 admission sheets;
2 observation charts;
3 patients' personal notes, as written or as dictated to the nurse;
4 progress notes, including interaction process recordings;
5 rating scales and graphs.

Admission is a detailed procedure in itself and is covered separately, in Chapter 17.

Rating scales

Downing, Francis and Brockington (1980) review the history of nurse-rating scales, noting that the outcomes of trials of pharmacological treatment are often assessed by data accumulated by such scales. Wilkinson (1979) provides a note of caution in her account of a double-blind study of behaviour change in a ten-year-old boy, the required observations being carried out by nurses. There was a good deal of difficulty in achieving consistency between nurses' ratings of even highly visible behaviour such as gait. Having tested a selection of rating scales Downing and Brockington (1978, p. 560) are cautious in recommending them for assessment of individual patients.

However, carefully documented and repeated use of a rating scale with individual patients, together with evaluation of its results against actual outcomes for those patients, can gradually provide the psychiatric nurse

with evidence of the worth of the scale in the assessment process.

The assessment process

The assessment process can be divided into three stages. The first stage involves observation of the patient's behaviour in as wide a variety of settings as possible, and checking out findings with the patient, his or her significant others, and other staff. The second involves agreeing with the nursing and multidisciplinary teams which of the patient's behaviours are to be selected with a view to change, before going on to more detailed observation and measurement. The third stage involves defining, observing and measuring target behaviours or responses as specifically as possible.

FIRST STAGE OF ASSESSMENT

1 Observe the patient's behaviour in as wide a variety of settings as possible (there might be a need to set up situations to evoke responses, e.g. talking/walking with the patient; family meetings; attending ward groups).
2 Record the observations.
3 Decide in what ways the everyday behaviour of the patient's peers, friends, family coincides with or differs from that of the patient.
4 Establish whether the patient's significant others, employer, people in society at large, friends or hospital staff think that his or her behaviour is a problem.
5 Establish whether the patient agrees with these accounts. Items 3, 4 and 5 are to do with establishing some sort of validity for the objectives and interventions that will be planned with the patient. The other reason for attending to the settings for a person's behaviour is that deviation from the behaviour that is usually accepted in specific settings such as offices or shops is used as evidence that someone is psychologically disturbed (Weick, 1985, p. 612).
6 Discuss the observations with other members of the nursing and multidisciplinary teams.

SECOND STAGE OF ASSESSMENT

1 Agree with the nursing and multidisciplinary teams which of the patient's behaviours are to be selected with a view to change.
2 .Choose the instruments and methods by which these behaviours will be observed and measured.
3 Ensure that observations are made and recorded systematically and consistently.

THIRD STAGE OF ASSESSMENT

1 Define the target behaviours as specifically as possible.

2 Observe and measure the behaviour as accurately as possible in order to establish a baseline for comparison after any interventions.
3 Identify and record the antecedents of or stimuli for the patient's behaviour.
4 Identify and record the consequences of the behaviour.
5 Select the methods for measuring and recording observations, e.g. will only overt behaviour be measured or will self-report (e.g. headaches, tension, hallucinations) and physiological (e.g. pulse, blood pressure) measures be used?

Avoid the use of global concepts such as withdrawn, depressed, uncommunicative, or overactive. Instead observe and specify the behaviours which lead nurses to infer that the patient is depressed or overactive. During the planning and implementation stages nurses will identify specific objectives in order to direct nursing care. Global concepts promote vagueness rather than specificity.

GUIDELINES: ASSESSMENT OF PATIENT

Action

Rationale

1 Observe the patient's behaviour in as wide a variety of settings as possible.

To identify antecedents and effects of the behaviour.

2 Decide in what ways the patient's behaviour is similar to or different from friends, relatives or other patients.

To establish validity for any subsequent nursing interventions to change the behaviour.

3 Establish whether the patient, his or her friends and relatives, and the staff think the patient's behaviour is a problem.

To work out a rationale for subsequent nursing interventions.

4 See whether the patient agrees with the findings from 1–3 above.

It will be necessary to gain the patient's consent to any treatment programme.

5 Discuss all observations with other members of the multidisciplinary clinical team (MDCT).

In order to validate the assessment as far as is possible.

6 Agree with the patient and the MDCT which of the patient's behaviours will be chosen with a view to change.

In order to start the second phase of the assessment process.

7 Choose the instruments and methods by which these behaviours will be observed and measured.

So that they will be assessed as accurately as possible.

8 Ensure that observations are made and recorded systematically and consistently.

In order that subsequent changes can be accurately measured.

9 Define the target behaviours as specifically as possible.

In order to start the third stage of the assessment process.

10 Select the methods for measuring and recording observations.

So that target behaviours will be specified and differentiated, for example between motor activity and physiological activity.

11 Avoid the use of global terms such as withdrawn, depressed, uncommunicative.

Global concepts hinder specificity in subsequent plans.

12 Complete the front sheet of the nursing record in accordance with central medical records policy.

In order to record key information such as next of kin, status under the Mental Health Act 1983, address.

13 File the front sheet at the beginning of the nursing record.

So that it is easily accessible for frequently used information and for admission baselines.

14 File an index to the nursing record containing the headings of the patient's individual charts, scales and graphs.

To facilitate access and information retrieval.

15 Update the index as necessary.

To facilitate access and information retrieval.

16 Complete two missing persons forms.

(a) So that if needed they are not completed from memory.
(b) If they are needed, a copy may be supplied to the police and a copy retained in the nursing record.

17 File the missing persons forms after the front sheet.

So that they are in a consistent place from patient to patient and from ward to ward.

18 Record the patient's weight on a graph at least once a week.

(a) Weight is often an index to pathology.
(b) So that fluctuations may be seen at a glance.

19 File the observation charts in an order such as from A–Z.

(a) Because easy reference is required to many different kinds, depending on the individual patient. Examples include behaviour charts, fluid balance charts, sleep charts, weight charts, depression inventory graphs and premenstrual assessments.
(b) So that there is a simple system which is the same from ward to ward.

20 At a predetermined interval, say weekly, plot on a simple graph the results of individual rating scales. See Figure 1.1 for an example of scales for self-report measures. Of the many possible types, examples are visual analogue scales of symptoms or complaints, as well as pre-printed inventories.

So that fluctuations may be summarized and seen at a glance.

21 File the progress notes in date order, the last sheet in the file bearing the current date.

(a) To be consistent with conventional practice.
(b) Because it is usual to use books reading front to back and left to right.

22 File the progress notes after the care plans, occupational therapy programmes and pass forms.

So that the nursing record follows the stages of assessment, planning, implementation and evaluation.

23 Maintain a minimum of daily, nightly and weekly progress notes.

(a) Legal recommendations are for daily entries in the nursing record.
(b) Collation of information on a weekly basis helps evaluation and monitors progress.

24 Start each entry in the progress notes with the date in figures and words, and the time using the twenty-four-hour clock.

(a) To pinpoint changes accurately.
(b) To avoid confusion between day and night when referring retrospectively to the notes.

ANALOGUE SCALES   Hospital No. ....

Patient ....   Primary Nurse ....

Construct to be rated:

0	1	2	3	4	5	6	7	8	9	10
not at all					definitely					extremely

Date/Time:

Construct to be rated:

0	1	2	3	4	5	6	7	8	9	10
not at all					definitely					extremely

Date/Time:

Construct to be rated:

0	1	2	3	4	5	6	7	8	9	10
not at all					definitely					extremely

Date/Time:

Construct to be rated:

0	1	2	3	4	5	6	7	8	9	10
not at all					definitely					extremely

Date/Time:

Construct to be rated:

0	1	2	3	4	5	6	7	8	9	10
not at all					definitely					extremely

Date/Time:

Figure 1.1 Example of scales for self-report measures

25 Each entry is signed in full with the time and date it was made. If the signature is illegible, it is accompanied by block capitals.

(a) To ensure accountability.
(b) To facilitate information retrieval.
(c) To facilitate audit.

26 Start each daily or nightly progress note with an account of any discussion with the patient at the beginning of the shift.

(a) It is desirable to negotiate in advance any work to be done with patients.
(b) The way in which such negotiation is carried out influences the degree to which patients are prepared to go along with it.

27 Record objectives for the shift, agreed with the patient wherever possible. If the objectives are the same as those already recorded in the care plan, refer to them and to the date of the care plan.

To provide the basis for audit of nursing care.

28 If an interaction takes place during the span of duty, write process recordings using a format which includes the following:
  (i) pre-interaction target;
  (ii) setting for the interaction;
  (iii) summary (of the main points and the patient's demeanour);
  (iv) verbatim account (of the essential parts of the interaction);
  (v) evaluation.

(a) To facilitate information retrieval.
(b) To facilitate clinical supervision.
(c) To facilitate evaluation and audit.

29 At the end of the shift, record the outcome of the objectives set at the beginning.

(a) To evaluate immediately.
(b) To provide the basis of any retrospective evaluation.

30 Complete each shift's entry in the progress notes by a concise summary using one or more of the headings summarized in 31–37.

To provide a quickly scanned basis for fuller summaries written for case discussions or weekly progress notes.

31 When writing weekly summaries, classify material in the following categories:
  (A) physical state;
  (B) psychological state;
  (C) social circumstances;
  (D) values and preferences;
  (E) behaviour;
  (F) safety.

(a) To facilitate information retrieval.
(b) To speed up the process of memorizing the headings.
(c) To ensure consistent organization of information from patient to patient and from ward to ward.
(d) So that the same core of information is available regardless of the nursing model used.

32 Include the folowing material under
  (A) physical state:
  (i) appetite
  (ii) diet;
  (iii) hygiene;
  (iv) libido;
  (v) self-care;
  (vi) sleep;
  (vii) weight;
  (viii) menses.

As for 31.

33 Include the following material under
  (B) psychological state:
  (i) attention;
  (ii) concentration;
  (iii) affect;
  (iv) memory;
  (v) mood;
  (vi) perception;
  (vii) speech and thoughts;
  (viii) orientation;
  (ix) level of consciousness;

As for 31.

(x)   level of awareness of environment.

34   Include the following material under   As for 31.
        (C)   social circumstances:
        (i)   employment status;
        (ii)   involvement outside hospital;
        (iii)   significant others;
        (iv)   social competence (formally and informally);
        (v)   visitors.

35   Include the following material under   As for 31.
        (D)   values and preferences:
        (i)   the patient's view of his or her nursing needs;
        (ii)   the patient's view of his or her own capabilities;
        (iii)   the patient's view of care and changes that are
                occurring.

36   Include the following material under   As for 31.
        (E)   behaviour:
        (i)   the patient's ways of occupying him- or herself;
        (ii)   recreational skills (depending on the availability of,
                say, occupational therapy);
        (iii)   social interaction with other patients, staff, visitors,
                family and friends.

37   Include the following material under   As for 31.
        (F)   safety:
        (i)   safety to self;
        (ii)   safety to others.

38   Once full notes have been written under a given   (a)   To ensure brevity.
        heading, anything that remains unchanged in   (b)   To maintain clarity.
        subsequent assessments need not be repeated.

39   Refer to dates of previous entries when referring to   To facilitate information retrieval.
        aspects of the patient that are unchanged.

40   Record the patient's own account as often as nursing   (a)   To ensure that the patient's own experiences are at the
        summaries are made.   centre of the nursing record.
                                                                  (b)   To facilitate comparison between nurses' and patients'
                                                                         views.

41   Offer the patient paper to write his or her own notes.   So that the patient's self-report can be studied along with
                                                                     the nurses' notes.

42   Record notes that the patient dictates.   Patients are not necessarily prepared to write their own
                                                          notes.

REFERENCE MATERIAL
References

Altschul, A. (1978) A systems approach to the nursing process, *Journal of Advanced Nursing*, Vol. 3, pp. 333–40.

Ashworth, P. *et al.* (1987) *People's Needs for Nursing Care: A European Study*, WHO, Copenhagen.

Barker, P. (1985) *Patient Assessment in Psychiatric Nursing*, Croom Helm, Beckenham.

Cronenwett, L.R. (1983) Helping and nursing models, *Nursing Research*, Vol. 32, no. 6, pp. 342–6.

De la Cuesta, C. (1983) The nursing process: from development to implementation, *Journal of Advanced Nursing*, Vol. 8, pp. 365–71.

Downing, A.R. and Brockington, I.F. (1978) Nurse-rating of psychotic behaviour, *Journal of Advanced Nursing*, Vol. 3, pp. 551–61.

Downing, A.R., Francis, A.F. and Brockington, I.F. (1980) A comparison of information sources in the study of psychotic illness, *British Journal of Psychiatry*, Vol. 137, pp. 38–44.

DSM–III (rev) (1987) *Diagnostic and Statistical Manual of Mental Disorders* (3rd edn, revised) DSM–III–R, American Psychiatric Association, Washington DC.

ICD–9 (1978) *Manual of the International Statistical Classification of Diseases, Injuries, and Causes of Death*, WHO, Geneva.

Lang, P.J. (1968) Fear reduction and fear behaviour: problems in treating a construct, in J.M. Schlien (ed.) *Research in Psychotherapy*, Vol. 3, American Psychological Association, Washington DC.

Levin, G. *et al.* (1976) *The Dynamics of Human Service Delivery*, Ballinger, Cambridge, Mass.

Ludwig, A.M. (1980) *Principles of Clinical Psychiatry*, Free Press, New York.

Nelson, R.O. and Hayes, S.C. (1981) Nature of behavioural assessment, in M. Hersen and A.S. Bellack (eds.) *Behavioural Assessment: A Practical Handbook*, Pergamon Press, New York.

Riehl, J.P. and Roy, C. (eds.) (1980) *Conceptual Models for Nursing Practice*, Appleton-Century-Crofts, Norwalk.

Walton, I. (1986) *The Nursing Process in Perspective: A Literature Review*, University of York.

Weick, K.E. (1985) Systematic observation methods, in G. Lindzey and E. Aronson (eds.) *Handbook of Social Psychiatry*, Random House, New York.

Whyte, L. and Youill, G. (1984) The nursing process in the care of the mentally ill, *Nursing Times*, 1 Feb. 1984, pp. 49–51.

Wilkinson, T. (1979) The problems and the values of objective nursing observations in psychiatric nursing care, *Journal of Advanced Nursing*, Vol. 4, pp. 151–9.

Further reading

Altschul, A.T. *et al.* (1980) *Psychiatry under Review*, Macmillan Journals, London.

Barlow, D.H. (ed.) (1981) *Behavioural Assessment of Adult Disorders*, Guilford, New York.

Binnie, A. *et al.* (1984) *A Systematic Approach to Nursing Care: An Introduction*, Open University, Milton Keynes.

DHSS (1977) *The Role of Psychologists in the Health Service: Report of the Sub-Committee*, HMSO, London.

Dingemans, P.M. *et al.* (1986) A cross-cultural study of the factorial dimensions of the NOSIE: a follow-up note, *Journal of Clinical Psychology*, Vol. 42, no. 3, pp. 479–84.

Garrick, T.R. and Stotland, N. (1982) How to write a psychiatric consultation, *American Journal of Psychiatry*, Vol. 139, no. 7, pp. 849–55.

Gerson, S. and Bassuk, E. (1980) Psychiatric emergencies: an overview, *American Journal of Psychiatry*, Vol. 137, no. 1, pp. 1–11.

Hall, J.N. (1977) The content of ward-rating scales for long-stay patients, *British Journal of Psychiatry*, Vol. 130, pp. 287–93.

Hall, J.N. (1979) Assessment procedures used on long-stay patients: a survey of papers published in the *British Journal of Psychiatry*, *British Journal of Psychiatry*, Vol. 135, pp. 330–5.

Hartmann, D.P., Roper, B.L. and Bradford, D.C. (1979) Some relationships between behavioural and traditional assessment, *Journal of Behavioural Assessment*, Vol. 1, no. 1, pp. 3–21.

Hawkins, R.P. (1979) The functions of assessment, *Journal of Applied Behaviour Analysis*, Vol. 12, pp. 501–16.

Hefferin, E.A. and Hunter, R.E. (1975) Nursing assessment and care plan statements, *Nursing Research*, Vol. 24, no. 5, pp. 360–6.

Johnston, M. (1982) Recognition of patients' worries by nurses and by other patients, *British Journal of Medical Psychology*, Vol. 21, no. 4, pp. 255–61.

Kasch, C.R. (1984) Interpersonal competence and communication in the delivery of nursing care, *Advances in Nursing Science*, Vol. 6, no. 2, pp. 71–88.

Katz, S. *et al.* (1963) The index of ADL: a standardized measure of biological and psychosocial function, *Journal of the American Medical Association*, Vol. 185, no. 12, pp. 914–19.

Krause, K. (1983) Documentation of the physical, psychological and social needs of the patient/client, in E. Hamrin (ed.) *Research: A Challenge for Nursing Practice*, Swedish Nurses Association, Stockholm.

Kuhn, M.H. (1982) The interview and the professional relationship, in A.M. Rose (ed.) *Human Behaviour and Social Process*, Routledge & Kegan Paul, London.

Lamonica, E.L. (1979) *The Nursing Process: A Humanistic Approach*, Addison Wesley, Menlo Park, Calif.

Manthey, M. (1980) *The Practice of Primary Nursing*, Blackwell, Oxford.

Palmateer, L.M. and McCartney, J.R. (1985) Do nurses know when patients have cognitive deficits?, *Journal of Gerontological Nursing*, Vol. 11, no. 2, pp. 6–16.

Parsonson, B.S. and Baer, D.M. (1978) The analysis and presentation of graphic data, in T.R. Kratochwill (ed.) *Single Subject Research: Strategies for Evaluating Change*, Academic Press, New York.

Philip, A.E. (1977) Cross-cultural study of the factorial dimensions of the NOSIE, *Journal of Clinical Psychology*, Vol. 33, no. 2, pp. 467–8.

Smith, D.W., Hogan, A.J. and Rohrer, J.E. (1987) Activities of daily living as quantitative indicators of nursing effort, *Medical Care*, Vol. 25, no. 2, pp. 120–30.

Smith, L. (1986) Talking it out, *Nursing Times*, Vol. 82, no. 13, pp. 38–9.

Stanitis, M.A. and Ryan, J. (1982) Noncompliance: an unacceptable diagnosis? *American Journal of Nursing*, Vol. 82, pp. 941–2.

Steckel, S.B. (1976) The use of reinforcement contracts to increase written evidence of the nursing assessment, *Nursing Research*, Vol. 25, no. 1, pp. 58–61.

Sundeen, S.J. *et al.* (1985) *Nurse–Client Interaction: Implementing the Nursing Process*, Mosby, St Louis, Mo.

Vaughn-Wrobel, B.C. and Henderson, B.S. (1982) *The Problem-Oriented System in Nursing*, Mosby, St Louis, Mo.

WHO (1977) *The Nursing Process*, WHO, Copenhagen.

WHO (1980) *Nursing Process Workbook*, WHO, Copenhagen.

Williamson, Y.M. (1978) Methodologic dilemmas in tapping the concept of patient needs, *Nursing Research*, Vol. 27, no. 3, pp. 172–7.

Wood, D.D. *et al.* (1979) In-patient behavioural assessment with a problem-oriented psychiatric logbook, *Journal of Behaviour Therapy and Experimental Psychiatry*, Vol. 10, pp. 229–35.

Yule, W. and Carr, J. (eds.) (1987) *Behaviour Modification for People with Mental Handicaps*, Croom Helm, Beckenham.

2

Nursing Care Planning

DEFINITIONS

Problem
In a given situation or setting, an activity or aspect that is undesired from the point of view of the problem-owner, who is also the person concerned with identifying such activities or aspects.

Need
From the point of view of a need-owner, some necessary element, internal or external, which is required for a stated condition or objective to be achieved.

Target
The overall end product desired by the problem- or need-owner.

Objective
The specific end to which effort by the problem- or need-owner is directed.

Nursing intervention
The description of the nursing actions required to assist a problem- or need-owner to reach a given objective.

Patient action
The description of the actions required of a patient as a problem- or need-owner to reach a given objective.

Evaluation
Comparison of the outcomes of nursing interventions and patient actions with the objectives they were designed to achieve.

Numerous definitions of the components of performance goals or objectives exist. They have in common the requirement of the nurse to take account of constraints on the performance of the person attempting to achieve the objective, and to be specific about the desired behaviour.

DISCUSSION

In contrast to the complexity of the assessment process, the planning stage is most effective if its documentation is kept simple. It can be assumed that each plan is specific to an individual patient. However, the planning process itself is not so simple. Davies and Crisp (1980, p. 383) acknowledge that 'setting performance goals is an admittedly time consuming, complex and sometimes tedious procedure, even when the performance concerned itself takes place over a short time span'.

The first component of planning is to formulate specific problems out of situations which often remain unstructured even though the assessment stage of the nursing process will have attempted to order the available information about the patient. Another main component of planning is the statement of the objectives designed to improve or resolve the identified problems.

According to a social policy view of planning, defining a problem is a way of testing the world in order to correct mistakes. The ability to solve problems and correct mistakes is thought to be a major component of effectiveness.

Educational research suggests that broadly stated educational objectives may be as effective as narrowly stated ones (Davies, 1976). Research into goal-setting by nurses has been performed by clinical psychologists (Davies and Crisp, 1980). Thinking about actions leads to the construction of reasons, which are also hypotheses, as is the nursing assessment performed before implementation of interventions.

According to one view of the multidisciplinary team, a prerequisite for a treatment programme to succeed is that all those involved will co-operate with one another. The price for smooth implementation of a plan is negotiation of the interventions required and, possibly, lowering the aims to those which everyone can guarantee to meet. Mason (1984) demonstrates just how complex is this process of agreeing and writing standards for interventions.

Writing objectives as a nursing practice skill was described by Smith (1971). Sparrow and Pearson's paper (1985) adds little new technically, but is a helpful model of how to write objectives consistently and systematically.

Berger and Luckmann (1967) propose that human activity may be viewed both as 'conduct in the material environment and as externalization of subjective meanings' (p. 68). Much nursing literature seems to be based on a view of the nursing process as being conducted solely in a material environment whose stability and comprehensibility remain unaffected by nurses' manipulation of it. It is suggested that problems are intellectual constructs derived from consultation between the nurse and the patient, rather than objectified entities which exist 'out there', ready for use.

Where possible, problems are expressed using the patient as the subject of the main verb of the sentence which states the problem. That is, the patient is, whenever possible, the owner of the problem being described. The term 'problem-owner' will be used. To be consistent and coherently applicable to problems, objectives are stated in terms of action by the subject of the problem (the patient or problem-owner) not another person. If objectives cannot sensibly be written so that the problem-owner takes the action him- or herself, the problem is reformulated until the patient can agree with the construction being made from his or her predicament.

The use of terms such as problem-owner and objectives builds the patient's consent into the care plan. This is necessarily an approach based on interaction between the nurse and the patient. Wherever possible, the nurse refrains from unilaterally pronouncing the problem or objective, and refrains from taking action independently of any patient action on a given problem. The only exception to this rule is when the patient's safety is thought to be at risk. Just as some forms of mental disorder invalidate a person's capacity to consent, so they may interfere with the patient's capacity to keep him- or herself safe. When a patient will not or cannot negotiate a care plan, the nurse will always implement a plan which is directed to keeping him or her safe.

Nursing diagnosis

The move towards nursing diagnosis is an aspect of an approach where classification is used to determine systematically a nursing care option from all those available. The open-ended nature of most problem situations faced by psychiatric patients and their nurses means that an individualized interactional approach is generally more useful. In this approach, if objectives are correctly written, they provide effective performance measures by which outcomes can be assessed.

Targets

The fundamental ingredient of a plan is the statement of its time frame. That is, the time by which the objective is expected to be achieved. Targets, which are overall statements of ends to which effort is directed, are useful only if they are staged in clearly defined steps with objectives leading to them in the shorter term. In day-to-day planning, targets are unlikely to be used until a patient's condition is fairly stable.

In the procedure which follows, it is implied that problem definition precedes the definition of objectives. However, patients and nurses may have clearly defined objectives they wish to achieve, but anticipate problems in doing so. In this case the original objective becomes a target, until the objectives to resolve such problems have been achieved.

Evaluation

Aspects of evaluation are covered in this chapter, because the recording of the outcome of a plan takes place on the plan itself. Evaluation is discussed in detail in Chapter 4.

GUIDELINES: PLANNING CARE

Action

1   In the planning section of the nursing record, file the nursing care plans, occupational therapist programmes and pass forms in date order, left to right, classified alphabetically.

2   Care plans comprise the following headings:
 (i) date formulated;

Rationale

(a) To facilitate access and information retrieval.
(b) So that they are in a consistent place from patient to patient and ward to ward.

(a) The signature of the first-level nurse signifies direction of nursing care in accordance with the Nurses Rules

(ii)   date to be evaluated;

(iii) signatures of the patient, the primary and associate nurses, and a first-level nurse;

(iv)   problem or need;

(v)   target (if used);

(vi)   objective;

(vii) nursing intervention;

(viii) patient action;

(ix)   outcome of objective;

(x)   reasons for outcome;

(xi)   evidence for reasons.

(S.I. 1983/873).

(b) The signature of the patient signifies his or her agreement with the objectives.

(c) The last three items constitute the evaluation process.

3 Write the date on which the plan is written in words and numbers. For example: 21 November 1989.

To facilitate audit and other evaluation.

4 Write the date on which the plan is to be evaluated: 28 November 1989.

So that the time frame for achieving the objective is known.

5 Obtain the signature of a first-level nurse.

To demonstrate compliance with the Nurses Rules (S.I. 1983/873).

6 Write signatures in full.

(a) To demonstrate accountability.

(b) To facilitate information retrieval.

(c) To facilitate audit.

7 Accompany each signature with the time and date it was made. If the signature is illegible, it is accompanied by block capitals.

(a) To ensure accountability.

(b) To facilitate information retrieval.

(c) To facilitate audit.

8 Write a problem using the following components:

(i)   The point of view or perspective of the problem-owner.

(ii) The problematic behaviour (what is undesired in a given situation).

(iii) The given situation (the setting where the problematic or undesired activity occurs).

(iv) The time frame.

For example: William wishes to kill himself because he feels he has no future. He feels worse on his own.

So that it is clear to both patient and nurse exactly what the plan is intended to tackle.

9 Write a need using the following components:

(i)   The point of view or perspective of the need-owner.

(ii) The expectation by the need-owner that the lack or deficiency should be supplied.

(iii) What is lacking.

(iv) Where the need occurs.

(v)   The time frame.

For example: Mrs Brown, who wakes early every morning, would like to take her sleeping tablets at midnight instead of 22.00.

(a) So that a health or other need is distinguished from problems, diagnoses or concepts.

(b) In order to address the patient's needs as perceived by him- or herself.

10 Write a target using the following components:

So that, because a target is less specific than an

(i)   The person who will achieve it. That is, the need- or problem-owner.

(ii) The desired outcome.

(iii) The conditions in which the target will be reached.

(iv) The standard by which the target will be measured.

(v)   The date for evaluation.

For example: By 15 December 19— William will have remained free from serious self-injury while in the care of Ward X.

objective, it is clear to both patient and nurse what is to be achieved, by whom, and by when.

11 Write an objective using the following components:

(i)   The person who performs the necessary action. That is, the need- or problem-owner.

(ii) The actual behaviour or action to be performed.

(iii) The conditions in which the objective will be reached.

(iv) The standard by which the objective will be measured.

(v)   The time frame.

For example: William will meet with his nurse at the beginning of each shift for not more than ten minutes in order to negotiate a compromise between remaining safe and being intruded upon.

So that it is quite clear to both patient and nurse exactly what will be achieved, and by when it will be achieved.

12 Write a nursing intervention in the form of an instruction. For example: William's nurses will accompany him each time he leaves the ward.

If one of William's nurses is not on duty the nurse in charge of the ward will ensure that interventions are carried out.

So that it is clear to nurses who have not necessarily negotiated the plan, but will carry it out, what they are responsible for doing.

13 Write the patient action in the form of an instruction. For example: William will leave the ward only if accompanied by a nurse or responsible friend or relative.

William will approach one of his nurses or the nurse in charge of the ward if he feels distressed.

So that it is clear to the patient what he or she is responsible for doing.

14 Give the patient a copy of his or her care plan.

(a) So that he or she can use it as a reminder.

(b) In order to demonstrate patient-centred care.

(c) To motivate him or her to be involved in negotiating his or her care.

15 Word the outcome in similar words to the objective. For example: William met (did not meet) with his nurses at the beginning of each shift.

If the objective is written as a closed performance goal, the outcome serves as the performance measure.

16 The reasons for the outcome may be obvious or may have to be inferred from discussion between the patient and the nurses.

For example: William said that there was no point in meeting his nurses as he had nothing to talk about.

Reasons are discussed because they are likely to affect how the next objective is devised.

17 The evidence for the reasons may be obvious or may have to be inferred from discussion between the patient and the nurses.

For example: William told the morning group that talking to nurses at the beginning of shifts was a waste of time.

Because the reasons for an outcome will possibly be used to change the direction or emphasis of the nursing care, the evidence for them is carefully documented.

18 The notes on the care plan are kept brief. The progress notes are used to amplify the discussion.

(a) In order to make the relationship between outcomes and objectives clear.
(b) To facilitate reworking of the plan.

19 The occupational therapy programme is kept up to date by discussions between primary nurses and occupational therapists.

To maintain interprofessional communication.

20 Any pass form is updated at intervals of not more than seven days by the primary nurse in discussion with the patient, the nursing and multidisciplinary care teams.

(a) To maintain interprofessional communication.
(b) To provide agreed safety criteria for the care plans.

21 The pass form is countersigned, if necessary, by a first-level nurse.

To demonstrate that care is directed in accordance with the Nurses Rules (S.I. 1983/873).

REFERENCE MATERIAL
References
Berger, P.L. and Luckmann, T. (1967) *The Social Construction of Reality*, Allen Lane, London.

Davies, A.D.M. and Crisp, A.G. (1980) Setting performance goals in geriatric nursing, *Journal of Advanced Nursing*, Vol. 5, pp. 381–8.

Davies, I.K. (1976) *Objectives in Curriculum Design*, McGraw-Hill, London.

Mason, E.J. (1984) *How to Write Meaningful Nursing Standards*, Wiley, New York.

Smith, D.M. (1971) Writing objectives as a nursing practice skill, *American Journal of Nursing*, Vol. 71, pp. 319–32.

Sparrow, S. and Pearson, A. (1985) Teach yourself goal setting, *Nursing Times*, Vol. 81, no. 42, p. 24–5.

Further reading
Barnett, D. (1982) Planning patient care 1–4, *Nursing Times*, Vol. 78, no. 13, Supplement, pp. 1–16.

Barnett, D. (1985) Making your plans work, *Nursing Times*, Vol. 81, no. 2, pp. 24–7.

Bevvino, C.A. *et al.* (1984) Planned change: an innovative nursing rehabilitation model, *Perspectives in Psychiatric Nursing Care*, Vol. 22, no. 4, pp. 149–58.

Binnie, A. *et al.* (1984) *A Systematic Approach to Nursing Care: An Introduction*, Open University, Milton Keynes.

Chapman, C.M. (1980) The rights and responsibilities of nurses and patients, *Journal of Advanced Nursing*, Vol. 5, pp. 127–34.

Clarke, M. (1978) Planning nursing care, *Nursing Times*, Vol. 74, no. 5, pp. 17–20.

Cormack, D.F.S. (1980) The nursing process: an application of the SOAPE model, *Nursing Times*, Vol. 76, no. 9, pp. 37–40.

Fisher, R. and Ury, W. (1982) *Getting to Yes*, Hutchinson, London.

Fuhr, Sr M.T. (1978) *Clinical Experience Record and Nursing Care Planning*, Mosby, St Louis, Mo.

Hefferin, E.A. and Hunter, R.E. (1975) Nursing assessment and care plan statements, *Nursing Research*, Vol. 24, no. 5, pp. 360–6.

King, I. (1981) *A Theory for Nursing*, Wiley, New York.

Kreger, S.M. and Whealon, R.C. (1981) A procedure for goal-setting: a method for formulating goals and treatment plans, *Rehabilitation Nursing*, Vol. 6, no. 2, pp. 23–6.

Mager, R.F. (1975) *Preparing Instructional Objectives*, Pitman, Belmont, Calif.

Malloy, J.L. (1976) Taking exception to problem-oriented nursing care, *American Journal of Nursing*, Vol. 76, pp. 582–3.

McGilloway, F.A. (1980) The nursing process: a problem-solving approach to patient care, *International Journal of Nursing Studies*, Vol. 17, pp. 79–90.

Mead, G.H. (1934) *Mind, Self and Society*, University of Chicago Press.

Nezu, A. and D'Zurilla, T.J. (1981) Effects of problem definition and formulation on decision making in the social problem-solving process, *Behaviour Therapy*, Vol. 12, pp. 100–6.

Nurses, Midwives and Health Visitors Rules Approval Order (S.I. 1983/873), HMSO, London.

Parsons, P.J. (1986) Building better treatment plans, *Journal of Psychosocial Nursing and Mental Health Services*, Vol. 24, no. 4, pp. 9–14.

Peplau, H. (1952) *Interpersonal Relations in Nursing*, Putnams, New York.

Sanders, J.B. and Du Plessis, D. (1985) An historical view of right to treatment, *Journal of Psychosocial Nursing and Mental Health Services*, Vol. 23, no. 9, pp. 12–17.

Schröck, R. (1980) Planning nursing care for the mentally ill, *Nursing Times*, Vol. 76, no. 16, pp. 704–6.

Swearingen, D. *et al.* (1977) Improving patient care through measurement: goal importance and achievement scaling, *Journal of Psychiatric Nursing*, Vol. 15, no. 9, pp. 30–5.

Teasdale, K. (1987) Partnership with patients?, *The Professional Nurse*, Vol. 2, no. 12, pp. 397–9.

Yule, W. and Carr, J. (eds.) (1987) *Behaviour Modification for People with Mental Handicaps*, Croom Helm, Beckenham.

3

Implementation of the Care Plan

DEFINITIONS

Implementation

To implement is to carry out the interventions required to achieve the objectives stated in the nursing care plans.

Interventions

Interventions are the nursing actions to be taken to help a patient achieve the objective stated in a care plan. They are written in the form of instructions.

DISCUSSION

Hayward (1986, p. 22) remarks that: 'It is perhaps regrettable that the term "implementation" has come to be used in two ways: firstly, as the widespread adoption of the nursing process; secondly, as the stage of the nursing process which involves carrying out the care plan.'

Implementation is less easy to identify as a discrete stage than the other three stages – assessment, planning and evaluation – partly because it demonstrates the dynamic nature of the nursing process, and partly because it is both a statement of what nursing actions are proposed and a word standing for particular kinds of nursing actions which are not easy to define.

Cormack (1980) suggested that difficulties in implementation result from having no model for implementation and no framework for assessment. He asserts, like Kasch (1984), that the nursing process necessarily leads to individualized patient care. However, Flaskerud *et al.* (1979) suggest that to make a closer relationship with a patient, the nurse must tolerate a certain absence of control. Anxiety results, and to avoid the anxiety, nurses both avoid the close relationship and attempt to set limited clearly defined objectives for nursing activities. Setting patient-centred, specific behavioural objectives does not imply limits on nursing interventions, but rather tests nurses' creativity in designing facilitative rather than controlling plans of care.

Implementation in the context of the nursing process

Crow (1977, p. 4), like the RCN Association of Nursing Practice (RCN, 1979), describes the nursing process in terms of stages: 'the nurse first obtains the relevant information . . . then she interprets [it] . . . The next stage is drawing up a care plan . . . The final stage is evaluating the care plan once it has been implemented.' However, a systems view adapted from Levin *et al.* (1976) provides the diagram shown in Figure 3.1.

The rate of change for each of the elements in Figure 3.1 is often very different. For instance, plans may change faster than assessments, but slower than events. Events and phenomena often change faster than perceptions. Assessments change more slowly than perceptions. The effect of these changes on implementation is to make it susceptible to sudden, possibly unpredicted influences.

Implementation as success or failure

Objectives and decisions do not therefore proceed inevitably to implementation. The act of implementing and thinking about a plan may well bring about a change in the plan itself. Implementation may change the objectives stated in a plan, so that evaluation begins at the same time as implementation. An implementation failure is an outcome which does not meet the standards stated in the objective. It is not possible to know it is a failure unless the pre-existing standards are known. But it is possible to imagine that a successful outcome to a plan might be one which resulted from the patient's or the nurse's recognition that the plan was ill-conceived. It may be that in actually implementing the objectives as stated the nurse and patient realize they will have unsatisfactory results. Rather than just abandoning the plan they might be more creative by altering it as they go along.

Implementation is contained within the nursing inter-

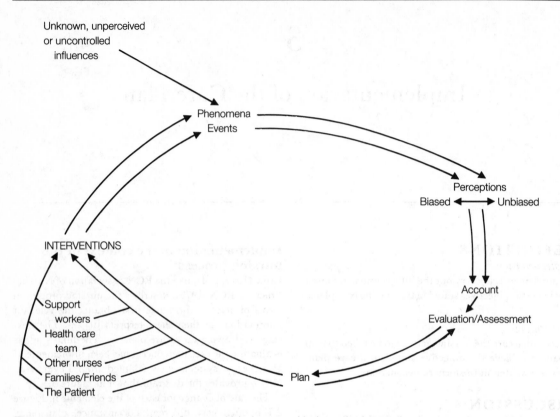

Figure 3.1   A dynamic view of the influences which shape psychiatric nursing interventions

ventions of the nursing care plans, but because it contains the possibility of its own change within it, it appears in much more detail in the progress notes of the day-to-day interaction of nurses with patients. It overlaps to a large extent with the assessment stage, but aspects of it are kept distinct under the heading of implementation in order to facilitate cross-reference to the procedures of assessment and planning.

Interventions

Mason (1984) makes a nursing intervention synonymous with a procedure. She conceptualizes the nursing process as being one where the nurse synthesizes into units of nursing care all the data concerning the client and his or her family or significant others. Definition of the units of nursing care results from the conceptual framework held by the nurse. Five types of nursing care units are, according to Mason:

1 nursing diagnosis;
2 health problems;
3 health needs;
4 concept;
5 medical diagnosis.

Each unit of nursing care contains, Mason says, the specific interventions required to achieve it. The choice of intervention is more or less flexible depending on the framework that has been adopted. A nursing or medical diagnosis is likely to involve less choice by the nurse as to appropriate interventions, whereas a health problem, health need, or concept will require negotiation or selection from a number of alternative actions, depending on the assessment and the data available.

Examples of health problems include deafness, hemiparesis, delirium, malnutrition. Examples of health needs include elimination, sleep and hygiene. Examples of concepts include safety, confusion, aggression, hallucinations, delusions and paranoia. Examples of medical diagnoses include schizophrenia, manic-depressive psychosis and presenile dementia.

EXAMPLE

This example shows a written form of intervention, as defined at the beginning of this chapter.

Need

Mr Brown needs to become more independent as the time for his discharge approaches.

Objective
Mr Brown will stay in his flat alone for one night during the weekend of 5–6 October.

Nursing interventions
1 Mr Brown's primary nurse (George Green) will accompany him to the shops on Friday to buy milk, tea, and other food for supper, breakfast and lunch at his flat.
2 George will write down his hours of duty so that Mr Brown can ring him if necessary from his flat.
3 Mr Brown's associate nurse (Carol Smith) will meet him when he returns from his flat on Sunday in order to hear how he got on.
4 George will let the welfare officer know that Mr Brown is on leave, so that he will receive the correct benefit payment.

Patient actions
1 Mr Brown will make a shopping list before he goes to the shops with George.
2 Mr Brown will ring his neighbour during the week to let her know he will be at home during the weekend.
3 During the week Mr Brown will check if there are any engineering works that will affect his getting the train back on Sunday.
4 Mr Brown will ring the ward at any time if he feels he would like to speak to a nurse.
5 Mr Brown will meet Carol when he returns to the ward on Sunday.

GUIDELINES: IMPLEMENTING CARE

Action	Rationale
1 Document implementation on care plans in the form of 'nursing interventions' and 'patient actions'.	So that both the patient and the nurse are clearly aware of their respective responsibilities.
2 After negotiating objectives with a patient that are additional to existing care plans, write the nursing interventions and patient actions in the progress notes.	To record a negotiated activity that does not require a care plan as it is a one-off event such as going to the shops to buy stamps and personal items.
3 Write nursing interventions and patient actions in the form of instructions.	So that it is clear to both the nurse and the patient what they are each responsible for doing.
4 Write in the progress notes how a nursing intervention is actually carried out.	To facilitate exploration of the reasons for outcomes to objectives.
5 If possible, ask the patient to record what he or she actually does, and file it in the progress notes.	(a) To facilitate exploration of the reasons for outcomes to objectives. (b) So that the patient retains influence over the process.
6 Write in words and figures the dates on which the implementation is carried out and recorded. For example, 23 November 1989.	To facilitate audit and other evaluation.
7 Write the time the implementation was carried out using the twenty-four-hour clock.	(a) To pinpoint changes accurately. (b) To avoid confusion between day and night when referring retrospectively to the notes.
8 Each entry is signed in full with the time and date it was made. If the signature is illegible, it is accompanied by block capitals.	(a) To ensure accountability. (b) To facilitate information retrieval. (c) To facilitate audit.

9 Obtain the signature of a first-level nurse if necessary.

To demonstrate compliance with the Nurses' Rules (S.I. 1983/873).

REFERENCE MATERIAL
References

Cormack, D.F.S. (1980) The nursing process: an application of the SOAPE model, *Nursing Times*, Vol. 76, no. 9, pp. 37–40.

Crow, J. (1977) *The Nursing Process*, Macmillan Journals, London.

Flaskerud, J. *et al.* (1979) Avoidance and distancing: a descriptive view of nursing, *Nursing Forum*, Vol. 18, no. 2, pp. 158–74.

Hayward, J. (ed.) (1986) *Report of the Nursing Process Evaluation Working Group*, King's College, University of London.

Kasch, C.R. (1984) Interpersonal competence and communication in the delivery of nursing care, *Advances in Nursing Science*, Vol. 6, no. 2, pp. 71–88.

Levin, G. *et al.* (1976) *The Dynamics of Human Service Delivery*, Ballinger, Cambridge, Mass.

Mason, E.J. (1984) *How to Write Meaningful Nursing Standards*, Wiley, New York.

Royal College of Nurses (RCN) (1979) *Implementing the Nursing Process*, RCN, London.

Further reading

Anderson, M.L. (1983) Nursing interventions: what did you do that helped? *Perspectives in Psychiatric Care*, Vol. 21, no. 1, pp. 4–8.

Bandura, A. (1977) Self-efficacy: toward a unifying theory of behavioural change, *Psychological Review*, Vol. 84, no. 2, pp. 191–215.

Binnie, A. *et al.* (1984) *A Systematic Approach to Nursing Care: An Introduction*, Open University, Milton Keynes.

Kasch, C.R. and Lisneck, P.M. (1984) Role of strategic communication in nursing theory and research, *Advances in Nursing Science*, Vol. 7, no. 1, pp. 56–71.

Kogan, H.N. and Betrus, P.A. (1984) Self-management: a nursing mode of therapeutic influence, *Advances in Nursing Science*, Vol. 6, no. 4, pp. 55–73.

McMorrow, M.J., Cullinan, D. and Epstein, M.H. (1978) The use of the Premack Principle to motivate patient activity attendance, *Perspectives in Psychiatric Care*, Vol. 16, no. 1, pp. 14–20.

Pressman, J.L. and Wildavsky, A. (1984) *Implementation*, University of California Press, Berkeley.

Sayre, J. (1978) Common errors in communication made by students in psychiatric nursing, *Perspectives in Psychiatric Care*, Vol. 16, no. 4, pp. 175–87.

Schroder, P.J. (1979) Nursing intervention with patients with thought disorder, *Perspectives in Psychiatric Care*, Vol. 17, no. 1, pp. 32–9.

Streiff, L.D. (1986) Can clients understand our instructions? *Image*, Vol. 18, no. 2, pp. 48–52.

Yule, W. and Carr, J. (eds.) (1987) *Behaviour Modification for People with Mental Handicaps*, Croom Helm, Beckenham.

4

Evaluation of Nursing Care

DEFINITION
Evaluation is defined as comparing outcomes with the objectives defined in the planning stage; and recording the reasons, along with relevant evidence, for the effects of nursing interventions and patient actions.

DISCUSSION
The nursing process comes closest to the scientific method in the evaluation stage. Evaluation consists of comparing observed phenomena in the 'real world' with abstract concepts such as intentions, predictions, objectives or standards.

Evaluation may have immediately useful results, or it may have results that are useful over varying lengths of time. The results of evaluation may indicate where different kinds of investigation are required, as in the suicide rate of a hospital; or evaluation may lead directly to further planning. Thinking about evaluation of health care has been largely shaped by Donabedian in a series of influential papers starting in the mid-1960s.

In those papers Donabedian set the scene for evaluation of medical care. He recommended that during any evaluation procedure the distinction between values and the elements of structure, process and outcome is recognized and maintained; that values, structure, process and outcomes are examined equally critically; that the gathering and interpretation of information, which are a large part of the medical care process itself, are researched; that how physicians function in the medical care process should be investigated; and that patient–physician interaction should be investigated (Donabedian, 1966, pp. 193–6). If the words 'nurse' and 'nursing process' are substituted for the words 'physician' and 'medical care process', Donabedian provides a clear programme for nurses who wish to evaluate the care they provide to patients.

Figure 4.1 shows this process diagrammatically.

Types of evaluation
When futher actions are required, as they generally are, it is useful to classify different kinds of evaluation and to identify its components in order to choose rationally between alternatives and where to make interventions. It can be seen that although evaluation owes a good deal to scientific method, it may lead into areas which are not immediately quantifiable, and call for qualitative judgements. For this reason, it is important to be clear about the kind of evaluation being used.

FORMATIVE EVALUATION
The purpose of formative evaluation, as implied by its label, is to examine the forms in which given activities are carried out. For example, nursing care of psychiatric patients is delivered in community or hospital settings. Formative evaluation looks at systems of care in order to decide how priorities should be set and to identify activities where modification is desirable, and is based on an assumption that systems of care are ongoing. Formative evaluation is therefore designed to facilitate further development of services, whether provided by an individual or by a group.

SUMMATIVE EVALUATION
The purpose of summative evaluation is to examine (summarize) the results or outputs of given activities. It assumes that an activity is at a stage where conclusions can be made about its continuation, cessation or transformation.

Structure, process and outcome
Three areas or dimensions have been identified where evaluation is performed. They are structure, process and outcome.

FOCUS AND ASSUMPTION
Within each area of structure, process and outcome, two

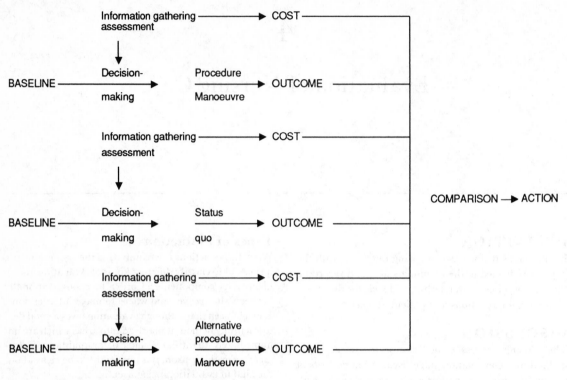

Figure 4.1 Evaluation (adapted from Donabedian, 1966)

AREA or DIMENSION	FORMATIVE or SUMMATIVE	FOCUS	ASSUMPTION [VALUE BASE]
Structure Considerations such as organizational systems, hierarchies, staffing levels	Formative or summative	Specific kinds of organization, grades of staff, numbers of staff etc.	Ratios of trained to untrained staff etc.
Process Activities performed by the elements or components of a given system	Formative rather than summative	CONCURRENT or RETROSPECTIVE Specific actions, staff and client attitudes and knowledge, efficiency	Utilization of resources, cost-effectiveness
Outcome Results [output] of a given system	Summative or formative	Concurrent or retrospective results	Standards, costs, conditions, criteria
The nursing process	Tends to be summative	Outcomes	Nurses *negotiate* with patients
	Formative evaluation also required	To utilize the documentation of the nursing process itself	To identify actual or potential deficiencies in delivery of nursing care to individual patients

Figure 4.2 Nursing evaluation

Patient . . . .   Hospital No. . . . .

Date/Time . . . .   Primary nurse . . . .

Problems/Needs

Choose a number from the scale below to show how much you are troubled by each problem or need listed and write the number in the box opposite.

0	1	2	3	4	5	6	7	8	9	10
not at all					definitely troubled					very greatly troubled

Problem/Need . . . .

Problem/Need . . . .

Problem/Need . . . .

Other problem or need . . . .

Date/Time _____

Objectives

Choose a number from the scale below to show how far towards each of your objectives you have progressed.

0	1	2	3	4	5	6	7	8	9	10
not at all					definite progress					very great progress

Objective . . . .

Objective . . . .

Objective . . . .

Date/Time _____

Figure 4.3 Evaluation of problems/needs/objectives

further constituents need to be made explicit for evaluation to be effective: focus and assumption. Another term for assumption is value base.

STRUCTURE

Structure involves considerations such as organizational systems, hierarchies, staffing levels. Evaluation may be focused on specific kinds of organization, grades of staff or numbers of staff. Value bases will include assumptions to do with, for instance, ratios of trained to untrained staff. Structural evaluation may be formative or summative.

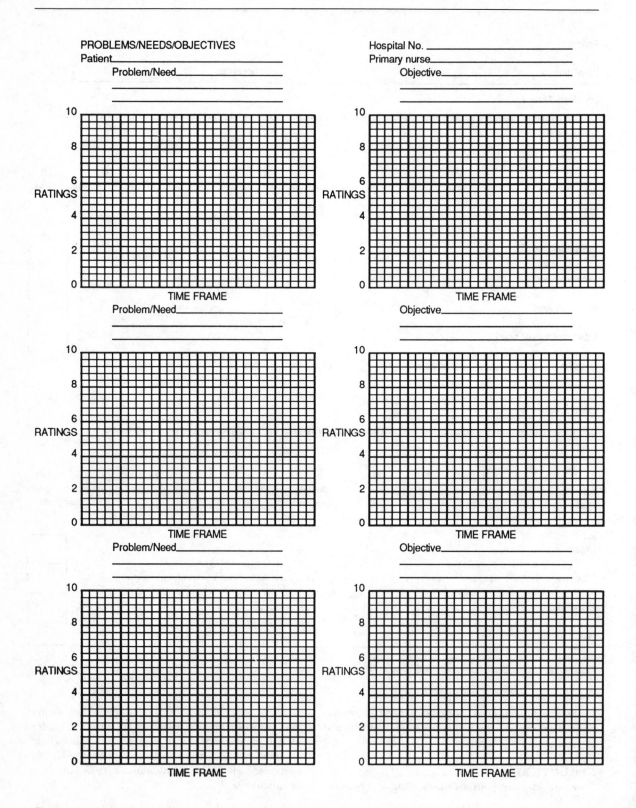

Figure 4.4 Cumulative evaluation of problems/needs/objectives

PROCESS

Process involves the activities performed by elements or components of a given system. Evaluation may be focused on specific actions, staff and client attitudes and knowledge, or efficiency. It may be performed concurrently (in the here and now) or retrospectively. Its value bases will include assumptions to do with, say, utilization of resources and cost-effectiveness. It is formative rather than summative evaluation.

OUTCOME

Outcomes involve the results or outputs of a system. Evaluation may be performed concurrently or retrospectively. Its value bases will include assumptions to do with standards, costs, conditions and criteria. Outcome evaluation may be summative or formative.

The nursing process

Because these procedures concerning the nursing process are based upon defined objectives, evaluation tends to be summative, focused on outcomes, and assuming that nurses negotiate with patients. However, formative evaluation is also required in order to utilize the documentation of the nursing process itself to identify actual and potential deficiencies in the delivery of nursing care to individual patients.

Figure 4.2 summarizes diagrammatically structure, process, outcome and the nursing process.

Recording evaluations

As the definition at the beginning of the chapter implies, evaluation may be recorded in two ways. The first, graphic way is influenced by examples from behavioural

psychologists and nurse therapists (Marks *et al.*, 1986), and is particularly useful for problems and objectives which have been defined in measurable, behavioural terms. It provides an example of summative evaluation. The comparison may be performed by the nurse and the patient using the form illustrated in Figure 4.3. The nurse asks the patient to use the analogue scale to rate how troublesome the problems or needs are as listed on the care plan. The ratings are recorded on the form. On the same form, the patient is then asked to rate the progress that he or she has made towards the objectives as stated on the care plan. The nurse transfers these ratings to another form (Figure 4.4) in order to provide a cumulative record which shows the changes over time. The time frame may be over hours, days or weeks, as agreed by the nurse and patient.

The second way of recording the evaluation is a written account which interprets and discusses the reasons for the changes recorded on the graphs and in other descriptive, qualitative or quantitative records. It is an example of formative evaluation, and is necessary beause of the different ways in which apparently objectively recorded data can be interpreted. The nurse records his or her reasoning in order to justify decisions made using the graphs and other records as evidence. This kind of evaluation also makes explicit its focus and assumptions. Observable behaviour is an example of one kind of focus; psychodynamic process is an example of another kind of focus. As Figures 4.3 and 4.4 indicate, an assumption is that the nurse negotiates with the patient. The evaluation will make explicit how this negotiation is carried out, or if a more directive, controlling approach is used, this will be made explicit.

GUIDELINES: EVALUATING CARE

Action	Rationale
1 Document summative outcome evaluations directly next to objectives.	So that comparison between outcome and objective can be made at a glance.
2 Document formative, process-focused evaluations in the progress notes.	In order to facilitate discussion and because more space is available in the progress notes.
3 Write the date on which the evaluation is performed in words and figures. For example: 28 November 1989.	(a) So that it is clear that the evaluation is being made on the date stated in the objective. (b) To facilitate audit of the nursing process records.

4 Obtain the signature, if necessary, of a first-level nurse.

To demonstrate the care is delivered in accordance with the Nurses' Rules (S.I. 1983/873).

5 Write signatures in full.

(a) To demonstrate accountability.
(b) To facilitate information retrieval.
(c) To facilitate audit.

6 In summative evaluation, use similar wording for the outcome as for the objective.

(a) So that it is clear whether the objective was achieved or not.
(b) So that specific reasons for the outcome can be identified.

7 Remember that reasons may be self-evident or may need to be inferred. State if they are inferred, and on what evidence the inference was based.

So that the nature of the reasons is made clear when documentation of them takes place.

8 Document the evidence for the reasons stated for the outcome.

The reasons may have been inferred from material other than that which is in the nursing interventions and patient actions.

9 Amplify summative evaluations in the progress notes if necessary.

In order not to crowd the evaluation of specific objectives with less immediately relevant material.

10 In formative evaluation, focus on the ways in which the stages of the nursing process are performed.

(a) To audit the process.
(b) To monitor quality.
(c) To identify necessary changes and improvements.
(d) To confirm whether the supervision of nurses' work with patients is adequate.

REFERENCE MATERIAL
References

Donabedian, A. (1966) Evaluating the quality of medical care, *Milbank Memorial Fund Quarterly*, Vol. 44, no. 2, pp. 166–203.

Marks, I.M. *et al.* (1986) *Behavioural Psychotherapy: Maudsley Pocket Book of Clinical Management*, Wright, Bristol.

Further reading

Aggleton, P. and Chalmers, H. (1984) Rogers' unitary field model, *Nursing Times*, Vol. 80, no. 50, pp. 35–9.

Binnie, A. *et al.* (1984) *A Systematic Approach to Nursing Care: An Introduction*, Open University, Milton Keynes.

Burgoyne, J.G. and Cooper, C.L. (1975) Evaluation methodology, *Journal of Occupational Psychology* Vol. 48, pp. 53–62.

Burton, M. (1986) What do we mean by evaluation?, *Health Service Journal*, 17 July 1986, pp. 954–5.

Chang, B.L. (1980) Evaluation of health care professionals in facilitating self-care: a review of the literature and a conceptual model, *Advances in Nursing Science*, Vol. 3, no. 1, pp. 43–58.

Elbeik, M.A.H. and McGill, B. (1985) Nursing audits: pragmatic evaluation and assessment, *Dimensions*, Vol. 62, no. 2, pp. 34–5, 38.

Farrell, P. and Scherer, K. (1983) The Delphi technique as a method for selecting criteria to evaluate nursing care, *Nursing Papers*, Vol. 15, no. 1, pp. 51–60.

Hegedus, K.S. (1979) A patient outcome criterion measure, *Supervisor Nurse*, Vol. 10, no. 1, pp. 40–5.

Hegyvary, S.T. (1979) Nursing process: the basis for evaluating the quality of nursing care, *International Nursing Review*, Vol. 26, no. 4, pp. 113–6.

Lillesand, K.M. and Korff, S. (1983) Nursing process evaluation: a quality assurance tool, *Nursing Administration Quarterly*, Vol. 7, no. 3, pp. 9–14.

MacRae, J. (1986) Developing a nursing audit, *Australian Nurses Journal*, Vol. 15, no. 9, pp. 44–61.

Openshaw, S. (1984) Literature review: measurement of adequate care, *International Journal of Nursing Studies*, Vol. 4, pp. 295–304.

Openshaw, S. (1985) Evaluation of the effectiveness of nursing care, *Nursing Research Abstracts*, Vol. 7, no. 1, p. 20.

Parker, S.O. (1983) A conceptual model for outcome assessment, *Nurse Practitioner*, Vol. 8, no. 1, pp. 41–5.

Stanley, B. (1984) Evaluation of treatment goals: the use of goal attainment scaling, *Journal of Advanced Nursing*, Vol. 9, pp. 351–6.

Strain, M. (1987) Evaluating the practice of care: interests and methods, *Nurse Education Today*, Vol. 7, pp. 253–7.

Summary report of a working group on the evaluation of inpatient nursing practice (1978) *Journal of Advanced Nursing*, Vol. 3, pp. 413–15.

Waters, K. (1986) Cause and effect, *Nursing Times*, Vol. 82, no. 5, pp. 28–30.

Webb, D. (1984) Quality in nursing: three major components, *Dimensions*, Vol. 61, no. 8, pp. 14, 19.

Wilson-Barnett, J. (1986) A measure of care, *Nursing Times*, Vol. 82, no. 33, pp. 57–8.

Wing, J. and Häfner, H. (eds.) (1973) *Roots of Evaluation*, Nuffield Provincial Hospitals Trust, London.

Wiseman, J. (1983) Health quality assurance, *Nursing Times*, Vol. 79, no. 1, pp. 16–17.

Wright, D. (1984) An introduction to the evaluation of nursing care: a review of the literature, *Journal of Advanced Nursing*, Vol. 9, pp. 457–67.

Yule, W. and Carr, J. (eds.) (1987) *Behaviour Modification for People with Mental Handicaps*, Croom Helm, Beckenham.

Zimmer, M.J. *et al.* (1974) Guidelines for development of outcome criteria, *Nursing Clinics of North America*, Vol. 9, no. 2, pp. 317–21.

Part Two

Therapeutic Milieu

5

Nurse–Patient Relationships

DEFINITIONS
Professional relationships
A professional relationship is one between a member of a profession and his or her client, or between members of different professions. Relationships between health care professionals are dealt with in Chapter 6 for the role of the nurse in the multidisciplinary clinical team.

Professions
A profession may be defined as a self-monitoring and self-perpetuating body which regulates the provision of specific services by accrediting as practitioners only those individuals who meet its criteria, and by advancing the study of its subject. A professional body controls and disciplines its members by means of a code of conduct which defines their duties to society in general and to their clients in particular.

DISCUSSION
The United Kingdom Central Council for Nursing, Midwifery and Health Visiting (UKCC) is the professional and statutory body created by the Nurses, Midwives and Health Visitors Act 1979. The UKCC exercises the powers conferred by the 1979 Act to set standards, issue qualifications to practise, and to monitor discipline and welfare of nurses, midwives and health visitors. Its Code of Professional Conduct (UKCC, 1984) is designed to give guidance to nurses on standards of practice and on their responsibilities to patients as well as to each other.

UKCC Code of Conduct
The UKCC Code of Conduct (UKCC, 1984) is a valuable and useful statement which provides a set of broad guidelines (see Appendix A). It could be described as a foundation upon which a procedure manual builds a firm structure.

The values which inform individual professional practice may derive from different ethical and philosophical standpoints. Although it can be argued that the primary task of the UKCC is to register nurses, with the purpose of protecting the public, the Code uses a vague and paternalistic clause, speaking of 'safeguard[ing] the interests of individual patients and clients'. In contrast, each nurse is expected to 'uphold and enhance the good standing and reputation of the profession' (UKCC, 1984, p. 2).

PROFESSIONAL CONDUCT
Professional conduct is a set of actions based on professional knowledge, skills and judgement. All these are measurable by the systems of written and practical assessment which lead to state registration, and, subsequently, by peer judgement. The procedure described here makes three additions to the UKCC Code of Conduct. The first, and one which can be argued as encompassing the other two, is the absolute requirement to ensure that patients have consented to treatment. The Mental Health Act 1983 emphasizes this aspect. The other two may be described as desirable principles, but are not legally binding in any way. The second principle is veracity: the requirement to tell the truth to patients (Bok, 1980). The third is the requirement to ensure the patient's privacy.

The Code is least ambiguous in its statements on accountability, safety, competence, and confidentiality. It is far less explicit on questions of multidisciplinary teamwork, religion, conscientious objection and gifts. A separate leaflet issued by the UKCC (1985) deals with advertising (see Appendix B).

ACCOUNTABILITY
The Nurses, Midwives and Health Visitors Act 1979 empowers the UKCC to define professional knowledge, expertise and judgement. The Nurses Rules (S.I.

1983/873) lay down that nurses qualified in Parts 1, 3, 5 and 8 of the register are responsible for directing the work both of students in training for those parts of the register and of nurses qualified in Parts 2, 4, 6 and 7. Accountability refers to the responsibility of a nurse for work that is appropriately delegated to him or her. That is, delegated along with the necessary authority and in the belief that the nurse has the competence to carry it out. The UKCC (UKCC, 1989) have issued a framework to assist nurses, midwives and health visitors to consider ethical aspects of professional practice (see Appendix A).

Thus the patient can expect that nurses will not fail in their duty of care. Seniors can expect nurses to undertake specific responsibilities and tasks which constitute a given job and which a nurse has a duty to perform. Colleagues can expect that nursing care and treatment plans will be implemented and evaluated by the nurses allocated to do so.

Accountability as defined above means that the nurse must be competent (in the terms of the Nurses Rules) to carry out the work delegated to him or her and that he or she fulfils his or her duties in five senses of the word duty.
1 The principle that patients' rights entail specific duties.
2 To this end there are duties defined by the procedures and policies of the service within which the nurse works.
3 The duties defined in the Nurses Rules.
4 The duties defined by the Code of Conduct laid down by the UKCC, the statutory body responsible for standards of professional practice.
5 The duties as defined by the common law or more specific legislation such as the Abortion Act 1967, the Children and Young Persons Act 1969, the Suicide Act 1971, the Race Relations Act 1976, the Mental Health Act 1983.

SAFETY
The duty not to do harm is strongly stated in the Code. Negligence is most likely to become an issue in relation to safety. A negligent act may be one the nurse carelessly or wilfully carries out, or one that the nurse carelessly or wilfully fails to carry out. The basic standard at which the nurse is required to practise is that expected of a competent qualified nurse.

Mental Health Act 1983
Section 139 of the Mental Health Act 1983 sets out the expectation that nurses along with other staff act in good faith and with reasonable care. The test of good faith is that the nurse acts according to his or her duty of care to the patient. The duty of care is based on criteria of safety as defined in the practical assessments for the examina-

tion leading to the qualification of RMN. The tests of reasonable care are threefold.
1 The standards of competence defined by representatives of the psychiatric nursing profession and by the criteria for inclusion on the register.
2 Adherence to the standards of the Mental Health Act.
3 The nurse's familiarity with the law related to his or her work.

The implications are that nurses performing duties related to the provisions of the Mental Health Act 1983 must have been instructed and found competent to do so. That is, they are Registered Mental Nurses (RMN) or Registered Nurses for the Mentally Handicapped (RNMH), and they carry out specifically nursing duties as defined in the Act and agreed by the management team of officers of their health authority.

These nursing duties include participating only with consent in treatment of patients admitted either informally or compulsorily for assessment; maintaining nursing records on detained patients which may be accessible to any person authorized by the Mental Health Act Commission (MHAC); ensuring that patients know their rights according to the Act and the MHAC Code of Practice; judging what represents the minimum restraint and intervention for patients not subject to detention or treatment; judging when it is reasonable to search certain patients and their belongings; if appointed, inspecting the mail of certain patients; and treating patients detained under the Mental Health Act 1983 strictly in accordance with the provisions of the Act.

DUTIES TOWARDS COLLEAGUES
The question of professional loyalty to colleagues whose practice jeopardizes safe standards presents particular difficulties because a conflict sometimes appears to exist between the nurse's duty of care to the patient and professional loyalty. The UKCC Code of Conduct does not make clear the extensive confidential advisory and welfare services available to nurses in trouble. A duty of all nurses is to ensure that their colleagues are competent to practise, but it is not made explicit in the Code.

COMPETENCE
The competence of nurses is defined in the Nurses Rules. A student who is preparing for Parts 1, 3, 5 or 8 of the register must be directed by a nurse who is qualified in one or more of these parts of the register, a first-level nurse. The first-level nurse is also responsible for organizing the care of groups of patients and for directing the work of second-level nurses: those qualified in Parts 2, 4, 6 and 7 of the register. Competence implies an ability to carry out each step of the nursing process as well as to

supervise the practice of other nurses.

CONFIDENTIALITY
Privacy and confidentiality are closely related. The nurse–patient relationship necessitates a sense of physical and emotional intimacy, a position which must be held in respect and confidence. It is a privilege and its abuse is absolutely prohibited. The provision to patients of psychological privacy necessitates an understanding by the nurse that all he or she learns about a patient is professional information of the highest order. It is to be transmitted only on a professional basis to colleagues directly involved in the patient's care. The UKCC (UKCC, 1987) have published guidelines on the subject of confidentiality (see Appendix D).

CONSENT TO TREATMENT
The right to agree or withold consent and the right to be told the truth are closely linked with the concept of informed consent: the right to be truthfully informed. Chapter 40, 'Ethical issues', and Chapter 10, 'Consent to treatment', consider the question of consent in detail.

VERACITY
It is argued that there is never any justification for lying to patients. The professional relationships of nurses are subject to a particular kind of risk whereby someone who has power over another person may abuse that power. Although psychiatric patients may have disorders which can severely impair their judgement about what may be harmful to them, it is an abuse of the nurse's power to use impaired judgement as a reason for lying. This does not mean that the nurse is obliged to answer every question a patient asks. It may benefit the patient to obtain the information in different ways. Asking a nurse may conceal reluctance to confront another person. If the nurse is alert to such possibilities and takes advice from colleagues before acting, it may be possible to avoid telling untruths.

PRIVACY
Bok (1986) argues that if inquiries are to be made into people's private feelings and behaviour, their consent is required. In the UKCC Code of Conduct the relationship between nurse and patient is described as privileged, one which allows privileged access to the patient's home, belongings and workplace. The UKCC Code of Conduct does not mention the fourth aspect of the patient to which the nurse has privileged access: his or her body. There is an absolute prohibition on sexual relations between psychiatric nurses and patients.

OTHER MATTERS
Multidisciplinary teamwork
This is discussed in Chapter 6.

Religious practice
This is discussed in Chapter 11.

Conscientious objection
This is discussed in Chapter 40.

Advertising
The UKCC (1985) has issued a supplementary leaflet explaining how nurses are prohibited from using their qualifications in advertisements.

Supervision
The following procedure focuses on supervision, because the aspects of nurses' relationships which have been discussed will generally become visible to others through the supervision process. The supervisory system is essential in order to monitor professional relationships. It is also part of the process of training and development in nursing.

Supervision by nurses of one another's practice provides a system of checks and balances to ensure that there can be positively no abuse of the privileged relationship between nurse and patient.

GUIDELINES: CONDUCT WITHIN NURSE–PATIENT RELATIONSHIPS

Action

1 Each nurse ensures that he or she receives systematic supervision in accordance with the procedure for carrying out supervision.

Rationale

So that on-the-job training in professional relationships is available for each member of the nursing team.

2 The charge nurse ensures that students preparing for Parts 1, 3, 5 or 8 of the register are supervised by nurses qualified in those parts.

To comply with the Nurses Rules (S.I. 1983/873).

3 The charge nurse ensures that nurses who are qualified in Parts 2, 4, 6 or 8 of the register are supervised by nurses who are qualified in Parts 1, 3, 5 or 8.

To comply with the Nurses Rules (S.I. 1983/873).

4 The charge nurse bases supervision on the guidelines laid down in the nursing policy manual.

Although charge nurses are free to develop some of the criteria for supervision and evaluation, the nursing policy manual determines the specific components of each job description.

5 The charge nurse delegates to each first-level nurse the supervision of the student nurses in the ward or department.

(a) The charge nurse is responsible for supervising the first-level nurses.
(b) The charge nurse's supervision of the first-level nurses includes formal and regular monitoring of their work with the untrained staff in the ward.

6 The charge nurse agrees with each first-level nurse his or her plans for supervision.

The plans provide individually based criteria for supervising nurses.

7 The charge nurse conducts regular meetings of all ward supervisors.

In order that each supervisor has the opportunity to discuss professional relationships and ethical issues.

8 Each supervisor agrees with individual supervisees a timetable for supervisions and appraisal interviews.

(a) So that performance may be continuously monitored.
(b) So that objectives can be set within the agreed time frame.

9 Each supervisor arranges the time of a supervision session at least a week in advance, preferably at the end of each supervision.

So that each member of the nursing team knows and can discuss the limits of his or her responsibility.

10 The supervisor confirms after such a supervision that both participants agree about what has taken place.

So that there is no misunderstanding about conclusions reached in the supervision sessions.

11 The supervisor keeps a confidential record of all supervisions.

An up-to-date record is necessary for subsequent evaluation of professional relationships.

12 The supervisor bases supervision of professional relationships on consideration of the following headings:
  (i)   accountability;
  (ii)   safety;
  (iii) competence;
  (iv)   confidentiality;
  (v)   consent to treatment;
  (vi)   veracity;
  (vii) privacy;
  (viii) multidisciplinary teamwork.
  (ix)   religion;
  (x)   conscientious objection;
  (xi)   advertising.

(a) This is in accordance with the UKCC Code of Conduct.
(b) To ensure congruence between patients' rights and nurses' actions.

13 When supervising a nurse's work with individual patients the supervisor ensures that the nurse's documentation in the nursing record reaches the standards specified in the procedures for the nursing process.

(a) For a nurse's accountability for his or her work to be monitored the evidence of what has been done must be available.
(b) The nursing record is the means by which nurses render account for work which has been delegated to them.

14 The shift rota is compiled in such a way that supervisees and supervisors work shifts together.

(a) In order that the supervisor can systematically induct a supervisee to the safety procedures.
(b) So that the supervisor can continuously monitor a supervisee's practice in relation to safety.

The nurse's duty of care centres on the issue of the safety of the patient.

15 Supervisors continuously evaluate supervisees' knowledge and practice of procedures for:
    (i)   fire;
    (ii) suicidal behaviour;
    (iii) violence;
    (iv) health and safety;
    (v)   drug administration.

16 Staffing levels are regulated so that supervision by nurses of the necessary competence is not compromised by staff shortages.

The Nurses Rules place a legal obligation on nurse managers to ensure that students and nurses qualified in Parts 2, 4, 6 and 7 of the register are directed by nurses qualified in Parts 1, 3, 5 and 8 of the register.

17 Each supervisor ensures that his or her supervisees are thoroughly familiar with the following procedures:
    (i)   confidentiality;
    (ii)   the nurse's role in the multidisciplinary clinical team;
    (iii) the chaplaincy;
    (iv)   ethics;
    (v)   depot injections;
    (vi)   ECT;
    (vii) injecting a patient without consent;
    (viii) consent to treatment.

In order that they know where to find guidance on the relevant professional issues.

18 Nurses refrain from any kind of financial transaction with patients.

(a) There is a risk of potentially abusing the nurse's privileged access to details about the patient's financial circumstances.
(b) However well intentioned a nurse might be (for example, promising money for knitting materials used by a patient to make a garment for the nurse), unforeseen circumstances such as illness or accident could prevent the nurse from honouring the transaction.

19 A nurse is truthful towards patients in all situations.

Veracity is essential for a patient to be able to make informed choices about treatment.

20 The obligation to be truthful does not imply that the nurse will give direct and immediate answers to questions.

(a) Many situations require nurses to take advice before acting.
(b) It is important to find out what a patient knows already before supplying a too-ready answer.

21 The patients' information booklet might specify that if patients wish to show their appreciation of their treatment while in a particular ward, they can make a gift via the hospital administrator, nominating the ward or unit for which the gift is intended.

Since nurses are not paid directly by patients for their work, the acceptance of personal gifts may be interpreted as an infringement of the nurse's privileged access to patients.

22 Primary nurses ensure that each patient has a key with which to lock his or her personal storage facilities.

The Welsh Standards Document (DHSS, 1980) specifies that all patients should have access to lockable private storage facilities co-located with their sleeping space.

23 Nurses ensure that both psychological and physical privacy are available for patients when necessary.

So that patients have the opportunity to use rooms in wards for activities such as reading, listening to music with headphones, or board games, and are not obliged to lie on their beds in order to achieve privacy.

24 Nurses assess carefully the degree of intrusiveness experienced by individual patients in relation to history-taking and interviews.

(a) People, regardless of whether they are patients or not, have a right not to disclose private areas of their lives.
(b) It is notoriously difficult, when assessing certain mental states, to distinguish between a normal and abnormal extent of secretiveness.
(c) Intrusiveness may provoke angry, frightened or psychotic reactions in certain patients.

25 Nurses refrain under all circumstances from initiating or responding to offers to initiate social or sexual relationships of any kind with patients.

To participate in such a relationship is to abuse the nurse's privileged access to areas of the patient's life which would otherwise be inaccessible.

REFERENCE MATERIAL
References

Bok, S. (1980) *Lying: Moral Choice in Public and Private Life*, Quartet, London.

Bok, S. (1986) *Secrets: On the Ethics of Concealment*, Oxford University Press.

DHSS (1980) *Organizational and Management Problems of Mental Illness Hospitals*, DHSS, London.

Nurses, Midwives and Health Visitors Act (1979), HMSO, London.

Nurses, Midwives and Health Visitors Rules Approval Order (S.I. 1983/873), HMSO, London.

UKCC (1984) *Code of Professional Conduct for the Nurse, Midwife and Health Visitor*, 2nd edn, UKCC, London.

UKCC (1985) *Advertising*, UKCC, London.

UKCC (1987) *Confidentiality*, UKCC, London.

UKCC (1989) *Exercising Accountability*, UKCC, London.

Further reading

Austin, R. (1978) Professionalism and the nature of nursing reward, *Journal of Advanced Nursing*, Vol. 3, pp. 9–23.

Baly, M. (1984) *Professional Responsibility*, Wiley, Chichester.

Bottorff, J.L. and D'Cruz, J.V. (1984) Towards inclusive notions of 'patient' and 'nurse', *Journal of Advanced Nursing*, Vol. 9, pp. 549–53.

Brazier, M. (1987) *Medicine, Patients and the Law*, Penguin, Harmondsworth.

Chapman, C.M. (1980) The rights and responsibilities of nurses and patients, *Journal of Advanced Nursing*, Vol. 5, pp. 127–34.

Countryman, K.M. and Gekas, A.B. (1980) *Development and Implementation of a Patient's Bill of Rights in Hospitals*, American Hospital Association, Chicago.

Dawson, J.D. *et al.* (1977) Discussion of the RCN code of professional conduct, *Journal of Medical Ethics*, Vol. 3, no. 3, pp. 115–23.

Finch, J. (1981) The Arthur judgement, *Nursing Mirror*, Vol. 153, no. 21, pp. 12–13.

Griffin, A.P. (1983) A philosophical analysis of caring in nursing, *Journal of Advanced Nursing*, Vol. 8, pp. 289–95.

Gutierrez, J.L. and Ruiz, J. (1978) A comparative study of the psychiatric nurses' attitude towards mental patients, *International Journal of Social Psychiatry*, Vol. 24, no. 1, pp. 47–52.

Henry, B.M. *et al.* (1980) The hospitalized rich and famous, *American Journal of Nursing*, Vol. 80, pp. 1426–9.

Heslop, A. (1985) Establishing therapeutic relationships, *Nursing Mirror*, Vol. 160, no. 22, pp. 28–9.

Jones, B.E. and Miles, J.E. (1976) The nurse and the hospitalized mentally ill physician, *American Journal of Nursing*, Vol. 76, no. 8, pp. 1314–17.

Kitson, A.L. (1987) A comparative analysis of lay-caring and professional (nursing) caring relationships, *International Journal of Nursing Studies*, Vol. 24, no. 2, pp. 155–65.

Lego, S. (1980) The one-to-one nurse–patient relationship, *Perspectives in Psychiatric Care*, Vol. 18, no. 2, pp. 67–89.

Marshall, P.D. (1985) Nursing patients: an enjoyable task?, *Journal of Advanced Nursing*, Vol. 10, pp. 429–34.

Martin, A.J. (1978) Wills and gifts, *Nursing Times*, Vol. 74, no. 15, p. 625.

McGilloway, F.A. (1976) Dependency and vulnerability in the nurse–patient relationship, *Journal of Advanced Nursing*, Vol. 1, pp. 229–36.

McIntosh, J.B. (1979) The nurse–patient relationship, *Nursing Mirror*, Vol. 148, no. 4 (supp.), pp. i–ii, iv–v, vii, x–xx.

Meize-Grochowski, R. (1984) An analysis of the concept of trust, *Journal of Advanced Nursing*, Vol. 9, pp. 563–72.

Mills, V.H. (1977) Mutuality in nursing leads to vulnerability for patient and nurse in a psychiatric setting, *Journal of Advanced Nursing*, Vol. 2, pp. 21–8.

MIND (1985) *Your Rights in Hospital*, National Association for Mental Health, London.

National Staff Committee for Nurses and Midwives (1985) *Nurses with Alcohol and Drug Abuse Problems: Guidelines for Managers*, National Staff Committee for Nurses and Midwives.

Pembrey, S. (1984) Nursing care: professional progress, *Journal of Advanced Nursing*, Vol. 9, pp. 539–47.

Philpott, M. (1985) *Legal Liability and the Nursing Process*, Saunders, Toronto.

Pyne, R. (1982) Professional discipline, *Nursing*, Vol. 1, no. 36, pp. 1540–1.

Pyne, R. (1987) The UKCC Code of Conduct, *Nursing*, Vol. 3, no. 14, pp. 510–11.

Pyne, R. (1987) A professional duty to shout, *Nursing Times*, Vol. 83, no. 42, pp. 30–1.

Rea, K.M.J. (1982) Professional care, *Nursing*, Vol. 1, no. 36, pp. 1553–4.

Resolution on a European charter on the rights of patients (1984) *Office Journal of the European Communities*, C.46/104.

Roach, M.S. (1980) *Code of Ethics: An Ethical Basis for Nursing in Canada*, Canadian Nurses Association.

Schröck, R. (1980) A question of honesty in nursing practice, *Journal of Advanced Nursing*, Vol. 5, pp. 135–48.

Semin, G.R. and Manstead, A.S.R. (1983) *The Accountability of Conduct: A Social Psychological Analysis*, Academic Press, London.

Winslow, G.R. (1984) From loyalty to advocacy: a new metaphor for nursing, *Hastings Center Report*, Vol. 14, no. 3, pp. 32–40.

Yeaworth, R.C. (1985) The ANA Code: a comparative perspective, *Image*, Vol. 17, no. 3, pp. 94–8.

Yuen, K. (1986) The nurse–client relationship: a mutual learning experience, *Journal of Advanced Nursing*, Vol. 11, no. 5, pp. 529–33.

6

The Multidisciplinary Clinical Team

DEFINITION

The Royal Commission on the National Health Service (1979) defined a multidisciplinary clinical team as 'a group of colleagues acknowledging a common involvement in the care and treatment of a particular patient' (p. 171). The Commission used the abbreviation MDCT, which is also used in this procedure.

In the setting of the ward or inpatient unit of a hospital, an MDCT consists of all the professionals working in the ward with a consultant. In general, such a team includes some or all of the following, in addition to the nursing staff and the consultant: a senior registrar, a registrar or trainee psychiatrist, a clinical psychologist, a social worker and an occupational therapist. Sometimes the clinical psychologist, social worker and occupational therapist may have trainees working with them. In the same way, nursing and medical students take their places within the team. The hospital chaplains, teachers and art therapists may also be part of the MDCT.

DISCUSSION

Discussion of health care teams dates back to the early days of the National Health Service (NHS). Yet in 1984 Duncan's opinion (Duncan and McClachlan, 1984) was that there were many problems to be resolved in multidisciplinary teamwork. Aspects of the history of the NHS help to explain the problem.

History

The reorganization of the NHS in 1974 was designed to tackle the problems of long-term illness and handicap and of 'inadequate leadership, inefficient management, muddled organization' which had been identified by Schuster (1959). The three parts of the NHS (hospitals, local authorities and general practitioners) were to be integrated. Reorganization was to be achieved 'without infringing the clinical autonomy' of consultants and 'without interfering with the professional standards [and judgement] of the health-care professions' (DHSS, 1972a, p. 10). The apparent incompatibility of these two aims is at the base of many of the problems encountered by members of MDCTs.

The professional standards and organization of the main professions working within the NHS were examined by a number of reports in the 1960s and 1970s. The Cogwheel Reports (Ministry of Health, 1967; DHSS, 1972b, 1974) addressed the organization of the work of hospital doctors. By 1974 medical staff approached the multi-professional management arrangements of the reorganized NHS from a position of strength. The proposals of the Salmon Report strengthened the hierarchical structure of nursing management, but isolated clinical nurses (Report, 1966). In the same year, a report, *Psychiatric Nursing: Today and Tomorrow* (Ministry of Health, 1968), indicated that there was too little research on multi-professional teamwork, and on the roles of nurses in different settings. This lack made it difficult for the committee to make specific recommendations other than for urgent research. The Seebohm Report's proposals for unified local authority social service departments called into question the administration and function of hospital-based psychiatric social work services (Report, 1968). The remedial professions, including occupational therapists, were dismayed by the Tunbridge Report on Rehabilitation (DHSS Welsh Office, 1972; DHSS, 1973) which, they felt, did not acknowledge their autonomy, and did not consider their contributions to the multi-professional team. The Trethowan Report (DHSS, 1977), on the role of psychologists in the health services, recommended that interprofessional relationships should be based on multidisciplinary teamwork which, the report argued, reconciles the two principles of clinical and medical responsibility by recognizing that each member shares responsibility for patient care, while retaining professional independence. The report helped to consolidate the position of psychologists.

In 1982 a further reorganization of the NHS took place, designed to arrange services below district level into units of management: units being defined either in geographical terms or in terms of client care services. The Report of the NHS Management Inquiry (Griffiths, 1983) recommended urgent action to implement clearly defined general management with, according to HC(84)13, 'one person (at each level) who would take personal responsibility for securing action' (DHSS, 1984). General management was to complement multi-professional consensus management in order to ensure 'effective and timely management action'. It was proposed that clinicians would receive the necessary management training for them to advise and decide about the most effective use of resources. Since MDCTs were already variable in their strength and effectiveness, it remained to be seen whether unit and general management would strengthen or weaken multi-professional teamwork.

The lack of definition between the professions of leadership, autonomy and responsibility, as illustrated in the preceeding outline of the history of teamwork, required MDCTs at ward level to negotiate carefully their procedures for co-operation. A series of publications indicated that many MDCTs did not.

In 1975 the White Paper, *Better Services for the Mentally Ill* (DHSS, 1975), was published with many reservations about the possibility of funding the kind of long-term changes required to implement its recommendations. It described in some detail the concept of multi-professional teamwork, but said little about the specific role of psychiatric nurses within the MDCT. Continuing inquiries and reviews demonstrating 'grave inadequacies in individual hospitals' prompted the Secretary of State to set up in 1977 a working group to examine and make recommendations regarding the organization and management problems of mental illness hospitals (DHSS, 1980a, 1980b). In a critical review of the report, Towell (1980) suggested that many of its recommendations would not be implemented unless staff were prepared and able to 'adopt new approaches to their planning and management responsibilities' (p. 89). But as Towell indicated, the very problems which caused the working group to be set up in the first place were those which prevented staff from changing their ways of working. Related to the difficulties of implementing change is the lack of research to show the way.

Research

Temkin-Greener (1983) confirms that little research into teamwork exists, and criticizes the amount of prescriptive literature that has been published. Among other problems she identifies the conflicting goals of medicine and nursing. Davies (1979) comments on the wide differences in the history and contemporary settings of nursing in the USA and the UK, resulting in problems when American ideas are adapted to the British context. In particular, the idea of collegial teams has proved difficult to transplant.

Collegiality

Collegial teams are those in which members are not differentiated by hierarchy. Campbell-Heider and Pollock (1987) define collegiality as 'interdependent practice between physicians and nurses' (p. 421). They suggest that while doctors exercise most authority, nurses 'possess great informal power' (p. 423). It is suggested that the discrepancies in professions' authority and power relations can result in serious difficulties in implementing collegial teamwork. Another factor is the nature of the tasks and problems facing a team. A hierarchical structure can allow rapid decision-making and implementation, but may impede the co-ordination and balancing of the various contributions required for tackling complex, open-ended problems. Feiger and Schmitt's study (1979) of four teams caring for elderly diabetic patients in a nursing home demonstrated that collegiality of the teams was significantly associated with a positive outcome for patients. Teams which are undifferentiated by hierarchy are discussed in the extensive therapeutic community literature, which documents both the benefits and risks of non-differentiation.

Collaboration

Koerner, Cohen and Armstrong (1986, p. 40) define collaborative practice as a 'planned system through which members of the medical and nursing professions, together with other related health care disciplines, work to assure consistent, quality patient/family care'. Elpern *et al.* (1983) see collaborative practice as the historical successor to hierarchical practice. Weiss and Davis (1985) tested collaborative practice scales in order to determine the elements of collaborative practice between nurses and doctors. They recommend further research in the area because of the inconclusiveness of their results.

Communication

Several writers on teamwork cite communication paradigms (Pozgar, 1983; Deyne, 1985; McConnell, 1985; Wessel, 1985). Attempts to improve multidisciplinary practice have been based on human relations theories (Main, 1957, Revans, 1978). Engström (1986) identifies education in problem-solving strategies as being a key to nurses' improving their abilities to co-ordinate communication and decision-making in team conferences.

Conflict

Williams *et al.* (1978) argue that the lack of opportunity for nurses and social workers to interact during their training programmes leads to poor collaboration in the hospital setting. Furnham, Pendleton and Manicom (1981) conclude from their study of the perception of different occupations that adverse stereotypes based on prejudice decrease the likelihood of health teams functioning effectively. Guy (1986) concludes that conflict is associated with the degree of organizational complexity surrounding a team: the more complex a unit the more conflict there is likely to be. Hausman (1982) used a case study to argue that interdisciplinary conflicts often mask individuals' responses to threat in the form of change, whether imposed from outside or from within, say by the appointment of a senior member of a team.

Clinical responsibility

Clinical responsibility refers to the duty of care of each professional towards each patient. Dimond (1987a, 1987b) suggests that the issue comprises three aspects of professional care, management responsibilities and patient rights. She notes that no professional can plead that he or she carried out an illegal action under orders from another person. Nurses must be familiar with all relevant legislation in order to ensure that their actions always comply with the law regardless of orders from other nurses or health care colleagues. Criminal negligence can include the administration of incorrectly prescribed drugs. In some cases, a nurse cannot justify an action by saying he or she was ordered to carry it out if that action is contrary to the professional code of conduct and accepted professional practice. Management responsibilities are those to the nurse's employer. Dimond argues, for instance, that the administration of electroconvulsive therapy (ECT) is an example of the nurse's responsibility to carry out instructions, not of a doctor, but of an employer. Patients' rights are more problematic, since there is not a strong tradition of attention to the rights of health care consumers in the UK.

It is often supposed that the consultant is solely responsible for the patients in his or her care. This is not the case. Each member of the team can be called to account for the fulfilment of his or her responsibility for any delegated component of a treatment programme. Once a team member's responsibility is defined and agreed with the team and, if necessary, a qualified supervisor, in accordance with hospital policies, then he or she is deemed to be accountable for carrying out that part of the treatment programme. If an unsatisfactory treatment programme is decided upon jointly by the team members, they are all liable to be called to account. If a satisfactory treatment programme is decided jointly, but carried out negligently by one person, that person is liable, not the team.

Leadership

The Royal Commission (1979) concluded that each health professional was likely to have the last word on matters which were within his or her professional competence. Batchelor (Batchelor and McFarlane, 1980) was quite clear that if doctors were no longer to be seen as leaders of an MDCT, such a change should be determined by patients' needs and that nurses or psychologists who undertook to lead an MDCT should be educated for that role. Kane (1975) provides a number of questions to ask about leadership which are helpful for nurses attempting to clarify the role:

1 By what process is the leader selected?
2 Is there a leader at all?
3 Does leadership change according to the situation?
4 Is leadership geared to aims or process?
5 To what hierarchy do members belong outside the unit?

Margerison and McCann (1986) say that leaders of 'high performing teams' facilitate the use by team members of their skills rather than exact obedience from them.

Cameron *et al.* reported (1985) on the effect of Griffith reorganization on a psychiatric hospital where a highly structured project to change management teams 'never tackled directly' MDCTs at clinical level. Carlyn and Stoffelmeyer (1981) concluded from their study that clinical staff at the bottom of the administrative hierarchy not only had very different goals from administrators but also exerted a strong influence on organizational goals.

Human relations

Attention to the human relations of teams has been seen as a way out of the difficulties resulting from the constant implementation of change. Observation of cases has led to reports of deterioration of relationships within teams which has led to adverse consequences for individual members, and, it is claimed, for the well-being of patients (Stanton and Schwartz, 1954; Main, 1957; Hausman, 1982). Others have not seen the relevance of teamwork or doubt the need for human relations training (Appleyard and Maden, 1979; Batchelor and McFarlane, 1980). What has been repeatedly documented, however, is the difficulty that psychiatric MDCTs have in agreeing among themselves (Dick, 1981).

Margerison and McCann (1986) use Belbin's (1981) work in identifying key roles and activities of members of teams:

1 linking;

2 advising;
3 organizing;
4 explaining;
5 controlling.

They argue that in order to function effectively team members must be skilled in these activities. They suggest that individuals are able to adopt a number of roles which utilize these skills so that balanced team management results from the interplay of roles derived from the skills possessed by individuals in different degrees. They argue that self-assessment and feedback are necessary for each individual to maintain and improve standards.

Margerison's and McCann's model of teamwork (1986) requires fairly intensive education and training of team members. Stoelwinder (1984) suggests that such a model becomes established only in settings where teamwork is an accepted tradition. Evers' (1981) examination of MDCTs in geriatric wards concluded that co-operation between colleagues was more a matter of co-ordinating routines of work within the hierarchies of the respective professions than of collaboration. Stoelwinder (1984) suggests that teamwork is likely to decrease as each profession attempts to achieve and maintain autonomy.

Role of the nurse

Evers (1977) studied the place of the learner in the MDCT in the hospital ward. She concluded that total patient care is a precondition for integrated teamwork. Anderson and Finn (1983) reached a similar conclusion, that primary nursing facilitates collaboration and communication, which take place directly between assigned nurses and other disciplines. Evers (1977) also concluded that the ward sister has central responsibility for integrating and strengthening interprofessional relationships and communication.

GUIDELINES: WORKING AS A MULTIDISCIPLINARY CLINICAL TEAM

Action

Rationale

1 The trained nurses participate with other team members in drawing up the professional operating procedures, the ward objectives and the operational plan for the ward or department in conjunction with hospital policies.

(a) Consultation within and between levels of a hierarchy is essential for the acceptance and implementation of plans and procedures.
(b) Unless they conform to hospital policy they could be unsafe.

2 The professional operating procedures, ward objectives and operational plans are made available to all MDCT members.

(a) To orient new members.
(b) To ensure consistent practice.

3 The trained nurses agree on their allocation to the MDCTs in the ward.

In order that accountability and responsibility can be defined.

4 The charge nurse co-ordinates communication between team members.

(a) In order to remain fully informed.
(b) In order to disseminate information consistently and reliably.

5 The charge nurse publishes a timetable of all ward and MDCT activities, ensuring that all meetings are clearly timetabled.

(a) To orient new members.
(b) To facilitate attendance by members.
(c) To assist scheduling of other appointments.

6 The MDCT agrees the membership and purpose of each meeting. For example:
   (i) ward round;
   (ii) management round;
   (iii) inter-shift report.

So that each member knows what his or her responsibilities are in relation to each meeting of the MDCT.

7 The trained nurses attend consistently all the scheduled meetings of their assigned team.

    (a) To monitor nursing care.
    (b) To monitor face-to-face contact with other team members.

8 The charge nurse ensures a location for all scheduled meetings of the MDCT, as free from interruption as is consistent with safety.

    (a) To motivate members to attend.
    (b) To avoid disruption of decision-making processes.

9 The charge nurse ensures that the internal and external telephones are to hand during meetings.

    (a) To maintain communication with other staff and departments.
    (b) So that bleeps can be answered.
    (c) To be able to respond to emergencies.

10 Each member of the MDCT is responsible for arriving for meetings on time and helping to complete business on time.

    (a) So that everyone participates in the communication of information.
    (b) So that meetings do not go over time, and thereby interfere with work that is due to follow.
    (c) To help the conductor of the meeting fulfil his or her responsibility to monitor progress of all patients.

11 Team members miss scheduled meetings of the MDCT only in unavoidable circumstances, and, where possible, having given notice.

So that any problems can be anticipated and contingency plans agreed by the team.

12 In addition to patient-centred meetings, the MDCT holds regular sessions, say once a month, to:
    (i) evaluate performance;
    (ii) review procedures and objectives;
    (iii) plan changes;
    (iv) discuss current issues.

So that team members can review their own and their colleagues' work in a setting which does not confuse such review with issues of patient management.

13 Primary nurses attend all management meetings for their assigned patients.

    (a) To be the patient's advocate.
    (b) To give an account of their use of delegated responsibility.
    (c) So that other professionals deal directly with the nurses responsible for carrying out nursing care of individual patients.

14 The charge nurse monitors delegation to nurses by the team, ensuring that decisions are agreed and documented.

    (a) To ensure that only appropriate delegation of responsibility takes place.
    (b) To ensure that nurses receive appropriate supervision.

15 The charge nurse maintains a 'Who is Who' system in the ward.

So that new staff immediately have a reference for identifying the names and functions of the other members of the MDCT.

REFERENCE MATERIAL
References

Anderson, O.J. and Finn, M.C. (1983) Collaborative practice: developing a structure that works, *Nursing Administration Quarterly*, Vol. 8, no. 1, pp. 19–25.

Appleyard, J. and Maden, J.G. (1979) Multidisciplinary teams, *British Medical Journal*, Vol. 2, no. 170, p. 6200.

Batchelor, I. and McFarlane, J. (1980) *Multidisciplinary Clinical Teams*, Kings Fund Centre, London.

Belbin, R.M. (1981) *Management Teams*, Heinemann, London.

Cameron, D. *et al.* (1985) The way we do things round here – organizational change in a psychiatric hospital, *Hospital and Health Services Review*, Vol. 87, no. 2, pp. 65–8.

Campbell-Heider, N. and Pollock, D. (1987) Barriers to physician–nurse collegiality: an anthropological perspective, *Social Science and Medicine*, Vol. 25, no. 5, pp. 421–5.

Carlyn, M. and Stoffelmeyer, B. (1981) Diversity of goals in a state mental hospital, *Administration in Mental Health*, Vol. 9, no. 1, pp. 57–66.

Davies, C. (1979) Comparative occupations' roles in health care, *Social Science and Medicine*, Vol. 13A, no. 5, pp. 515–21.

Deyne, A.L. (1985) The importance of good communication among hospital personnel, *World Hospitals*, Vol. 21, no. 3, pp. 67–72.

DHSS (1972a) *Management Arrangements for the Reorganized National Health Service*, HMSO, London.

DHSS (1972b) *Second Report of the Joint Working Party on the Organization of Medical Work in Hospitals*, HMSO, London.

DHSS (1973) *The Remedial Professions*, HMSO, London.

DHSS (1974) *Third Report of the Joint Working Party on the Organization of Medical Work in Hospitals*, HMSO, London.

DHSS (1975) *Better Services for the Mentally Ill*, HMSO, London.

DHSS (1977) *Role of Psychologists in the Health Service* (Trethowan Report), HMSO, London.

DHSS (1980a) HC(80)8, *Structure and Management*, DHSS, London.

DHSS (1980b) *Organizational and Management Problems of Mental Illness Hospitals*, DHSS, London.

DHSS (1984) HC(84)13, *Implementation of the NHS Inquiry Report*, HMSO, London.

DHSS Welsh Office (1972) *Rehabilitation*, HMSO, London.

Dick, D. (1981) The medical contribution to the management of mental illness services, *Bulletin of the Royal College of Psychiatrists*, Vol. 5, no. 7, pp. 119–21.

Dimond, B. (1987a) Your disobedient servant, *Nursing Times*, Vol. 83, no. 4, pp. 28–31.

Dimond, B. (1987b) Doing the right thing, *Nursing Times*, Vol. 83, no. 5, p. 61.

Duncan, A.S. and McClachlan, G. (eds.) (1984) *Hospital Medicine and Nursing in the 1980s*, Nuffield Provincial Hospitals Trust, London.

Elpern, E.H., Rodts, M.F., DeWald, R.L. and West, J.W. (1983) Associated practice: a case for professional collaboration, *Journal of Nursing Administration*, Vol. 13, no. 10, pp. 27–31.

Engström, B. (1986) Communication and decision-making in a study of a multidisciplinary team conference with the registered nurse as conference chairman, *International Journal of Nursing Studies*, Vol. 23, no. 4, pp. 299–314.

Evers, H.K. (1977) The patient care team in the hospital ward: the place of the nursing student, *Journal of Advanced Nursing*, Vol. 2, pp. 589–96.

Evers, H.K. (1981) Multidisciplinary teams in geriatric wards: myth or reality?, *Journal of Advanced Nursing*, Vol. 6, pp. 205–14.

Feiger, S.M. and Schmitt, M.H. (1979) Collegiality in interdisciplinary health teams: its measurement and its effects, *Social Science and Medicine*, Vol. 13A, pp. 219–29.

Furnham, A., Pendleton, D. and Manicom, C. (1981) The perception of different occupations within the medical profession, *Social Science and Medicine*, Vol. 15E, no. 4, pp. 289–300.

Griffiths, R. (1983) *NHS Management Inquiry*, DHSS, London.

Guy, M.E. (1986) Interdisciplinary conflict and organizational complexity, *Hospital and Health Services Administration*, Vol. 31, no. 1, pp. 111–21.

Hausman, W. (1982) Interdisciplinary conflicts – the realities and illusions: a case report, *Administration in Mental Health*, Vol. 9, no. 4, pp. 250–6.

Kane, R.A. (1975) *Interprofessional Teamwork*, Syracuse University, New York.

Koerner, B.L., Cohen, J.R. and Armstrong, D.M. (1986) Professional behaviour in collaborative practice, *Journal of Nursing Administration*, Vol. 16, no. 10, pp. 39–43.

Main, T. (1957) The ailment, *British Journal of Medical Psychology*, Vol. 30, no. 3, pp. 129–45.

Margerison, C. and McCann, D. (1986) High performing management teams, *Health Care Management*, Vol. 1, no. 1, pp. 26–31.

McConnell, C.R. (1985) The supervisor's central role in organizational communication, *Healthcare Supervisor*, Vol. 3, no. 2, pp. 77–86.

Ministry of Health (1967) *First Report of the Joint Working*

Party on the Organization of Medical Work in Hospitals, HMSO, London.

Ministry of Health (1968) *Psychiatric Nursing: Today and Tomorrow,* HMSO, London.

Pozgar, G.D. (1983) Perceptive communications, *Healthcare Supervisor,* Vol. 1, no. 4, pp. 1–13.

Report (1966) *Report of the Committee on Senior Nursing Staff Structure* (the Salmon Report), Ministry of Health, London.

Report (1968) *Report of the Committee on Local Authority and Allied Personal Social Services (Seebohm Report),* HMSO, London.

Revans, R.W. (1978) Action learning takes a health cure, *Education, Training,* November–December, pp. 1–3.

Royal Commission (1979) *Royal Commission on the National Health Service,* HMSO, London.

Schuster, G. (1959) Creative leadership in a state service, in *Creative Leadership in a State Service: A General Survey,* Acton Society Trust, London.

Stanton, A.H. and Schwartz, M.H. (1954) *The Mental Hospital,* Basic Books, New York.

Steel, J.E. (1981) Putting joint practice into practice, *American Journal of Nursing,* Vol. 81, pp. 964–7.

Stoelwinder, J.U. (1984) Managing patient care on the ward, *Australian Health Review,* Vol. 7, no. 3, pp. 180–90.

Temkin-Greener, H. (1983) Interprofessional perspectives on teamwork in health care: a case study, *Milbank Memorial Fund Quarterly,* Vol. 61, no. 4, pp. 641–58.

Towell, D. (1980) Large institutions reconsidered: an approach to the management of transition, *Hospital and Health Services Review,* Vol. 76, no. 3, pp. 87–9.

Weiss, S.J. and Davis, H.P. (1985) Validity and reliability of the collaborative practice scales, *Nursing Research,* Vol. 34, no. 5, pp. 299–305.

Wessel, F. (1985) Communication: getting the best from your staff, *Hospital and Healthcare,* Vol. 16, no. 4, pp. 8–10.

Williams, C.C. *et al.* (1978) Social work and nursing in hospital settings, *Social Work in Health Care,* p. 322.

Further reading

Badawi, M. (1982) The role of the hospital social worker, *Nursing Times,* Vol. 78, no. 38, pp. 1601–3.

Benfer, B.A. (1980) Defining the role and function of the psychiatric nurse as a member of the team, *Perspectives in Psychiatric Care,* Vol. 18, no. 4, pp. 166–77.

Black, E., Whitehead, T. and Moore, R. (1983) New from old, *Nursing Mirror,* Vol. 157, no. 23, pp. 33–5.

Bouras, N., Trauer, T. and Watson, J.P. (1982) Ward environment and disturbed behaviour, *Psychological Medicine,* Vol. 12, pp. 309–19.

Carter, R. *et al.* (1984) *Systems, Management and Change,* Harper & Row, London.

Chacko, T.I. and Wong, J.K. (1984) Correlates of role conflict between physicians and nurse practitioners, *Psychological Reports,* Vol. 54, no. 3, pp. 783–9.

Coser, R.L. (1979) *Training in Ambiguity,* Free Press, New York.

Dartington, T. (1986) *The Limits of Altruism: Elderly Mentally Infirm People as a Test Case for Collaboration,* King Edwards Hospital Fund, London.

DHSS (1972) *Report of the Working Party on Medical Administrators,* HMSO, London.

DHSS (1974) *Third Report of the Joint Working Party on the Organization of Medical Work in Hospitals,* HMSO, London.

DHSS (1980) *Organizational and Management Problems of Mental Illness Hospitals,* DHSS, London.

Feldman, R., Cousins, A. and Grimaldi, D. (1981) The development phases of the nurse/patient relationship on an in-patient psychiatric unit, *Perspectives in Psychiatric Care,* Vol. 19, no. 1, pp. 31–9.

Goren, S. and Ottaway, R. (1985) Why health-care teams don't change: chronicity and collusion, *Journal of Nursing Administration,* Vol. 15, nos. 7–8, pp. 9–17.

Jaques, E. (1978) *Health Services: Their Nature and Organization, and the Role of Patients, Doctors and Nurses and the Complementary Professions,* Heinemann, London.

Keddy, B. *et al.* (1986) The doctor–nurse relationship: an historical perspective, *Journal of Advanced Nursing,* Vol. 11, no. 6, pp. 745–53.

Kucera, W.R. (1980) A defining of terms: collaboration versus supervision, *American Association of Nurse Anaesthetists,* Vol. 48, no. 6, pp. 547–8.

Lowe, J.I. and Herraness, M. (1981) Understanding teamwork: another look at the concepts, *Social Work in Health Care,* Vol. 7, no. 2, pp. 1–11.

Martin, A.J. (1976) Duty of care, *Nursing Times,* Vol. 72, no. 36, p. 1379.

Miller, M.H. (1975) PSROs–boon or bust for nursing? *Hospitals,* Vol. 49, no. 19, pp. 81–4.

Milne, M.A. (1980) Training for team care, *Journal of Advanced Nursing,* Vol. 5, pp. 579–89.

Ministry of Health (1952) *Report on Co-operation between Hospitals, Local Authority and General Practitioner Services,* HMSO, London.

Ministry of Health (1954) *Report of the Committee on the Internal Administration of Hospitals,* HMSO, London.

Ministry of Health (1963) *Communication between Doctors, Nurses and Patients: An Aspect of Human Relations in the Hospital Service,* HMSO, London.

National Health Service Act 1977, HMSO, London.

Nockin, M.S. (1983) Collaboration and communication, *Nursing Administration Quarterly,* Vol. 8, no. 1, pp. 1–7.

Report (1956) *Report of the Committee of Inquiry into the Cost of the National Health Service*, HMSO, London.

Report (1968) *Report of the Committee on Local Authority and Allied Personal Social Services*, HMSO, London.

Report (1972) *Report of the Committee on Nursing*, HMSO, London.

Report (1975) *Report of the Committee of Inquiry into the Regulation of the Medical Profession*, HMSO, London.

Roberts, C.A. (1985) Viewpoint: the multidisciplinary team in psychiatry, *Psychiatric Journal of the University of Ottowa*, Vol. 10, no. 3, pp. 147–152.

Ruch, M.D. (1984) The multidisciplinary approach: when too many is too much, *Journal of Psychosocial Nursing and Mental Health Services*, Vol. 22, no. 9, pp. 18–23.

Sanders, J.B. and Du Plessis, D. (1985) An historical view of right to treatment, *Journal of Psychosocial Nursing and Mental Health Services*, Vol. 23, no. 9, pp. 12–17.

Snyder, M. (1981) Preparation of nursing students for health care teams, *International Journal of Nursing Studies*, Vol. 18, no. 2, pp. 115–22.

Stoffelmayr, B.E., Lindsay, W. and Taylor, V. (1979) Maintenance of staff behaviour, *Behaviour Research and Therapy*, Vol. 17, no. 3, pp. 271–3.

Thompson, T., Labeck, L. and Zimmerman, R. (1980) Nursing staff adjustment as a function of psychiatric treatment modalities, *Journal of Behaviour Therapy and Experimental Psychiatry*, Vol. 11, no. 3, pp. 209–14.

Turnbull, E.N. (1982) Interdisciplinarism: problems and promises, *Journal of Nursing Education*, Vol. 21, no. 2, pp. 24–31.

Von Schilling, K. (1982) The consultant role in multidisciplinary team development, *International Nursing Review*, Vol. 29, no.3, pp. 73–5, 96.

Weinman, M.L. *et al.* (1979) Organizational structure and effectiveness in general hospital psychiatry departments, *Administration in Mental Health*, Vol. 7, no. 1, pp. 32–42.

Williams, R.A. and Williams, C. (1982) Hospital social workers and nurses: interprofessional perceptions and experiences, *Journal of Nursing Education*, Vol. 21, no. 5, pp. 16–21.

Wolfe, D.E. and Bushardt, S.C. (1985) Interpersonal conflict: strategies and guidelines for resolution, *American Medical Record Association Journal*, Vol. 56, no. 2, pp. 18–22.

Ziegfeld, C. and Jones, S. (1987) An innovative strategy to facilitate nurse–physician interaction, *Journal of Continuing Education in Nursing*, Vol. 18, no. 2, pp. 47–50.

7

Working Groups

DEFINITION

A working group is defined as a group within an organization which meets in order to specify and carry out tasks, solve problems, identify and achieve agreed objectives, and to make and implement decisions.

DISCUSSION
History

Hare (1976) identifies three original schools of small group research.

Sociometry

Sociometry was devised by J.L. Moreno in the 1930s and 1940s, and developed into socio- and psychodrama. Psychodrama is now part of a well-established field of humanistic approaches to training and personal experience in groups.

Group dynamics

The study of group dynamics was developed by Kurt Lewin in the 1930s and 1940s. He used applied research to study scientifically aspects of group process, including leadership, decision-making, conformity and the establishing and changing of norms.

Small groups

R.F. Bales at first engaged in laboratory studies of problem-solving by small groups, from which he developed interaction process analysis and applied research into social relations within small groups in the 1950s and 1960s.

Theories about personal relationships and organizational structure overlap. Most present-day assumptions about the functioning of groups stem from the three schools mentioned, combined with borrowings from several disciplines. Examples include sociological approaches to social differentiation and structure which

have taken conflict, power or role as their focus; biological theory, such as general systems theory, which has been extended to technological fields in engineering and management; and psychological approaches such as social learning theory, behaviourism and psychoanalysis.

Theories of organizations

It is suggested that theories of organizations overlap to a large extent, and that they are rarely completely incompatible. However, four broad groupings may be identified. One grouping assumes that the activities of members of organizations are constrained by the nature of the organization itself. A second assumes that the activities of its members define the organization: that their interaction produces its structure. A third assumes that the 'structure of an organization is contingent on the environment in which it exists', so that a structure which works in one place will not necessarily work in a different place. The fourth grouping assumes that the activities of the members of an organization are determined by the nature of its goals, whether clearly defined or not (Bowey, 1972). The studies and reports cited in the procedure for the nurse's role in the multidisciplinary team indicate that all four approaches offer plausible explanations for the problems of NHS management.

This procedure attempts to reconcile the four approaches, recognizing that whatever one's viewpoint, certain group interpersonal tasks must be managed in order that its specific tasks can be addressed. Interpersonal tasks include constructive management of conflict, determining of leadership, distribution of responsibility, delegation, communication, goal-setting and evaluation. Specific tasks include diagnosis, planning and management of treatment, face-to-face meetings, discussion, reporting and teaching.

Working groups with which psychiatric nurses are involved include ward rounds, management rounds, between-shift reports, supervisions, planning meetings, evaluation meetings, case conferences and staff groups. It is essential to distinguish a working group from a therapeutic group. Working groups have tasks and objectives that can be defined quite differently from those of therapeutic groups of whatever level. The principal distinguishing feature is that the focus is not on the intrapsychic processes or personal adjustment of the participants, but on interpersonal processes between the members of the MDCT only *as they affect the management of patients' treatment programmes*. In groups or meetings such as ward and management rounds, between-shift reports, planning and evaluation meetings, the attention paid to interpersonal processes is subordinate to that paid to the clinical management tasks specified for each meeting. In staff groups and supervisions the nature of interpersonal processes is likely to affect the task of the meeting to a much greater extent.

TERMINOLOGY

The terminology of groups and meetings can lead to some ambiguity. The words 'group' and 'meeting' may both refer to planned events which convene regularly; or they may refer to the collection of people convened at a given moment in time; or to a one-off discussion. Ambiguity can be exploited to enhance interpersonal relations. Each member of the MDCT is responsible for being sensitive to and helping to sort out potential confusions. The procedure for the role of the nurse in the MDCT emphasizes that all nurses are responsible for actively participating on equal terms with members of the other professions in the management of patient care programmes. They are not passive observers.

GUIDELINES: ESTABLISHING A WORKING GROUP

Action	**Rationale**
1 The charge nurse attends all working groups of the MDCT of which he or she is a member.	(a) Consistency of attendance by the charge nurse is essential for continuity of the nursing contribution from meeting to meeting. (b) Fragmentation in attendance at meetings is associated with poor staff morale and disturbed behaviour by patients. (c) In order to monitor supervision of the nurses.
2 The targets and objectives of all working groups are agreed with the MDCT, documented in the professional operating procedures and ward objectives and reviewed at regular intervals by the MDCT as a whole.	(a) To ensure a consistent and harmonious approach by team members. (b) To set and monitor standards.
3 Nurses in training attend as many working groups as is practicable.	To learn how to accept delegated responsibility.
4 The purpose of all working groups is explained to new nurses as part of their induction and orientation to the ward or unit.	(a) So that nurses are aware from the beginning of their training that working groups are integral to teamwork. (b) To demonstrate a coherent rationale. (c) To reduce anxiety.
5 Other meetings are not scheduled at times which clash with regular working groups.	(a) Common courtesy. (b) To prevent conflict between staff.

6 Chosen models for the working groups are made explicit in the professional operating procedures, agreed with the MDCT.

(a) In order that nurses may be taught skills specific to the model.
(b) In order that evaluation and comparison of the model can be carried out.

7 The MDCT agrees and documents in its procedures how each working group will be led, and the method for selecting leaders for meetings.

To prevent the jockeying for control which can arise from ill-defined or ambiguous practice.

8 Before a meeting the nurses discuss the ward atmosphere and decide on any precautions to be taken regarding safety.

(a) So that problems may be anticipated.
(b) So that a plan may be prepared in order to cause least disruption to the working group, while maintaining patient safety.

9 A nurse member of the meeting arranges for the room to be prepared in which the meeting is to take place, if it is in the ward. Otherwise team members decide on the routine for preparing the room.

(a) The nursing staff are responsible for the hotel services of the ward.
(b) Preparation of the room signifies that the business of the meeting is taken seriously.

10 The leader of each meeting is responsible for timekeeping.

Meetings start and finish on time so that the rest of the ward timetable may be carried out effectively.

11 Each member is responsible for conducting the business succinctly, with regard for other members and for safe practice.

Responsibility for the professional conduct of the meetings lies with the members as well as the conductor.

12 Nurses refrain from leaving meetings unless there is an emergency.

Continuity of nursing input ensures continuity of attention to patients' management, and co-ordination of treatment programmes.

REFERENCE MATERIAL
References
Bowey, A.M. (1972) Approaches to organization theory, reprinted in M. Lockett and R. Spear (eds.) (1980) *Organizations as Systems*, Open University, Milton Keynes.

Hare, A.P. (1976) *Handbook of Small Group Research*, Free Press, New York.

Further reading
Argyle, M. (ed.) (1981) *Social Skills and Health*, Methuen, London.

Beachy, P. and Biester, D.J. (1986) Restructuring group meetings for effectiveness, *Journal of Nursing Administration*, Vol. 16, no. 12, pp. 30–3.

Campbell-Heider, N. and Pollock, D. (1987) Barriers to physician–nurse collegiality: an anthropological perspective, *Social Science and Medicine*, Vol. 25, no. 5, pp. 421–5.

Coser, R.L. (1979) *Training in Ambiguity*, Free Press, New York.

Deyne, A.L. (1985) The importance of good communication among hospital personnel, *World Hospitals*, Vol. 21, no. 3, pp. 67–72.

Elpern, E.H., Rodts, M.F., DeWald, R.L. and West, J.W. (1983) Associated practice: a case for professional collaboration, *Journal of Nursing Administration*, Vol. 13, no. 10, pp. 27–31.

Engström, B. (1986) Communication and decision-making in a study of a multidisciplinary team conference with the registered nurse as conference chairman, *International Journal of Nursing Studies*, Vol. 23, no. 4, pp. 299–314.

Furnham, A., Pendleton, D. and Manicom, C. (1981) The perception of different occupations within the medical profession, *Social Science and Medicine*, Vol. 15E, no. 4, pp. 289–310.

Glaser, I. and Horvath, K. (1979) A tool for dealing with nursing problems, *Supervisor Nurse*, Vol. 10, no. 4, pp. 46–52.

Hardin, S.B., Stratton, K. and Benton, D. (1983) The video connection: group dynamics onscreen, *Journal of Psychosocial Nursing and Mental Health Services*, Vol. 21, no. 11, pp. 12–21.

Heron, J. (1975) *Six Category Intervention Analysis*, HPRP and BPMF, Guildford.

Heron, J. (1977) *Dimensions of Facilitator Style*, HPRP and BPMF, Guildford.

Jacobs, M.K. (1979) Equilibrium theory applied to small nurse groups, *Advances in Nursing Science*, Vol. 1, no. 2, pp. 23–39.

Jerrell, J.M. and Kouzes, J.M. (1982) Organization development in mental health agencies, *Administration in Mental Health*, Vol. 10, no. 1, pp. 22–39.

Johnson, R.M. (1982) The professional support group: a model for psychiatric clinical nurse specialists, *Journal of Psychosocial Nursing and Mental Health Services*, Vol. 20, no. 2, pp. 9–13.

Koerner, B.L., Cohen, J.R. and Armstrong, D.M. (1986) Professional behaviour in collaborative practice, *Journal of Nursing Administration*, Vol. 16, no. 10, pp. 34–43.

Lowe, J.I. and Herranen, M. (1981) Understanding teamwork: another look at the concepts, *Social Work in Health Care*, Vol. 7, no. 2, pp. 1–11.

Menzies, I.E.P. (1970) *The Functioning of Social Systems as a Defence Against Anxiety*, Tavistock, London.

National Association of Health Authorities (1985) *NHS Handbook*, NAHA, Birmingham.

Notkin, M.S. (1983) Collaboration and communication, *Nursing Administration Quarterly*, Vol. 8, no. 1, pp. 1–7.

Randolph, B.M. and Bernau, K. (1977) Dealing with resistance in the nursing care conference, *American Journal of Nursing*, Vol. 77, pp. 1955–8.

Robson, M. (1982) *Quality Circles: A Practical Guide*, Gower, Aldershot.

Steel, J.E. (1981) Putting joint practice into practice, *American Journal of Nursing*, Vol. 81, pp. 964–7.

Stoffelmayr, B.E., Lindsay, W. and Taylor, V. (1979) Maintenance of staff behaviour, *Behaviour Research and Therapy*, Vol. 17, pp. 271–3.

Tropman, J.E. (1980) *Effective Meetings: Improving Group Decision-Making*, Sage, Beverly Hills, Calif.

Veninga, R.L. (1984) Benefits and costs of group meetings, *Journal of Nursing Administration*, Vol. 14, no. 6, pp. 42–6.

Von Schilling, K. (1982) The consultant role in multidisciplinary team development, *International Nursing Review*, Vol. 29, no. 3, pp. 73–5, 96.

Wolfe, D.E. and Bushardt, S.C. (1985) Interpersonal conflict: strategies and guidelines for resolution, *American Medical Record Association Journal*, Vol. 56, no. 2, pp. 18–22.

8

Criticisms and Complaints

DEFINITIONS
Minor criticisms
A minor criticism is 'any comment or misgiving voiced by patients' (DHSS, 1981, Annex I, p. i). Such comments may be made to any nurse. An answer which is acceptable to the patient may be given straightaway, especially if the patient feels the nurse is listening sympathetically to what he or she has to say. However, the nurse remains alert to any dissatisfaction which may persist. Formal complaints can arise from misunderstandings and lapses in communication about apparently minor criticisms.

Formal complaints
'A formal complaint, which may be written or oral, is one which the complainant wishes to have investigated by senior staff and on which he wishes to have either a written reply or an oral explanation from the member of staff concerned' (DHSS, 1981, Annex I, p. i). The investigation of formal complaints is the responsibility of the senior member of staff of the department which is the subject of the complaint. A complaint about nursing care will be investigated by the chief nurse. Nurses from charge nurse and below are expected to help with such investigations but not to conduct them.

DISCUSSION
People who wish to complain about hospital treatment have many problems. Although the Hospital Complaints Procedures Act was passed in 1985, it has not, at the time of writing, been brought into force by statutory instrument. This means that hospitals are not required by law to have a complaints procedure. Despite the report of the Davies Committee on hospital complaints and a health circular, hospitals who do have a procedure do not have to standardize it (DHSS Welsh Office, 1973; DHSS, 1981). As will be seen, the present system is slow because it depends on moving complaints through the

clinical and administrative hierarchies (Consumers Association, 1978).

The Hospital Complaints Procedures Act 1985
This Act started life as a private member's bill put forward by an MP who had been seriously ill in an NHS hospital, and who found how difficult it was to have criticisms, comments and complaints answered. The Act was designed to ensure that health authorities implement effective complaints procedures so that patients' complaints can be dealt with more directly and quickly than they are at present. The Act proposes that each hospital employs its own ombudsman to deal with patients' complaints and to monitor care using accepted standards and procedures (Brazier, 1987).

The DHSS code of practice
MIND has been concerned for some years that psychiatric patients do not use their right to complain, and in 1987 published a booklet (Sinclair, 1987) designed to help patients through the labyrinth of procedures. Following the Davies Report (DHSS Welsh Office, 1973), the Department of Health issued a code of practice (DHSS, 1981). It distinguishes between 'minor criticisms' and 'formal complaints', and stresses that both types of complaint must be dealt with promptly. The annual reports of the Health Service Commissioner provide salutary evidence of the shortcomings of the implementation of many hospital procedures, including complaints.

The terminology of the DHSS guidelines (DHSS, 1981) is adopted here, bearing in mind that it would be much simplified by the statutory adoption of the Hospital Complaints Procedures Act. It is preferable to take a proactive rather than a reactive view of complaints. That is, anticipation and, where possible, prevention of patient-dissatisfaction will not only reduce the need for complaints, but will also assist any quality assurance programme. Patients' satisfaction with their care can be routinely assessed.

At present, management of patients' complaints is divided according to their content. Matters to do with clinical judgement, professional misconduct and the general quality of care are dealt with in different ways. This can be confusing and discouraging for patients, who become reluctant to pursue criticisms or complaints. The nurse who is primarily responsible for a patient's care is ideally placed both to monitor that person's and his or her relatives' and friends' views, and also to deal promptly with any problems as soon as they arise.

The procedure as stated here is based on the DHSS code of practice, which is recognized to be unwieldy. It is to be hoped that the consultation of health authorities concerning the appointment of their ombudsmen will result shortly in a streamlining both of policies and procedures.

Complaints by staff

The National Association of Health Authorities (1985) has issued a publication to guide staff who wish to make complaints on behalf of patients. Examples of the things which might prompt a nurse to complain include psychological or physical ill-treatment, loss or damage of a patient's property and deprivation of services or rights to which the patient is entitled.

The nurse can take the matter up with his or her line manager. Normally the line manager is expected to pursue the complaint until it is resolved but, if the nurse wishes, he or she can approach the unit general manager, director of nursing services, district general manager, or chairman of the health authority. In addition, the nurse may complain on behalf of a patient to the National Health Service Commissioner (about non-clinical matters) and to the Mental Health Act Commission (about detention of a patient under the Mental Health Act). In the process of investigation the nurse would be expected to produce evidence in support of his or her complaint.

GUIDELINES: DEALING WITH MINOR CRITICISMS

Action

1 If a patient or a friend or relative makes a comment about any aspect of the patient's care or treatment, invite them to speak in detail about what is concerning them.

2 Find out whether the person making the complaint wishes to have it investigated by senior staff; or if he or she wishes to have a written reply from a member of the health authority; or if he or she wishes for an explanation from a senior member of staff.

3 If the reply to 2 is 'Yes', turn to the Guidelines for dealing with formal complaints.

4 If the reply to 2 is 'No', give an explanation or answer straight away.

5 Regardless of the person to whom any comments are addressed, the charge nurse discusses the matter with his or her immediate nurse manager and, if thought appropriate, with the patient's consultant.

Rationale

(a) It is not usually necessary to ask the person to wait while a more senior nurse is found.
(b) It is important that the person making the complaint has an early opportunity to describe it in full.

In order to decide whether to follow the procedure for minor criticisms or the procedure for formal complaints.

In order to give a satisfactory answer as soon as possible.

(a) Some criticisms may easily be dealt with by comparatively inexperienced nurses.
(b) Even if a full answer cannot be supplied, some indication can be given of the likely course of events.

(a) In order to review the ward's practice and procedures in the light of the comments.
(b) In order to decide whether to conduct team discussions or to meet with individual members in order to review their practice.

6 If the matter concerns a person's treatment, arrange, via the charge nurse, if necessary, for the person to see the senior registrar or consultant without delay.

In accordance with HC/81/5.

7 Keep the person informed if there is any delay. For example, if the consultant or senior registrar is away for any reason.

So that it is clear that the matter has not just been shelved.

(i) Let the person know how long any delay is likely to be.

So that he or she knows when a response to the criticism may be expected.

(ii) Document in the nursing record the details of what has happened between the nurse and the person making the comments.

(a) For future reference.
(b) To record the details of the criticism and action taken in case the matter is pursued.

(iii) Inform the senior registrar or consultant via the charge nurse that the person wishes to see them.

The doctor concerned may wish to see the person alone or with another member of the multidisciplinary clinical team (MDCT).

(iv) Ask the person whether he or she is satisfied with the answer or explanation received.

In order to confirm that the staff have not merely paid lip service to the concerns expressed by the person making the comments.

(v) If the person expresses satisfaction, ask him or her to speak again if second thoughts occur.

Even apparently satisfactory responses to criticisms may leave doubts.

(vi) Document the details of what was said and done in the nursing record.

In order that evaluation and any review of practice necessary may take place.

(vii) Within two days, check with the person that he or she remains satisfied.

To ensure that the cause of the comments or criticism has not reappeared.

8 If the person is not satisfied with the answer, ask if he or she would like to meet with the nurse in charge of the ward. That is, the senior registered nurse on duty.

The nurse in charge will be able to direct the person making the complaint to another member of the MDCT, or to a manager.

(i) Arrange the meeting as soon as possible.

It is essential that criticisms are attended to promptly. Delay may otherwise seem like prevarication.

(ii) Keep the person informed if there is any delay. For example, if the nurse is away from the ward for any reason.

(iii) Tell the person how long any delay is likely to be.

So that he or she can ask to see somebody else if the delay seems too long.

(iv) Document in the nursing record the details of what has taken place.

(a) To inform others who are dealing with the person's criticisms what has been done so far.
(b) To provide documentation if the matter is investigated later.

9 The nurse in charge of the ward meets the person making the complaint and gives an explanation or answer.

At this point the nurse must have enough authority to make a decision as to further action, if necessary.

(i) The nurse in charge asks the person if he or she is satisfied with the answer or explanation.

In order to confirm that the staff have not merely paid lip service to the concerns expressed by the person making the comments.

(ii) If the person expresses satisfaction, he or she is asked to speak again if second thoughts occur.

Even apparently satisfactory responses to criticisms may leave doubts.

(iii) Document the details of what was said and done in the nursing record.

In order that evaluation and any review of practice necessary may take place.

(iv) Check with the person that he or she remains satisfied.

To ensure that the cause of the comments or criticism has not reappeared.

10   If the person is not now satisfied, ask if he or she now wishes to have the matter investigated by senior staff, or to have a written reply from the health authority, or to have an explanation from a senior member of staff.

In order to decide whether to follow the procedure for minor criticisms or the procedure for formal complaints.

11   If the reply to 10 is 'Yes', turn to the Guidelines for dealing with formal complaints.

In order to give a satisfactory answer as soon as possible.

12   If the reply to 10 is 'No', give an explanation or answer straight away.

Even if a full answer cannot be supplied, some indication can be given of the likely course of events, especially as this is the repeat of an earlier unresolved criticism.

13   Regardless of the person to whom any comments are addressed, the charge nurse discusses the matter with his or her immediate nurse manager and with the patient's consultant.

(a)   In order to review the ward's practice and procedures in the light of the comments.
(b)   In order to decide whether to conduct team discussions or to meet with individual members in order to review their practice.

14   (i)   If an answer or explanation cannot be given straight away, explain this to the person making the comments.

In order to give him or her the opportunity to request that the matter is dealt with by a senior member of staff or the health authority.

(ii)   If such a request is made, turn to the Guidelines for dealing with formal complaints.

In order to give a satisfactory answer as soon as possible.

15   If the person is willing to wait for an explanation or answer from another member of the ward team, ask if he or she will be satisfied with your finding out and bringing any answer.

In case the person making the criticism would prefer to speak directly to that other member of the team.

(i)   If 'Yes', keep him or her informed if there is any delay in finding an answer.

So that it is clear that the matter has not just been shelved.

(ii)   If 'No', ask if he or she wishes to write details of the complaint or whether it is acceptable for you to write them down.

A criticism is more likely to be accurately relayed to a third person if it is written down.

(iii)   When you have written two copies of what you understand the person's comments to be, leave the second copy with him or her, after checking that the wording is acceptable.

Once the criticism is in writing, the person who originated it keeps a copy to ensure that it is properly dealt with.

(iv)   If the person writes comments him- or herself, ensure that he or she delivers or posts it independently to the chosen member of the ward staff, and advise that a copy is kept by the complainant.

If a letter goes astray, the nurse who posted or delivered it for the patient will be at risk of being blamed for the loss.

(v)   Let the person know how long any delay is likely to be.

So that he or she knows when a response to the criticism may be expected.

(vi)   If the answer is directed to the nursing staff, convey it to the person making the comments as soon as is practicable.

To minimize delay.

(vii)   Ask the person whether he or she is satisfied with the answer or explanation received.

In order to confirm that the staff have not merely paid lip service to the concerns expressed by the person making the comments.

(viii)   If the person expresses satisfaction, ask him or her to speak again if second thoughts occur.

Even apparently satisfactory responses to criticisms may leave doubts.

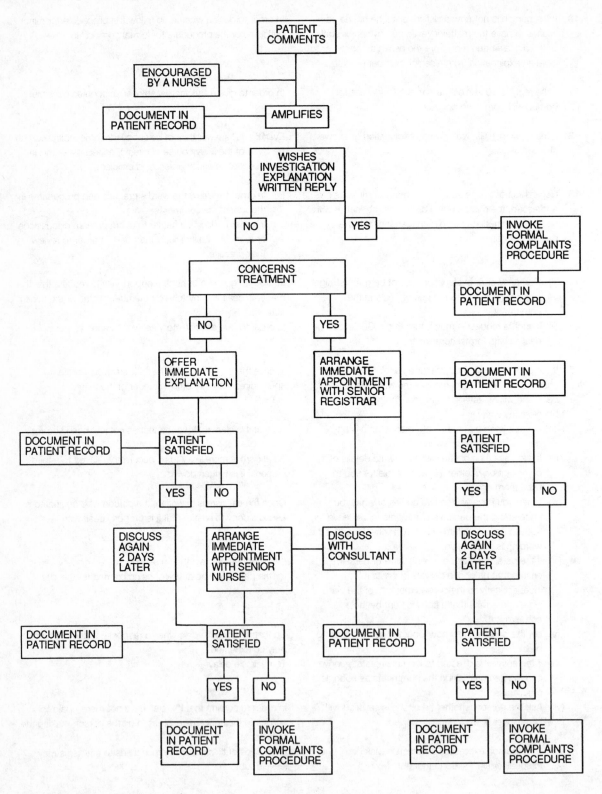

Figure 8.1   Minor criticisms procedure

(ix) Document the details of what was said and done in the nursing record.

In order that evaluation and any review of practice necessary may take place.

(x) Check with the person that he or she remains satisfied.

To ensure that the cause of the comments or criticism has not reappeared.

16 If the person is not satisfied, ask if he or she now wishes to have the matter investigated by senior staff, or to have a written reply from the health authority, or to have an explanation from a senior member of staff.

In order to decide whether to follow the procedure for minor criticisms or the procedure for formal complaints.

17 If the reply to 16 is 'Yes', turn to the Guidelines for dealing with formal complaints.

In order to give a satisfactory answer as soon as possible.

18 If the reply to 16 is 'No', arrange for a meeting of the multidisciplinary care team together with the nurse manager responsible for the ward or unit.

(a) To decide on the best course of action.
(b) To decide which member(s) of the team will continue to deal with the matter.
(c) It may be useful for the team itself to consult with a senior member of the hospital staff.

19 Regardless of the person to whom any comments are addressed, the charge nurse discusses the matter with his or her immediate nurse manager and with the patient's consultant.

(a) In order to review the ward's practice and procedures in the light of the comments.
(b) In order to decide whether to conduct team discussions or to meet with individual members in order to review their practice.

These guidelines are shown diagrammatically in Figure 8.1.

GUIDELINES: DEALING WITH FORMAL COMPLAINTS

Action

Rationale

1 Find out whether the complaint arises from a cause within the last twelve months.

Elapsed time of a year or more will affect investigation of the complaint.

2 Find out whether the person making the complaint wishes to have it investigated by senior staff; or if he or she wishes to have a written reply from the health authority or if he or she wishes for an explanation from a senior member of staff; or if the complaint concerns the person's treatment. (These alternatives are not necessarily mutually exclusive.)

(a) In order to direct the complaint to the right person as soon as possible.
(b) There may be only one opportunity for investigation and reply before the Health Service Commissioner is asked to intervene.
(c) If the complaint concerns a person's treatment the consultant is responsible for initiating any investigation.

3 If the complainant wishes to make a formal complaint the charge nurse takes over and carries out the following procedure without delay.

(a) To ensure close liaison between the senior member of staff investigating the complaint and nursing staff who may be asked to help the investigation.
(b) To ensure that both the complainant and any staff complained about are kept fully informed.
(c) In order to help the person make his or her complaint known without delay.

4 Ask the complainant if he or she wishes to write the complaint; or to make it orally; or to sign the complaint when it is written down by staff.

In order to facilitate the transmission of the complaint.

5 If the complainant wishes to write the complaint ask if he or she wishes to make it to a specific member of staff or to the health authority.

To ensure that the complaint is directed to the right person.

6 If the complainant wishes to write the complaint to a specific member of staff, advise him or her to do so without delay.

'All complaints should be investigated thoroughly and fairly and as quickly as circumstances permit. It should be remembered that the unsatisfactory handling of a complaint may become the cause of further complaint' (DHSS, 1981, Annex II, p. i).

7 If the complainant wishes to complain about the patient's treatment, ask whether he or she wishes to write to or meet with the patient's consultant.

(a) The consultant is likely to wish to begin his or her investigation as quickly as possible.
(b) The consultant may need to liaise with the patient's general practitioner as well as senior health authority staff and administrators.

8 Arrange for the complainant personally to mail or deliver the complaint to the member of staff he or she has designated, and to keep a copy.

If a letter delivered by a nurse subsequently goes astray, the nurse is open to allegations of interfering with it.

9 If the complainant wishes to make the complaint orally, arrange without delay for him or her to meet with the designated senior member of staff.

It may be possible for the senior member of staff to resolve the matter by discussion.

10 If the complainant wishes a nurse or another member of staff to write his or her complaint the charge nurse arranges without delay for the nurse or other staff member to meet with him or her and to write out two copies of the complaint.

In order to ensure that the complaint is promptly and accurately transmitted.

11 Regardless of the person to whom any complaint is addressed, the charge nurse discusses the matter with his or her immediate manager and with the patient's consultant.

In order to review the ward's practice and procedures in the light of the complaint, bearing in mind that this will not prevent disciplinary action if the complaint is upheld.

12 The charge nurse, together with his or her manager, advises any member of staff who is the subject of a complaint that he or she has the right to seek help and advice from a professional organization or trade union before making any statement.

As the representatives of the hospital organization the charge nurse or nurse manager may be involved in any subsequent disciplinary procedure.

13 All nurses who are asked to assist in investigating complaints are advised to seek advice or help from their professional organization or trade union.

Complaints which reveal defects in carrying out procedures could result in disciplinary action for the staff concerned.

14 The charge nurse informs the director of nurse education if a student nurse is the subject of a complaint.

(a) In case disciplinary action becomes necessary.
(b) In order to make educational use of the experience.
(c) In order that the student's personal tutor can provide support, guided by the DNE.

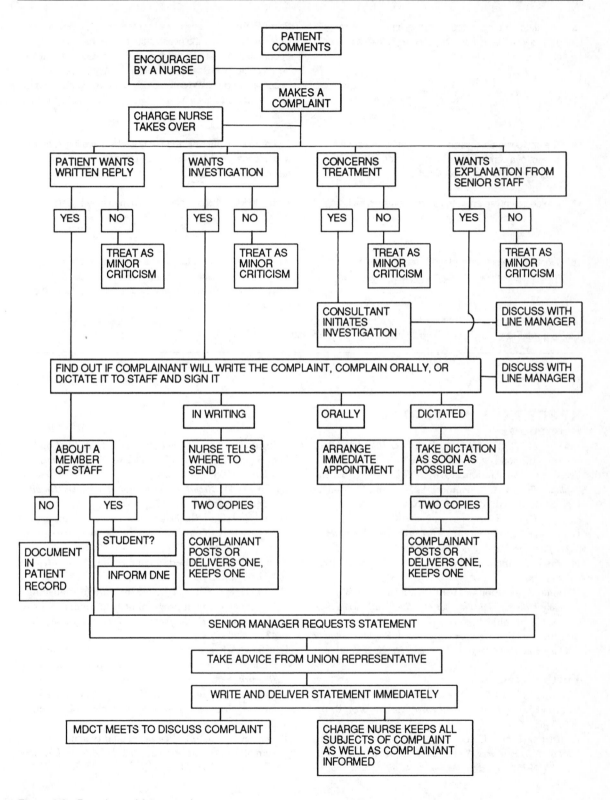

Figure 8.2 Formal complaints procedure

15 Any statement requested by the senior member of staff dealing with the matter is supplied as quickly as possible.

Because the complainant may apply to the Health Service Commissioner after the health authority has had one opportunity to deal with the complaint, it is essential that the health authority possesses as much information as necessary to complete satisfactorily any investigation and to give the complainant a full reply within a reasonable period of time.

16 The charge nurse ensures that any staff who are the subject of a complaint are kept fully informed about the progress and outcome of investigations.

Failure to keep staff informed may lead to lowering of morale and uncertainty about any disciplinary action which may result from the complaint.

17 The charge nurse ensures that the complainant is kept fully informed about the progress and outcome of investigations.

Failure to keep the complainant informed may be interpreted as evasion and prevarication.

18 Whatever the outcome of the complaint, the ward's multidisciplinary clinical team discusses the matter.

(a) In order to review the ward's practices and procedures.
(b) In order to make any changes necessary, bearing in mind that this will not prevent disciplinary action if the complaint is upheld.

These guidelines are shown diagrammatically in Figure 8.2.

REFERENCE MATERIAL
References

Brazier, M. (1987) *Medicine, Patients and the Law*, Penguin, Harmondsworth.

Consumers Association (1978) *A Report on NHS Complaints Procedures*, Consumers Association, London.

DHSS (1981) HC(81)5, *Health Service Complaints Procedure*, DHSS, London.

DHSS Welsh Office (1973) *Report of the Committee on Hospital Complaints Procedure*, HMSO, London.

Hospital Complaints Procedure Act 1985, HMSO, London.

National Association of Health Authorities (1985) *Protecting Patients: Guidelines for Handling Staff Complaints*, NAHA, Birmingham.

Sinclair, L. (1987) *Proper Channels: A Practical Guide to Complaints about Medical Treatment*, MIND, London.

Further reading

Altschul, A.T. (1983) The consumer's voice: nursing implications, *Journal of Advanced Nursing*, Vol. 8, pp. 175–83.

Armstrong-Esher, C.A. (1981) Standards of nursing care, *Nursing Times*, Vol. 77, no. 1, pp. 19–22.

DHSS (1975) *Report of the Committee of Inquiry into the Regulation of the Medical Profession*, HMSO, London.

DHSS (1976) HN(76)107, *Health Services Complaints Procedure*, DHSS, London.

DHSS (1980) *Report of the Review of Rampton Hospital*, HMSO, London.

Drew, N. (1986) Exclusion and confirmation: a phenomenology of patients' experiences with caregivers, *Image*, Vol. 18, no. 2, pp. 39–43.

Fautrel, F. (1977) Why don't nurses complain?, *Mindout*, Vol. 22, pp. 5–7.

Gould, E. and Glick, I.D. (1976) Patient–staff judgements of treatment programme helpfulness on a psychiatric ward, *British Journal of Medical Psychology*, Vol. 49, pp. 23–33.

Hinshaw, A.S. and Atwood, J.R. (1982) A patient satisfaction instrument: precision by replication, *Nursing Research*, Vol. 31, no. 3, pp. 170–5.

Inguanzo, J.M. and Harju, M. (1985) Consumer satisfaction with hospitalization, *Hospitals*, Vol. 59, no. 9, pp. 81–3.

Kitson, A.L. (1986) Indicators of quality in nursing care – an alternative approach, *Journal of Advanced Nursing*, Vol. 11, pp. 133–44.

Kucera, W.R. (1976) Legal problems with PSRO's, *Journal of the American Association of Nurse Anaesthetists*, Vol. 44, pp. 68–73.

Larson, E. (1983) Combining nursing quality assurance and research programmes, *Journal of Nursing Administration*, Vol. 13, no. 11, pp. 32–5.

Mangen, S.P. and Griffith, J.H. (1982) Patient satisfaction with community psychiatric nursing: a prospective controlled study, *Journal of Advanced Nursing*, Vol. 7, pp. 477–82.

Miller, G.A. (1976) Patient knowledge and nurse role strain in three hospital settings, *Medical Care*, Vol. 14, no. 8, pp. 662–73.

Miller, G.A. (1977) On knowledge and being a pest, *Medical Care*, Vol. 15, no. 4, pp. 351–3.

Miller, T.W. and Lee, L.J. (1980) Quality assurance: focus on environmental perceptions of psychiatric patients and nursing staff, *Journal of Psychosocial Nursing and Mental Health Services*, Vol. 18, no. 12, pp. 9–13.

Ministry of Health (1966) HM(66)15, *Methods of Dealing with Complaints by Patients*, Ministry of Health, London.

Moores, B. (1986) What 1357 patients think about aspects of their stay in British acute hospitals, *Journal of Advanced Nursing*, Vol. 11, pp. 87–102.

National Consumer Council (1983) *Patient's Rights*, HMSO, London.

Rayner, C. (1979) Reality and expectation of the British National Health Service consumer, *Journal of Advanced Nursing*, Vol. 4, pp. 69–77.

Thompson, A. (1986) A patient's eye view, *Nursing Times*, Vol. 82, no. 10, pp. 30–2.

Turner-Smith, A. and Thomson, I.G. (1979) Patients' opinions, *Nursing Times*, Vol. 75, no. 16, pp. 675–9.

Ventura, M.R. *et al.* (1982) A patient satisfaction measure as a criterion to evaluate primary nursing, *Nursing Research*, Vol. 31, no. 4, pp. 226–30.

Vousden, M. (1986) Removing labels, *Nursing Times*, Vol. 82, no. 48, pp. 18–19.

Watkin, B. (1976) Half a loaf, *Nursing Mirror*, Vol. 142, no. 11, p. 42.

9

Confidentiality

DEFINITION

The responsibility of the nurse for confidentiality in his or her dealings with patients relates to the privileged information to which he or she has access by virtue of his or her position. That is, the nurse is likely to hear much that the patient would be unlikely to divulge to anyone other than a health care professional.

DISCUSSION

The UKCC has issued an 'elaboration' of its Code of Conduct in order to provide 'a framework to assist individual professional judgement' (UKCC, 1987, p. 1, see Appendix A). The issues are complex and are laid out also as guidelines for doctors in the British Medical Association's *Handbook of Medical Ethics* (1981). There are four main exceptions to the general principle of confidentiality of all dealings with a patient: when a patient gives consent; when it is undesirable on medical grounds to seek a patient's consent; when the patient is the subject of medical research; when the information is required by due legal process. A number of statutes require disclosure by doctors of patients' treatment when relevant. They include the Abortion Act 1967, the Road Traffic Act 1972 and the Public Health Acts (Phillips and Dawson, 1985).

Since privileged information is divulged to the nurse in the context of his or her professional relationship with the patient, it follows that he or she will normally divulge it only in the context of professional activities as a member of a multidisciplinary clinical team (MDCT). The routine spread of information is therefore restricted to the nursing process documentation, the patient record, and the MDCT's meetings, which have as their objective the planning and evaluation of the care being given to the patient (Martin, 1978). This means that the nurse will avoid discussing a patient with any colleague who is not a member of the ward team. Even if a nurse establishes, for instance, that a general practitioner or

other professional colleague not in the ward team is making an inquiry, he or she will divulge no more than is absolutely necessary.

Case notes

The patient's personal notes are kept under lock and key in the ward or department office, together with the nursing process documentation. Only those personnel involved in the care of the patient have access to these records, the keys to which are held by the charge nurse or a designated deputy. To preserve confidentiality, to ensure continuity of patient management, and to ensure that case notes leave a ward or department for as short a time as possible, the charge nurse will implement a signing-out procedure to be followed by people who are authorized to remove case notes from the ward.

There are exceptions. Nurses in training may be asked to bring clinical material to classes by their tutors as part of the educational process. As long as the patient is not named in any written work used in the school of nursing, and such classes are held in private, not recorded on audio- or videotape, confidentiality remains intact.

The second exception concerns the duty of the nurse to pass on information when it seems likely that a crime has been or is likely to be committed, or that the patient has been involved in an accident (Martin, 1978). Protection for a criminal, even if only suspected, is not accepted professional practice.

The third exception concerns the liability of any nursing record to be subpoenaed as evidence in a court of law, including a coroner's court, investigations by the National Health Service Commissioner and the Mental Health Act Commissioners. The nurse may be required to give oral evidence in addition to the nursing record. To refuse to do so would risk being in contempt of court. The same liability applies to priests, lawyers, doctors and journalists who may acquire sensitive information from clients.

Where patients request secrecy before divulging information

Patients may ask nurses to keep secret information which they say they are about to divulge. Nurses must make it clear to patients that in the last resort this is not possible and ask the patient to consider whether he or she wishes to go ahead with disclosure. 'We can properly promise only that which is ours to give or what is right for us to do in the first place' (Bok, 1986, p. 152).

In the short term there is evidence to suggest that therapeutic programmes and working relationships within teams are jeopardized by attempts of individual members to keep secret aspects of their interaction with patients. The assumption by staff members of responsibility for something where that responsibility is not theirs to take leads to an attempt to defend an untenable position. The patient, meanwhile, is relieved of responsibility for determining a course of action to deal with the matter which he or she has passed on to the nurse. A nurse who is clear about his or her own position can more confidently assess the patient's position, maintaining a professional working relationship with that patient. The nurse who agrees to work with the patient on the patient's terms whatever their implications for his or her professional conduct is unlikely to be able to maintain a working relationship with that patient or with colleagues.

If a patient *does* ask a nurse to keep secret a piece of information before he or she divulges it, the nurse has the opportunity of exploring with the patient his or her motivations for making the request before saying what the constraints on the nurse are – taking care that the information itself is not inadvertently (or deliberately) disclosed during the discussion. If caught unawares the nurse can ask the patient not to continue, and to arrange to meet on another occasion. An example of a verbal intervention is: 'You shouldn't tell me anything personally that I cannot share with my colleagues.' The nurse then takes

advice from his or her colleagues within the nursing and multidisciplinary teams. The nurse may feel that he or she is being unhelpful or ungracious when refusing to be drawn into the patient's absolute confidence. Therefore he or she needs a practical repertoire for dealing with this, for example: 'I have no authority to accept your confidence; I can only listen to what you say as a member of a team of people who are trying to help you.'

Where patients request secrecy after divulging information

If the patient divulges the information to a nurse before asking him or her to keep it secret, it may be easier to examine with the patient why he or she took the risk of disclosure before checking whether the nurse would keep a secret. Many patients worry that their problems or needs deviate unacceptably from those of other people, and feel ashamed of talking about them. The shame is expressed in having second thoughts after making the disclosure. It can be a relief to hear the nurse acknowledge this experience, and to hear that the whole team and not just one person is at his or her disposal.

Retaining information within the MDCT

It is unusual for nurses to find that they have to disclose information given by a patient outside the MDCT. Whenever possible, such disclosure is done only with the consent of the patient, with the agreement of the MDCT and of senior colleagues. It follows that the nurse's obligation to retain the information within the MDCT precludes him or her from casual discussion during, say, meal breaks, social occasions, journeys on public transport and so on.

The patient's acknowledgement of the possibility of information going outside the MDCT does not imply agreement to the disclosure of information. It is a serious breach of confidentiality to allow this to happen without the patient's consent. It is necessary to obtain in writing the patient's consent to any disclosure of information as the result of an approach by a third party.

GUIDELINES: MAINTAINING CONFIDENTIALITY

Action

1 The ward keys are held only by a charge nurse or designated deputy.

Rationale

(a) Hospital policy.
(b) To ensure limited access to confidential material.

2 The nursing and medical notes are held in a locked cupboard in the ward or department office.	To ensure security of confidential information.
3 All staff wear their identification badges.	To ensure that only those who are authorized to do so have access to confidential material.
4 Any person requesting access to the patient records identifies him- or herself as a member of the ward team to the charge nurse and states the purpose for which the notes are wanted.	To prevent access to confidential material by unauthorized persons.
5 No information about a patient is given over the telephone unless the caller says who they are and permission is asked from the patient concerned to give information about him or her.	Where possible, the patient agrees to the nurse giving the patient's telephone number to the caller so that the patient and the person making the inquiry can speak together.
6 In the case of written requests for information concerning a patient, the member of the MDCT to whom the request is addressed secures the agreement of the patient.	Nurses do not carry out this task unless agreed with the charge nurse and the rest of the MDCT.
7 Recording of information in the nursing record takes place as soon after an interaction as possible and, so far as possible, quoting the patient directly.	In order that nurses distinguish between interpretations or opinions of a patient's behaviour and descriptions of the same behaviour.
8 If an opinion about a patient is recorded in the notes and is that of someone other than the person making the entry, he or she is named.	(a) So that opinions are clearly identified. (b) So that it is clear who within an MDCT holds a given opinion.
9 Process recordings of interactions for educational use outside the ward or department do not identify the patient concerned.	To ensure that confidentiality remains intact when nursing care is discussed outside the patient's MDCT.
10 The signed consent of the patient is obtained (the health authority may provide a printed form) before any audio- or videotaping or photography of that patient takes place.	(a) Informed consent of the patient is a prerequisite. (b) In order to allow him or her later to withdraw consent after reflection on the matter.
11 Audio- and video-recordings and photographs of patients are stored in locked facilities for that purpose.	(a) In order that any recordings used for teaching purposes can be borrowed and returned under secure conditions and within appropriate time limits. (b) In order to maintain catalogues and issue receipts as necessary.
12 A nurse to whom a patient discloses information which leads him or her to believe that a crime has been or will be committed seeks advice from the nurse manager responsible for the ward or department, and the patient's social worker.	In order that any action taken safeguards the patient's rights, as well as protects others.
13 Documentation of such information is scrupulously accurate.	The document may be regarded as evidence in the same way that the piece of paper bearing a car number written immediately after an accident is liable to be produced in court.

14 The procedures for the documentation of the nursing process are followed.

(a) Failure to follow procedures and policy risks the nurse's breaching his or her duty of care to the patient.
(b) Investigations of nursing care necessarily rely on the documentation of it.
(c) The nursing record may be required as evidence in any court case.

15 Practise patient-centred planning and evaluation.

The negotiations required to devise patient-centred plans make it less likely that patients will take nurses completely by surprise with requests to keep material confidential.

16 As soon as is practicable after first meeting a patient, the nurse clarifies with him or her the nurse's role within the MDCT.

In order to initiate and maintain an atmosphere of openness and confidence without secrecy.

17 The nurse proposes to a patient who requests secrecy for information already disclosed that he or she will continue the discussion at another (named) time. (Say, within an hour.)

(a) It is possible to take advice without disclosing the information itself.
(b) Such an action enables the nurse to declare immediately the limits on his or her ability to act independently of the MDCT.

(i) Return to the patient at the time agreed.

It is essential to appear to be reliable if the patient's confidence in the nurse is to be maintained.

(ii) Invite the patient to reconsider his or her request for secrecy.

Discussion of the patient's concerns about the information may lessen his or her anxiety about making it known to others.

(iii) Explain that the information has not yet been communicated to other members of the MDCT, but that the nurse has obligations of trust both to colleagues and patients.

It is essential to be open about the issues of trust which may seem to conflict.

(iv) Offer the patient a joint interview between you and another member of the MDCT of his or her choice.

(a) Allowing the patient time for reflection.
(b) If the patient can choose which member of the team to talk to, he or she is likely to feel more in control of whatever is concerning him or her.

18 If taken by surprise by a patient who requests secrecy for information not yet disclosed, the nurse invites the patient to consider whether he or she really wants to reveal such sensitive material.

In order to initiate as open a discussion as possible, as soon as possible.

(i) The nurse explains to the patient that a guarantee of secrecy is not possible.

So that the patient can choose whether to continue with the disclosure.

(ii) The nurse negotiates with the patient a course of action to deal with the worry he or she feels about the secrecy of the matter.

In order to focus on alleviating anxiety rather than on exposing shame.

(iii) As soon as possible, the nurse takes advice from others in the nursing team and the MDCT.

It is often the case that a patient has already disclosed the information, possibly having put another person under a similar ban of secrecy.

REFERENCE MATERIAL
References

Bok, S. (1986) *Secrets: On the Ethics of Concealment and Revelation*, Oxford University Press.

British Medical Association (1981) *Handbook of Medical Ethics*, BMA, London.

Martin, A. (1978) Confidentiality – its nature in law, *Nursing Times*, Vol. 74, no. 2, pp. 503–4.

Phillips, M. and Dawson, J. (1985) *Doctors' Dilemmas*, Harvester, Brighton.

UKCC (1987) *Confidentiality*, UKCC, London.

Further reading

Allen, H. (1981) Voices of concern: a study of verbal communication about patients in a psychiatric day unit, *Journal of Advanced Nursing*, Vol. 6, no. 5, pp. 355–62.

Anonymous (1981) A question of privilege, *Nursing Times*, Vol. 77, no. 8, p. 307.

Canadian Health Record Association (1978) Code of practice for safeguarding health information, *Canadian Nurse*, Vol. 74, no. 11, p. 9.

Commission for Racial Equality (1978) *Multiracial Britain: The Social Services Response*, CRE, London.

Cornwell, R. and Staunton, M. (1985) *Data Protection: Putting the Record Straight*, NCCL, London.

Curtin, L.L. (1981) Privacy: belonging to oneself, *Perspectives in Psychiatric Care*, Vol. 19, nos. 3 and 4, pp. 112–15.

Cushing, M. (1985) Incident reports: for your eyes only?, *American Journal of Nursing*, Vol. 85, pp. 873–4.

Downs, F.S. (1979) Whose responsibility? Whose rights?, *Nursing Research*, Vol. 28, no. 3, p. 131.

Ferguson, C.G. (1985) Quality assurance documentation – its legal disclosure rights, *Dimensions in Health Service*, Vol. 62, no. 2, pp. 27–8.

Finch, J. (1980) Not so strictly confidential, *Nursing Mirror*, Vol. 151, no. 14, pp. 28–9.

Finch, J. (1983) In confidence, *Nursing Mirror*, Vol. 156, no. 10, p. 43.

Finch, J. (1983) Time to speak out, *Nursing Mirror*, Vol. 156, no. 11, p. 37.

Havard, J. (1985) Medical confidence, *Journal of Medical Ethics*, Vol. 11, pp. 8–11.

Home Office (1978) *Report of the Committee on Data Protection* (Lindop Report), HMSO, London.

Kucera, W.R. (1976) Legal problems with PSRO's, *Journal of the American Association of Nurse Anaesthetists*, Vol. 44, pp. 68–73.

Martin, A. (1979) Confidentiality, *Nursing Times*, Vol. 75, no. 28, p. 1193.

National Consumer Council (1983) *Patients' Rights*, HMSO, London.

Newton, T. (1986) Protecting data, *Senior Nurse*, Vol. 4, no. 3, pp. 10–11.

NHS Information Management Centre (1988) *NHS Data Protection Handbook*, NHS Information Management Centre, Birmingham.

NHS Training Authority (1985) *Data Protection Act Resource Pack*, NHSTA, Bristol.

Rollin, H. (1978) Confidentiality in psychiatric practice, *Nursing Times*, Vol. 74, no. 28, pp. 1161, 1163.

Royal College of Nurses (1980) *Guidelines on Confidentiality*, RCN, London.

Simpson, R. (1980) Confidentiality in psychiatric nursing, *Nursing Times*, Vol. 76, no. 19, pp. 835–6.

Slack, P. (1983) On the record, *Nursing Times*, Vol. 79, no. 29, pp. 11–12.

Steering Group on Health Services Information (1984) *The Protection and Maintenance of Confidentiality of Patient and Employee Data* (Report from the Confidentiality Working Group), HMSO, London.

Wertheimer, A. (1986) Information retrieval, *Nursing Times*, Vol. 82, no. 50, pp. 31–3.

10

Consent to Treatment

DEFINITION

Consent must be real, and given without force, fear or deception, by a person who has (or is deemed to have) capacity to give a valid consent in the circumstances. Mere knowledge does not constitute consent. Consent is required for treatment which includes all investigations, tests, experiments, or research whether or not they involve physical contact.

DISCUSSION

Consent to treatment is governed both by the rules of common law and by statute law. Mental health legislation is an example of statutes being used to modify or replace certain rules of common law. The Mental Health Act 1959 was believed to offer too much scope for treatment of patients without their consent. The 1983 Act specified the circumstances in which treatment without consent may take place, and set up the Mental Health Act Commission (MHAC, whose address is Room 22, Hepburn House, Marsham Street, London SW1P 4HW; Tel: 01-217-6005/6006) to monitor the working of the Act. In Scotland, contact the Mental Welfare Commission, and for Northern Ireland, contact the Mental Health Commission for Northern Ireland. Nurses have a particular responsibility to ensure that patients are kept informed of visits by the Mental Health Act Commissioners.

Nursing duties

As well as participating only with consent in treatment of patients admitted either informally or compulsorily for assessment, nursing duties include: maintaining nursing records on detained patients which may be accessible to any person authorized by the MHAC; ensuring that patients know their rights according to the Act and related code of practice, judging what represents the minimum restraint and intervention for patients not subject to detention or treatment; judging when it is

reasonable to search certain patients and their belongings; if appointed to do so, inspecting the mail of certain patients; and treating patients detained under the Mental Health Act 1983 strictly in accordance with the provisions of the Act.

Treatment

The notion of treatment includes all investigations, tests, experiments or research whether or not they involve physical contact. Consent is required as much for psychometry and videotaping as for invasive procedures such as venepuncture or X-rays. What have been called 'touch treatments' entail privileged access to the patient's body. The slightest touch without consent and without other lawful justification is a battery. 'Non-touch treatments' include psychotherapy of all categories or levels, including in groups. Consent is required in the same way as for touch treatments.

Because touch treatments are generally prescribed by a doctor, nurses are obliged to confirm with the patient, before carrying out the treatment, that he or she consents. If the patient does not consent, the nurse is required to confirm that other lawful justification exists before carrying out the treatment.

Mental Health Act 1983

Consent to treatment is covered by Part 4 of the Mental Health Act. Consent to treatment is required for both informal and detained patients. The 1983 Act specifies that certain limited forms of 'medical treatment' may be given without consent to patients detained under sections of the Act which allow detention for the purposes of treatment. In practice such treatment is limited to the administering of drugs for a period of time not exceeding three months from the date they were first prescribed. Three months is also the maximum permissible time for administering drugs without consent in any one period of detention. If an order under a section of the Act is renewed, the total period counts as a single period of detention, and so three months remains the maximum permissible period of time for drug treatment of a patient without consent.

Legal justification for medical treatment of detained patients without consent will be found in section 3 of the Act, which covers the admission and detention of patients in hospital for the purposes of treatment. Under section 3, treatment may be without the patient's consent for a period of time not exceeding three months in any single period of detention.

For all other detained patients and for informal patients, as well as for those patients who have already had medical treatment for three months under section 3, other lawful justification must be found within the Act for treatment without consent. Sections 57, 59, 60 and 62 of the Mental Health Act 1983 refer both to patients detained under the Act and 'also to any patient who is not liable to be detained under the Act'.

Section 62 sets aside the requirement for the detained patient's consent to treatment in certain circumstances. It states that detained as well as informal patients need not consent to 'urgent treatment':

> (a) which is immediately necessary to save the patient's life; or
>
> (b) which (not being irreversible) is immediately necessary to prevent a serious deterioration of his condition; or
>
> (c) which (not being irreversible or hazardous) is immediately necessary to alleviate serious suffering by the patient; or
>
> (d) which (not being irreversible or hazardous) is immediately necessary and represents the minimum interference necessary to prevent the patient from behaving violently or being a danger to himself or others.

Gostin (1986, p. 141) emphasizes that the use of drugs to 'restrain and control' behaviour is not necessarily 'medical treatment' in terms of the Mental Health Act 1983, and that such use is not covered by sections 57, 59, 60 and 62 of the Act, which deal with the treatment without consent of informal and detained patients. A single health professional is unlikely to be able to decide reliably whether a patient's behaviour constitutes the kind of risk outlined above. Although the nurse in charge of a ward may have to decide to restrain and medicate a patient, he or she will consult as soon as possible with senior nursing colleagues and with other members of the multidisciplinary clinical team.

RESTRAINT

The definitions of restraint must be carefully considered. The definition of what is 'reasonable' force or restraint is strictly limited by the provisions of Part II of the Act, as well as by the professional standards of psychiatric nursing. The term may be applied to the restricting of a person's movements so that he or she is unable to leave a place such as a ward or department of a hospital. This may be achieved by locking doors. Mainly, restraint is the use of threatened or direct force against a person so as to prevent him or her from free movement. Tranquillizing medication used to control a person's free movement is a form of restraint, as is the threat to use such medication. A threat to lock doors if a person does not comply with requests to remain in a ward or department is a form of restraint. A threat to detain a person under a section of the Mental Health Act if he or she does not submit to staff control is a form of restraint.

Reasonableness

The amount of restraint used is that which is 'reasonable'. The concept of 'reasonableness' is one which limits actions that are permissible in specific circumstances. That is, nurses are required to discriminate and judge specific interventions related to the behaviour, history and nature of individual patients, within the limits and safeguards of Part II of the Act. In particular, section 139 of the Act refers to 'bad faith' and 'reasonable care'. The test of good faith is that the nurse acts according to his or her duty of care to the patient. The duty of care is based on criteria of safety as defined in the practical assessments for the examination leading to the qualification of RMN.

The tests of reasonable care are threefold. First, the standards of competence defined by representatives of the psychiatric nursing profession and by the criteria for inclusion on the register. Second, adherence to the MHAC Code of Practice (when finalized and published). Third, the nurse's familiarity with the law related to his or her work. It follows that the definition of what is 'reasonable' force or restraint is strictly limited by the provisions of Part II of the Act, as well as by the professional standards of psychiatric nursing.

FORCE

Direct force may be defined in several ways. It includes personal handling of, or contact (which may be minimal) with another person; the use of weapons against a person (which could include blankets, towels, chairs or other furniture); the use of mechanical restraints (e.g. straitjacket or lockable fetters); the use of medication without a person's consent. The use, without legal justification, of direct force, anywhere on a scale from the minimum to that which requires implements or a number of people to achieve compliance is a battery. The threat, without legal justification, to use such force is an assault. Both assault and battery are criminal offences and are subject to the award of civil damages.

The use of tranquillizing medication to control behaviour is a form of restraint in itself, as is the threat to use such medication. If medication is administered to a patient against his or her will, force is required. In addition to the issue of consent, two other issues must therefore be considered, one being the nature of the justification for the use of force, the other being the degree of force that is reasonable in the circumstances.

Circumstances justifying the use of restraint or force

The Act does not give nurses any more specific guidance about the circumstances which justify restraint. In fact, restraint of patients is permissible in very limited circumstances. These are:

1 When consent has been given (for instance to a treatment programme involving restraint as a response to specific behaviours). This consent must be written, and may be withdrawn at any time. (Clearly, if a patient was consenting to remain in hospital, while refusing other forms of restraint, a nurse would not need to use the holding power of section 5(4) – see Chapter 42.)
2 To *prevent*, using 'reasonable' force, a crime.
3 To *prevent*, using 'reasonable' force, a breach of the peace. The definition of a breach of the peace involves the threat of violence which is likely to harm another person or his or her property.
4 In self-defence, defence of the employer's property, or (more problematically) defence of another person.
5 To prevent, by the use of 'reasonable' force, harm to a person who appears to be so mentally disordered as not to be competent to keep him- or herself safe and who appears likely to cause harm to others.

The extent to which an injection of a tranquillizing drug constitutes 'reasonable' force is debatable, particularly since, when given without consent, some force is required to administer it in the first place (Gostin, 1985).

GOOD FAITH
Section 139 of the Mental Health Act 1983 sets out the expectation that nurses along with other staff act in good faith and with reasonable care. The test of good faith is that the nurse acts according to his or her duty of care to a person known as a patient.

ECT
In the case of detained as well as informal patients, consent must always be obtained for ECT (section 58(1)(b)). The circumstances in which ECT can be given without consent to detained patients are also limited by sections 58 and 62 (MHA (Hospital, Guardianship and Consent to Treatment) Regulations 1983,

regulation 16, and see DHSS, 1987). If the patient does not consent a second opinion is sought from a medical practitioner appointed by the MHAC. This doctor interviews the patient and consults with the responsible medical officer and two other members of the multi-disciplinary clinical team caring for the patient, one of whom must be a nurse, the second someone other than a doctor. The doctor appointed by the MHAC will decide that ECT is necessary if 'the patient is not capable of understanding the nature, purpose and likely effects of that treatment or has not consented to it' (section 58(3)(b)) and ECT 'will alleviate or prevent a deterioration of his condition'. The doctor completes Form 39, which is retained and flagged in the patient's notes.

Real consent
'Real' consent, as laid down by the common law, is based on the freedom of a person to choose whatever treatment he or she wishes. For mentally impaired and disordered people this means that a broad explanation of the nature of the treatment and its likely risks is adequate so long as they remain free to refuse or decline it once they have grasped the information. It has been suggested that real consent also depends on the patient's recognition of being ill, and on his or her recognition of the consequences of not having the proposed treatment (Gostin, 1985). The responsible medical officer is responsible for giving the explanation. This broad explanation, though limited in scope, must be based on up-to-date knowledge and be free from bias. The patient may not be coerced: for example, by threats of action to be taken if he or she withholds consent. The explanation must include a description of alternative treatments, and the patient's questions must be answered truthfully (Gostin, 1985).

CAPACITY TO CONSENT
A patient's capacity to consent may be invalidated by two main groups of mental disorder. The first includes organic conditions which result in global neurological deficits. The second group includes conditions which result in disorders of perception, judgement, decision-making and mood.

MINORS
A minor who is under eighteen but who is aged sixteen or over can consent in his or her own right to any kind of medical treatment. A minor who is under sixteen may have consent given on his or her behalf either by one or both parents or by an appointed guardian or by the local authority if he or she is in care.

PROFESSIONAL RELATIONSHIPS
Central to the issue of consent to treatment is the nature

of the professional relationship between the nurse and patient. The procedures for the conduct of professional relationships, confidentiality, the role of the nurse within the multidisciplinary team and the nursing process are designed to safeguard the patient by defining the professional skills required to fulfil the nurse's duty of care.

Information

As well as confirming the broad explanation required in order to obtain a patient's consent to a specific treatment the nurse is required to explain to the patient any plan of treatment in use and the likely effects of all treatments. Nurses share responsibility for ensuring that detained patients are informed about and understand their rights to appeal to the Mental Health Review Tribunal; to be discharged; to consent to treatment; to withdraw consent; which sections of the Mental Health Act 1983 apply to them, in addition to any section under which they may be detained (section 132(2)); to have access to the Mental Health Act Commissioners; to be kept informed along with their nearest relative of the exact provisions of any section of the Act under which they are detained.

Emergencies

When a nurse considers taking action without a patient's consent, a number of factors are relevant:
1   the extent and focus of any danger;
2   responsibility for people other than the patient;
3   the balance of the benefits and risks to the patient of carrying out an intervention without consent;
4   alternative courses of action;

5   availability of colleagues with whom to consult.

Informal patients

Provided that the patient agrees, a close relative or friend is consulted about any treatment by the MDCT. The responsible medical officer (RMO) discusses treatment plans with the rest of the MDCT. Where necessary, the RMO requests a second opinion from another consultant, or from a general practitioner who knows the patient well. The MHAC may be consulted in the same way as it would be for a detained patient. Discussions regarding surgery are carried out between the RMO, general practitioner, surgeon and close relatives or friends.

Forms 38 and 39

Form 38 is the document which certifies that the patient is capable of consenting to treatment and has done so. It is completed by the RMO when the patient consents to ECT. It is also completed when a detained patient consents to medication which is being continued beyond the three-month period which limits the administering of medication without consent. Form 38 is placed in the patient's notes and flagged for easy retrieval.

Form 39 is the document which certifies that treatment should be given to a patient who withholds consent, or who is incapable of giving consent. It is completed by the doctor appointed by the MHAC to give the second opinion on such patients. Form 39 is also placed in the notes and flagged for easy retrieval.

Forms 38 and 39 may be used to remind nurses of the need to obtain further consent or a second opinion for any new treatment or for treatment extending beyond the date stated in the forms as the limit of time.

GUIDELINES: ENSURING CONSENT TO TREATMENT

Action	Rationale
1 Each member of the nursing team ensures that he or she participates in treatment of detained and informal patients only with their consent, which has been obtained and recorded in accordance with the Mental Health Act 1983 (MHA).	The MHA regards nurses as accountable for ensuring that they obtain patients' consent to treatments they administer whether or not prescribed by medical staff.
2 Each member of the nursing team ensures that he or she participates in treatment of detained or informal patients without consent in strict accordance with the provisions of the MHA.	The MHA regards nurses as accountable for ensuring that they have lawful justification for administering treatments without consent, whether or not they have been prescribed by medical staff.

3 Each member of the nursing team is responsible for ensuring that researchers who request access to patients or patient records have done the following:
(i) provided an abstract of their research proposal;
(ii) obtained in writing the permission of the consultant responsible for the patient;
(iii) obtained the written consent of the patient;
(iv) obtained the agreement of the hospital ethical committee.

(a) Research is regarded as a form of treatment.
(b) As such it is subject to the same safeguards.

4 Each member of the nursing team is responsible for ensuring that written consent is obtained before any video- or audiotaping of patients takes place. The consent form is stored with the tapes, which are clearly marked with a warning to check the consent form before use.

The consent form allows the patient to state restrictions on the use of the tapes.

5 Each member of the nursing team is responsible for ensuring that consent is obtained from patients before investigations of any kind.
    The term 'investigation' includes a range of procedures from venepuncture through X-ray to psychometry.

Investigations are a form of treatment and subject to the same controls.

6 The primary nurse and nurse in charge of the ward are responsible for ensuring that a patient for whom ECT is prescribed has received an explanation of its nature and effects before signing any consent form.

(a) Both informal and detained patients must be free to choose whether to have ECT or not.
(b) Both informal and detained patients must give consent before ECT is given.
(c) Real consent involves the patient receiving and understanding a broad explanation of the treatment to be given.

7 When the patient consents to ECT the primary nurse and nurse in charge of the ward are responsible for ensuring that the responsible medical officer has completed Form 38.

To ensure that the patient is capable of understanding the nature, purpose and likely effect of ECT and has consented to it.

8 Ensure that the RMO has correctly completed with the patient a standard consent form and has prescribed the type, number and frequency of electroconvulsive treatments.

(a) So that the patient agrees to the administering of a general anaesthetic in order to carry out ECT.
(b) So that the patient agrees specifically to unilateral or bilateral ECT.
(c) So that the patient agrees to a specific number of treatments.
(d) So that the patient agrees to a specific frequency of treatment.

9 The primary nurse participates in any decision to request a second opinion for a patient who refuses to consent to ECT.

(a) To ensure that no patient is treated without consent until a second opinion has been given by a medical practitioner appointed by the MHAC.
(b) As part of his or her assessment this doctor will consult with a nurse who has been working with the patient.

10 The primary nurse ensures that the second doctor correctly completes Form 39 if he or she decides that the patient should be treated without consent.

Form 39 is flagged and retained in the patient record as the authority for administering ECT without consent.

11 When administering medicines each nurse checks that the number and date of any section under which the patient is detained are recorded on the prescription card.

Accurate recording of the dates of detention is meant to prevent the administering of medication for a time longer than three months in any one period.

12 Each nurse who administers medicines to patients ensures that the starting date of any medication prescribed during a period of detention appears on the prescription card.

In order that the three months can be accurately recorded.

13 Each nurse responsible for administering medicines ensures that the date of any transfer between wards is clearly recorded on the prescription cards.

So that the duration of any administering of medicines which started in another ward can be accurately recorded.

14 Primary nurses are responsible for ensuring that consent forms, and Forms 38 and 39 are clearly flagged in patients' records.

So that any nurse can easily and quickly check the status of any patient who may be asked to consent to treatment or investigations.

REFERENCE MATERIAL
References

DHSS (1987) *Mental Health Act 1983: Memorandum on Parts I to IV, VIII and X*, HMSO, London.

Gostin, L. (ed.) (1985) *Secure Provision*, Tavistock, London.

Gostin, L. (1986) *Institutions Observed*, King Edward's Hospital Fund, London.

Mental Health Act 1983, HMSO, London.

Further reading

Armitage, S. (1980) Non-compliant recipients of health care, *Nursing Times*, Vol. 76, no. 1, pp. 1–3.

Barkes, P. (1979) Bioethics and informed consent in American health care delivery, *Journal of Advanced Nursing*, Vol. 4, pp. 23–38.

Bean, P. (1980) *Compulsory Admissions to Mental Hospitals*, Wiley, Chichester.

Brown, M. (1985) Matter of commitment, *Nursing Times*, Vol. 81, no. 18, pp. 26–7.

Daes, E.I.A. (1986) *Principles, Guidelines and Guarantees for the Protection of Persons Detained on Grounds of Mental Ill-Health or Suffering from Mental Ill-Health or Suffering from Mental Disorder*, United Nations, New York.

Davidhizar, R. and Wehlage, D. (1984) Can the client with chronic schizophrenia consent to nursing research?, *Journal of Advanced Nursing*, Vol. 9, pp. 381–90.

Dunstan, G.R. and Seller, M.J. (1983) *Consent in Medicine: Convergence and Divergence in Tradition*, King Edward's Hospital Fund, London.

Dyer, A.R. and Bloch, S. (1987) Informed consent and the psychiatric patient, *Journal of Medical Ethics*, Vol. 13, pp. 12–16.

Editorial (1985) Doctor knows best?, *Nursing Mirror*, Vol. 160, no. 9, p. 3.

Farndale, W.A.J. (1979) *Law on Hospital Consent Forms*, Ravenswood, Beckenham.

Finch, J. (1983) Consent of minors to treatment, *Nursing Mirror*, Vol. 157, no. 6, pp. 37–8.

Gostin, L. (1986) *Mental Health Services: Law and Practice*, Shaw and Sons, London.

Gostin, L. and Rassaby, E. (1980) *Representing the Mentally Ill and Handicapped*, Quartermaine House, Sunbury.

Gostin, L., Rassaby, E. and Buchan, A. (1984) *Mental Health: Tribunal Procedure*, Oyez Longman, London.

Hammond, M. (1982) I was being fed false information, *Nursing Mirror*, Vol. 155, no. 14, p. 21.

Jones, R. (ed.) (1985) *Mental Health Act Manual*, Sweet & Maxwell, London.

Lidz, C.W. *et al.* (1984) *Informed Consent: A Study of Decision-Making in Psychiatry*, Guilford, New York.

Local Government Training Board (1984) *Admission of the Mentally Disordered to Hospital or Guardianship: A Guide for Social Workers*, Local Government Training Board.

Martin, A.J. (1977) Consent to treatment, *Nursing Times*, Vol. 73, no. 22, pp. 810–11.

Mawson, D. (1986) Seeking informed consent, *Nursing Times*, Vol. 82, no. 6, pp. 52–3.

Melia, K. (1986) Dangerous territory, *Nursing Times*, Vol. 82, no. 6, p. 27.

Mental Health Act 1983, HMSO, London.

Mental Welfare Commission for Scotland (1981) *Does the Patient Come First?*, HMSO, Edinburgh.

Piesse, B. (1986) What is informed consent?, *Australian Nurses Journal*, Vol. 15, no. 9, p. 52–3.

Pyne, R. (1986) Tell me honestly, *Nursing Times*, Vol. 82, no. 21, pp. 25–6.

Robb, S.S. (1983) Beware the 'informed' consent, *Nursing Research*, Vol. 32, no. 3, p. 132.

Trandel-Korenchuk, D.M. (1986) Concept development in nursing research, *Nursing Administration Quarterly*, Vol. 11, no. 1, pp. 1–9.

Turnquist, A.C. (1983) The issue of informed consent and the use of neuroleptic medications, *International Journal of Nursing Studies*, Vol. 20, no. 3, pp. 181–6.

Watson, A.B. (1982) Informed consent of special subjects, *Nursing Research*, Vol. 31, no. 1, pp. 43–7.

11

Pastoral Care

DEFINITION

Pastoral care is defined as the professional attention required to meet the spiritual needs of patients.

DISCUSSION

Religious beliefs exist in such a variety and number of forms that a brief survey cannot hope to do justice to the complexity of the emotional and intellectual factors comprising them. Moreover, spiritual needs are not the same as religious needs. However, it may be argued that as a holistic nursing approach requires liaison with the other professions comprising the multidisciplinary clinical team, so it requires liaison with the professions concerning themselves with aspects of patients' lives which are not easily placed in diagnostic and causal categories. The chaplaincy service of a hospital may be understood as a pastoral care team offering just this kind of concern.

Religious orders were the first organizations to offer systematic care to the sick. While religious observances might have been seen as the price to be paid for skilled attention, increasingly technological and mechanistic models of nursing and medical care have tended to divert attention from the problem of the nature of the interaction between mind and body. Spiritual care becomes another form of treatment.

Ascertaining religious needs

Religious needs are a principal element of the information about a patient required by nurses on admission. Especially important are the religious needs of patients from ethnic minorities.

Discussion of spiritual needs will hinge on the participants' world-view: how they understand human culture to be constructed. That is, whether personality and culture are seen as the product of instinctual needs which require satisfaction; or as the product of environ-

mental and social conditions; or as the product of some kind of combination of social conditions and psychological factors (Arieti, 1976). In 1930 Fromm identified modern Christianity with a 'socially harmless channel' (Fromm, 1963, p. 69) which gratified individuals' needs for authoritative guidance and maintained social conformity. The presence in hospitals of patients and staff from many non-Christian cultures means that attitudes of white Anglo-Saxon staff to the relationship of religion to medicine, race, authority, family structure, sexuality, gender, health and illness are likely to be suspect in ways in which they are not necessarily aware. The hospital chaplaincy service is geared to offer pastoral care in such conditions, and is notable for the number of women who work as chaplains, thereby challenging at least one traditionally sex-linked occupation.

Hospital chaplains

'An effort to escape from the anxiety of separation (and with it the terror of basic anxiety) can result in a fantasy of oneness, or fusion. But this can bring a fear of loss of identity. Avoidance of this danger can result in withdrawal and a fearful state of isolation' (Hobson, 1984, p. 224). Patients as well as staff often describe such wishes and fears in terms of religious belief. Hospital chaplains can especially help patients to sort out how much they are driven by fear and anxiety, and how much by religious faith. They are trained to tolerate the uncertainty of the interaction between symptoms, feelings and thoughts, in order to attend to the expressed needs of patients as perceived by patients themselves. That is: when approached by a patient who wishes to discuss what God says, a chaplain is unlikely to ask if God's voice is heard inside or outside a patient's head, whether he speaks to or about the patient, how long he has been talking to the patient, and to recommend medication in order to remove the voice.

FULL-TIME AND PART-TIME CHAPLAINS

Chaplains are employed by hospitals in full-time and part-time posts. Part-time chaplains are usually employed by a hospital on a sessional basis from local churches. Because the hospital and its catchment area are part of one or more parishes the chaplains represent an important link between the hospital and the community it serves. The link is distinct from that provided by clergy who visit their parishioners admitted to hospital.

Full-time chaplains are based in the hospital, available to both staff and patients, liaising with the local churches and co-ordinating religious services within the hospital. Although full-time chaplains usually represent one of the main Western or British Christian denominations such as the Church of England, the Catholic or Methodist Churches, they are ecumenical in outlook, regarding all Christian people as belonging to one Church. They also have wide knowledge about the religious beliefs of most cultures other than Christian ones and can act as resources of advice and understanding, perhaps liaising between patients and staff to make apparently unusual beliefs comprehensible. A nurse can expect the hospital chaplain to obtain help from a representative of a patient's religion if required.

THE CHAPLAIN'S ROLE

An important function of the chaplain is to provide an additional resource to people under stress, whether they be staff or patients. Most important events of people's lives, such as bereavement, accidents, natural disasters and physical illness happen independently of any mental disorder they may experience. These events, however, are associated with mental disorder. It is not clear whether mental disorder results from the life events in a person who is already vulnerable, or whether the life events render a person vulnerable to mental disorder. The assumptions of a medical or nursing model constrain their users to limited kinds of help which involve labelling the recipient as a patient or client. The chaplains, who are not constrained by pressure to make diagnoses and devise treatment programmes, are able to attend to the whole person in ways that are usually not available to other membres of medical and allied professions.

Because the pastoral care and multidisciplinary teams are linked in these ways, it is well to involve chaplains in ward teams in some structured way which recognizes both their particular role and their part in the whole of patient care (Foskett, 1986).

Chaplains are equipped by their education and training to provide guidance on ethical and moral issues. Such guidance is not in the form of moral precepts, but in an ability to facilitate discussion of the 'good' and the 'just', helping people to form ethically sound judgements about their own as well as other people's conduct.

This is especially important for British nurses, whose Code of Conduct outlines only sketchily some of the philosophical background to the formation of professional standards. As is noted in the chapters concerning consent to treatment, ethics, and nurse–patient relationships, hospital ethical committees can offer valuable help in problems of patient management. Although participation in such committees is not specifically a chaplain's role, he or she provides another perspective and several other dimensions of pastoral care.

Law, a hospital chaplain with wide experience of parish and clinical work in hospital and formal psychotherapeutic settings, writes:

> The therapeutic role and the spiritual role were not opposite ends of the pole, but part of a continuum. I no longer felt that I should work as a 'chaplain' or a 'therapist' but that the roles were intertwined. This synthesis enabled me to use my psychotherapeutic insight in looking with patients and staff at the different levels at which people function. That pastoral/spiritual counselling is not a matter of supplying answers, but rather exploring with the individual the often hidden meanings in his/her life.
>
> (Law, 1983, pp. 2–3)

GUIDELINES: PARTICIPATING IN PASTORAL CARE

Action   **Rationale**

1 The charge nurse ensures that the ward or department's professional operating procedures (incorporating the results of consultation within the ward and between the ward and the chaplains) describe how the liaison with the chaplains takes place.

In order that the procedures may be accepted and implemented.

2 The charge nurse ensures that the ward timetable includes the activities available through the hospital chaplaincy service.

So that both patients and staff know and can choose what to attend.

3 During the admission procedure for each patient his or her religion is recorded in a readily retrievable form, along with whether he or she would like to see a chaplain or representative of the patient's own religion.

So that chaplains of specific denominations who visit the ward can easily find new patients who have been admitted and who may not, despite the ward procedures, know that a chaplaincy service is available.

4 The ward needs: (i) religious representatives' telephone numbers; (ii) times when they are available; (iii) names of someone to contact in an emergency.

To ensure that the chaplains or other religious representatives can be contacted if needed.

5 The charge nurse nominates a first-level nurse who is a permanent member of the ward team to be the main contact person for each religious representative.

(a) So that each religious representative has a contact person.
(b) To facilitate liaison between patients and religious representatives.
(c) To ensure that people in the ward know what service is available from religious representatives.

6 The nurses responsible for liaising with religious representatives meet regularly with them.

(a) To ensure continuity of contact.
(b) To ensure that any problems are dealt with in good time.

7 Nurses take the initiative in consulting with the religious representatives as needed about religious, spiritual, ethical or cultural issues which arise in the course of their work.

Because religious representatives may not necessarily visit wards or units unless specifically asked to do so.

8 The charge nurse ensures that a nurse is available to accompany patients on request to any religious services in the hospital.

To facilitate the patients' maintenance of religious observance regardless of the nurses' beliefs.

9 The hospital chaplaincy service and the liaison between it and the ward or department is explained to all new staff and patients when they come to the ward.

So that all staff and patients know that the religious representatives are part of the multidisciplinary clinical team.

10 Meetings with religious representatives are scheduled so that they do not clash with other meetings.

(a) Common courtesy.
(b) To prevent any conflict between staff.

11 Nurses and religious representatives ensure that they adhere to hospital guidelines regarding professional relationships with patients.

Inexperienced mental health workers can mistake a conversational style of interaction for ordinary social contact.

REFERENCE MATERIAL
References

Arieti, S. (1976) *Creativity*, Basic Books, New York.

Foskett, J. (1986) The chaplain, in D. Steinberg (ed.) *The Adolescent Unit*, Wiley, Chichester.

Fromm, E. (1963) *The Dogma of Christ and Other Essays on Religion, Psychology and Culture*, Routledge & Kegan Paul, London.

Hobson, R.F. (1984) *Forms of Feeling*, Tavistock, London.

Law, M. (1983) Unpublished report on the role of the chaplain, Bethlem Royal and Maudsley Hospital Chaplaincy Service.

Further reading

Anderson, R.G. and Young, J.L. (1988) The religious component of acute hospital treatment, *Hospital and Community Psychiatry*, Vol. 39, no. 5, pp. 528–33.

Baldwin, W. (1981) The chaplain's role: strictly confidential, *Nursing Mirror*, Vol. 153, no. 9, pp. 26–8.

Carson, V.B. *et al.* (1986) The effect of didactic teaching on spiritual attitudes, *Image*, Vol. 18, no. 4, pp. 161–4.

Commission for Racial Equality (1976) *Mental Health Among Minority Ethnic Groups*, CRE, London.

Commission for Racial Equality (1978) *Mental Health among Minority Ethnic Groups: Research Summaries and Bibliography*, CRE, London.

Del Valle, S. (1980) Spiritual care and the nursing process, *Australasian Nurses Journal*, Vol. 9, no. 7, pp. 12–13.

Dettmore, D. (1987) Nurses' conceptions of and practices in the spiritual dimensions of nursing, in *Clinical Excellence in Nursing International Networking*, Department of Nursing Studies, Edinburgh University, p. 84.

Ellis, D. (1980) Whatever happened to the spiritual dimension?, *Canadian Nurse*, Vol. 76, no. 8, pp. 42–3.

Foskett, J. (1986) The chaplain, in D. Steinberg (ed.) *The Adolescent Unit*, Wiley, Chichester.

Graves, C.C. (1983) Religion: cause or cure? *Perspectives in Psychiatric Care*, Vol. 21, no. 1, pp. 27–38.

Hospital Chaplaincies Council (1983) *Our Ministry and Other Faiths*, Hospital Chaplaincies Council, London.

Hospital Chaplaincies Council (1986) *A Guide for Introducing Chaplaincy Visitors to Work in Hospital*, Hospital Chaplaincies Council, London.

Hospital Chaplaincies Council (1987) *A Handbook on Hospital Chaplaincy*, Hospital Chaplaincies Council, London.

Jimack, M. (1985) *Jewish Social Services: A Research Review*, Central Council for Jewish Social Service, London.

Khan, G.M. (1982) *Personal Hygiene in Islam*, Ta Ha Publishers, London.

Law, M., Hill, D. and Harries, C. (1978) Exploring the work of a hospital chaplain in a psychiatric hospital, *Nursing Times*, Vol. 74, no. 36, pp. 1478–82.

Leininger, M. *et al.* (1986) Ethical and theoretical care issues in transcultural nursing, in S.M. Stinson *et al.*(eds.) *New Frontiers in Nursing*, University of Alberta, Edmonton.

McGilloway, O. and Myco, F. (1985) *Nursing and Spiritual Care*, Harper & Row, London.

Mei-Li Lee Lo (1976) Folk beliefs of the Chinese and implications to psychiatric nursing, *Journal of Psychosocial Nursing and Mental Health Services*, Vol. 14, no. 10, pp. 38–42.

Rahula, W. (1959) *What the Buddha Taught*, Grove Press, New York.

Reform Synagogues of Great Britain (1983) *The Jewish Family Today and Tomorrow*, Reform Synagogues of GB, London.

Schnorr, M.A. (1983) Religion: cause or cure?, *Perspectives in Psychiatric Care*, Vol. 21, no. 1, pp. 26–35.

Simsen, B. (1986) The spiritual dimension, *Nursing Times*, Vol. 82, no. 48, pp. 41–2.

Swami Ananyananda (1979) *Essentials of Hinduism*, Ramakrishna Vedanta Centre, Bourne End.

Zohoori, E. (1985) *The Throne of the Inner Temple*, National Spiritual Assembly of the Bahá'ís of Jamaica, Kingston, Jamaica.

12

Meal Times

DISCUSSION

A survey of psychiatric patients' views about the meals and service in their hospitals (Raphael, 1977) showed a majority who were dissatisfied with their food. It was found that there was no relationship between per capita spending on food in hospitals and the ratio of favourable to critical comments. In 1978, Gregory (1979), conducting research for the Royal Commission on the National Health Service, found that of all hospital patients except maternity patients a quarter were dissatisfied with the times that meals were served. Three-quarters said they were satisified with the food itself. Where people did complain, they spoke of cold, unappetizing, badly cooked food. Vegetarian and religious preferences were not catered for.

Tredger (1982) describes feeding the patient as a team effort. She emphasizes the complexity of the system directed towards nourishing the patient. She identifies as the components of the system:

1 physician;
2 nurses;
3 dieticians;
4 catering managers;
5 portering staff;
6 ward orderlies;
7 housekeepers;
8 relatives and visitors;
9 laboratory staff;
10 pharmacists.

It is clear that each component of the system may act in a way that counters the efforts of another. A system of individualized patient care such as primary nursing means that the primary nurse can provide both a focus and co-ordination for the team effort, but also means that he or she has complex responsibilities that are not clear and may be impossible to fulfil given the structure of the organization.

Wilson (1986) identifies 'three major aims in the process of assisting the patient to eat and drink,

1 It should be aesthetic
2 It should be therapeutic
3 It should be functional' (that is, enhancing the nurse–patient relationship).

She identifies three principles of personal integrity, personal dignity and safety.

Safety in psychiatric hospitals is a complex matter involving prevention not only of accidents but also of acts of deliberate self-harm and assault. Pearson, Wilmot and Padi (1986) in their study of violent behaviour among inpatients found that meal times were a peak time for violence, as did Jones (1977), in a study of violence in hospital in the USA. Rix (1985) discusses the issue of personal dignity in relation to the dependence of patients on nurses to fulfil the basic need of eating, which 'places the patient in an inferior position and can lead to frustration, anger and violence' (p. 53).

The environment where meals are provided may be extremely provocative to patients who dislike being in crowded places or eating in public, or who think that their food has been interfered with. Käppeli's study (1986) of nurses' assistance of patients' performance of self-care in a medical ward of a general hospital found that the emphasis was on management and coercion rather than on assistance. One of the constraints she identified was an ideology of efficiency in task performance, which outweighed the stated philosophy of total patient care and holistic nursing.

Patients' meal times are very much constrained by the timetables of the hospital catering service and by other tasks which compete for nurses' time, for example administering medicines or reports between shifts. Wilson's aims and principles may be difficult to maintain in an environment where large numbers of people have to be catered for and where cost is a major constraint on, for example, the number of non-nursing staff available to transport and serve food.

O'Brien (1981, p. 18) found that in the area health authority which she studied 'no special facilities have been made to serve ethnic minorities'. Examples of patients' concerns include the following. Vegetarians doubt whether vegetable oil has been used to cook their food; vegans are served with ordinary vegetarian food. Patients are not necessarily told whether diets which conform to their religious beliefs are available. They are not told whether relatives may bring in food for them.

Norberg and Athlin (1987) extrapolate from theories about interpersonal interaction to suggest that patients with Parkinson's disease can be helped if nurses 'focus on the socio-economic content before and after feeding and on the task during feeding' (p. 549). The nurse thus balances the patient's needs for autonomy and assistance.

In a psychiatric hospital a patient who is less obviously disabled is likely to be left to get on with his or her meals. There is little research to guide nurses in their attention to the environment as distinct from the physiology of eating. Where a ward operates a system of primary nursing the task of supervising a person's meals is less likely to be left to whomever is around, while other tasks are carried out.

GUIDELINES: ASSISTING WITH MEALS

Action	Rationale
1 On admission the primary nurse establishes whether the patient has any special dietary requirements and whether translation will be necessary.	To ensure that these requirements are met.
2 If necessary the nurse discusses the patient's diet with his or her relatives.	So that if there is to be a delay in providing the correct diet relatives may be able to bring in food for the patient.
3 If a patient appears to have problems with hospital meals or wishes advice on diet, the primary nurse arranges for the hospital dietician to see him or her.	(a) To advise the patient. (b) In order to liaise with the hospital catering service. (c) In order to advise the patient's nurses.
4 The primary and associate nurses record carefully their observations of patients' behaviour at mealtimes.	(a) In order to assess any help which may be needed. (b) In order to assess attitudes to food and self-care generally. (c) In order to assess whether appetite for and pleasure in food relates to what is actually eaten.
5 Primary and associate nurses weigh all patients weekly.	Weight is a valuable indicator of general well-being and of changes in a person's state of mind which may not be apparent from observations of their eating.
6 The charge nurse nominates a person to be responsible for liaison with the hospital catering service.	So that there is consistency and continuity of communication between the ward and the caterers.
7 Primary nurses make known to the person responsible for ordering the patients' meals the dietary requirements of their patients.	(a) So that the correct diets can be reliably supplied. (b) So that changes can be made as necessary. (c) So that the catering service has the necessary notice of requests.

8 The person responsible for ordering meals bases orders on the known requirements of patients in the ward, encouraging primary nurses to take responsibility for negotiating with their patients the kinds of meals required.	To ensure that correct quantities are ordered.
9 Primary and associate nurses give patients full menus and bring to their notice choices which are not necessarily published daily.	To ensure that patients have the necessary information with which to make their meal choices.
10 Primary and associate nurses tell patients: (i) where meals are supplied; (ii) when meals are supplied; (iii) how meals are supplied; (iv) how meals out of hours are supplied, for example, during Ramadan; (v) how to make any temporary arrangements required for food to be brought in until diets have been supplied.	To enable patients who so wish to plan their time.
11 At least two nurses, one of whom is a registered mental nurse, supervises patients' meal times.	Safety of patients and nurses requires the presence of the trained nurse.
12 Primary and associate nurses take turns to supervise patients' meal times.	In order that individual patients' needs may be assessed.
13 During meal times, nurses: (i) avoid rush; (ii) offer choices; (iii) refrain from standing over patients or on the periphery of the dining area; (iv) refrain from calling to patients or other staff; (v) refrain from holding conversations with other staff in the patients' dining area.	In order to promote a relaxed atmosphere.
14 In the dining area, nurses: (i) check for dirt and smells; (ii) close doors; (iii) establish a non-smoking area or time or both.	To ensure that the environment is maintained to the required standard of hygiene and is free from noise and other pollution.
15 If patients need to be helped with eating, the nurse does so in an area where the patient can be relaxed and have some privacy.	So that the patient can maintain personal dignity.
16 If a patient with eating difficulties is learning to be independent, the primary and associate nurse ensures that he or she is given the necessary time to eat a meal.	So that time is not used as an excuse for the patient to evade responsibility for eating.
17 The primary and associate nurses ensure that other members of the nursing team know about circumstances which their patients find provocative at meal times.	(a) It will not always be possible for primary and associate nurses to be present at meal times. (b) Other members of the nursing team will provide privacy, space or time as necessary for patients who find meal times disturbing.

18 If there have been any administrative problems during a meal the first-level nurse responsible for supervising it records what they are.

So that the charge nurse or the person responsible for liaising with the hospital catering services will take the necessary action.

REFERENCE MATERIAL
References
Gregory, J. (1979) *Patients' Attitudes to the Hospital Service*, HMSO, London.

Jones, D.C. (1977) *Food for Thought*, RCN, London.

Käppeli, S. (1986) Nurses' management of patients' self-care, *Nursing Times*, Vol. 82, no. 11, pp. 40–3.

Norberg, A. and Athlin, E. (1987) The interaction between the Parkinsonian patient and his caregiver during feeding: a theoretical model, *Journal of Advanced Nursing*, Vol. 12, pp. 545–50.

O'Brien, M. (1981) *Hospital Food for Ethnic Minority Patients*, Haringey CHC, London.

Pearson, M., Wilmot, E. and Padi, M. (1986) A study of violent behaviour among in-patients in a psychiatric hospital, *British Journal of Psychiatry*, Vol. 149, pp. 232–5.

Raphael, W. (1977) *Psychiatric Patients and their Hospitals*, King Edward's Hospital Fund, London.

Rix, G. (1985) Compassion is better than conflict, *Nursing Times*, Vol. 81, no. 38, pp. 53–5.

Tredger, J. (1982) Feeding the patient – a team effort, *Nursing*, Vol. 2, no. 4, pp. 92–3.

Wilson, M. (1986) Eating and drinking, *Nursing*, Vol. 3, no. 7, pp. 265–7.

Further reading
Barnes, K.E. and Hodkinson, H.M. (1988) Quantification of dietary intake in long-stay geriatric patients: do we need seven days observation?, *European Journal of Clinical Nutrition*, Vol. 42, pp. 527–30.

Coates, V. (1985) *Are They Being Served?*, RCN, London.

Dickerson, J.W.T. (1986) Nutrition in health and illness, *Nursing*, Vol. 3, no. 8, pp. 303–7.

Goodinson, S.M. (1987) Anthropometric assessment of nutritional status, *The Professional Nurse*, Vol. 3, no. 12, pp. 388–93.

Holmes, S. (1984) Stress and nutrition, *Nursing Times*, Vol. 80, no. 38, pp. 53–5.

Jones, D.C. (1977) *Food for Thought*, RCN, London.

Melin, L. and Göttestam, K.G. (1981) The effects of rearranging ward routines on communication and eating behaviours of psychogeriatric patients, *Journal of Applied Behaviour Analysis*, Vol. 14, no. 1, pp. 47–51.

Parsonage, S. (1980) There's more to eating than food, *Nursing*, Vol. 1, no. 11, pp. 471–2.

Pittam, M. (1982) Nutritional assessment, *Nursing*, Vol. 2, no. 4, pp. 94–8.

Schultz, D. (1983) Hospital malnutrition – the nursing response, *Australian Nurses Journal*, Vol. 12, no. 7, pp. 49–51.

Wood, S. (1986) Nutritional support: an overview of general principles, *Nursing*, Vol. 3, no. 8, pp. 301–2.

13

Preventing Violence

DEFINITIONS
Aggression
'Aggression . . . involves the intention to hurt or . . . emerge superior to others [but] does not necessarily involve physical injury' (Siann, 1985, p. 14).

Violence
'Violence . . . involves the use of great force or physical intensity' (Siann, 1985, p. 14).

DISCUSSION
It is difficult to compare studies of violent people to arrive at a generally accepted definition of violence which stands up to the realities of disturbed behaviour. Bowden (Bowden *et al.*, 1978) distinguishes violence from aggression and from other fear-inducing behaviour, including verbal threats; physical contact such as pushing; throwing articles which do not hit anybody or do not break. He emphasizes that although much is known about certain social settings of violence and psychological characteristics of certain kinds of violent people, not enough is known to understanding the phenomenon in general. It is not known whether people who behave in fear-inducing ways are more or less likely to be violent in ways that cause injury or damage (Rossi *et al.*, 1986).

Aggression
The problem has been described as one involving a distinction between 'high visibility and low visibility violent patients' (Tanke and Yesavage, 1985, p. 1410). Theories of aggression provide little practical guidance for a clinical nurse to predict how aggressive and, as a result, how dangerous a patient might be. Two types of theory of aggression may be identified which at first sight run counter to each other. One is that aggression is an innate characteristic of human beings. This leads to the notion that a certain difficult-to-define aggression is

'normal' or 'benign' (Storr, 1970; Fromm, 1977). The other main theory is that aggression is a learned behaviour, a response which can be extinguished so that new behaviour may be learned (Bandura, 1973).

Aggression and violence
Siann (1985) makes a different distinction:

Aggression
(a) Involves the intention to hurt or
(b) emerge superior to others.
(c) Does not necessarily involve physical injury (violence).
(d) May or may not be regarded as being underpinned by different kinds of motives.
(e) Aggression is not always negatively sanctioned but is more likely to be so when one of the participants does not enter willingly into the interaction.
(f) Applying the label 'aggressive' in a pejorative manner to a person or persons is a matter of subjective judgement on the part of the labeller.
(g) The labeller will be affected both by his or her value system and by his or her perception of the extent to which the person or persons to whom the label is applied is acting provocatively or defensively.

Violence
(a) Involves the use of great force or physical intensity.
(b) While it is often impelled by aggressive motivation,
(c) may occasionally be used by individuals engaged in a mutual interaction which is regarded by both parties as intrinsically rewarding.
(d) Though the term 'violence' tends to be negatively sanctioned always, the use of great physical force is often legitimized. How and when the use of great physical force is legitimized or condemned will depend both on the values of the person making the judgement and the extent to which the use of force is seen as provocative (a first strike) or defensive.
(Siann, 1985, p. 14)

Siann gives two useful descriptions which draw together the disparate factors, thereby emphasizing the complexity of biological, social, psychological and philosophical elements comprised in the concepts of aggression and violence. Any attempt to reduce this complexity to a few guidelines carries the risk of misleading the user into interventions that may be not only unhelpful for the patient but also dangerous for the nurse.

Predictability

As suggested, a particular problem is the predictability of violence, of the kinds of patients most likely to be violent. It is not clear whether people with a history of making verbal threats or of causing actual bodily harm, or with a criminal record involving such offences as rape or armed robbery are more likely to be violent when they become clients of psychiatric services. Several studies demonstrate low rates of agreement between professional mental health workers on the nature of dangerousness and its prediction in relation to specific cases.

It is not clear whether a person who is diagnosed as psychotic or personality disordered is more likely to be labelled as violent than those with other diagnoses; or whether the person labelled as violent is more likely to be diagnosed as psychotic or personality disordered. Interpreting statistics is difficult. Because some acutely disturbed patients may be particularly prone to violence, the diagnosis of psychosis may be over-represented in statistics of violent patients. Non-psychotic patients may be more likely to repeat acts of violence. Studies disagree about the reliability of methods of prediction and about whether an actuarial approach based on demographic variables is superior to a clinical one based on identifying psychopathology. Two British studies indicate that 10–12 per cent of inpatients engage in violence (Fottrell, 1980; Pearson, Wilmot and Padi, 1986).

RISK FACTORS

It is possible to compile a list of risk factors, but caution is necessary because such a list derives from the collective conclusions of many different studies whose definitions of violence and whose conclusions are in many ways incompatible.

Therapeutic environment programming

Little is known about the kinds of hospital environment that encourage or reduce violent behaviour. Some studies have shown that staff in hospitals tend to rely on a single method of control for violent behaviour rather than selecting from a repertoire of methods (Whitman, Armao and Dent, 1976). A division exists between those who advocate the use of mechanical restraints and

physical restraint generally, and those who favour methods thought not to inflict physical pain but which include seclusion and medication. The evidence which suggests that violence is associated with psychosis or demonstrable abnormalities in brain functioning provides a rationale for the use of neuroleptic medication to prevent violent behaviour (Curtis, 1985; Rossi et al., 1986; Weller, 1986).

Divisions between staff tend to obscure the opportunities to prevent violence and to examine the ways in which staff may contribute to the occurrence of violent episodes. Prevention of violence requires detailed individual assessment of patients, close co-operation between multidisciplinary team members, attention to the methods of communication used by the patient and clearly defined systems for decision-making which allow the patient a degree of control.

There is no clear evidence of an association between staffing levels and violence. To use resources effectively, charge nurses will consult with their managers when difficulties arise. Such difficulties include the numbers and skill mix of nurses in a ward or department, the numbers and mix of patients, and the availability of medical and other staff. Crammer (1984) suggests that the relationship between self-injurious behaviour and disruption of staff routine and confidence requires investigation. Broken furniture, a dirty or shabby environment, staff nervousness and avoidance of interaction with patients may all be seen as evidence of such disruption, and therefore as necessitating investigation of their relationship to violence. A too rigid order and routine is likely to lead to violence both by staff and patients.

The prevention by nurses of violence is an important aspect not only of the treatment of individual patients but of creating and maintaining a therapeutic atmosphere in the ward or department. Scott (1977) suggests that violent behaviour represents a crucial step by an individual across a psychological barrier which, once taken, ensures that violence is likely to be repeated. Prevention of violence is both a matter of helping someone to learn behaviour that does not involve violence and of helping someone develop strategies which lead to outcomes that satisfy and which do not prompt him or her to violence. Such a view implies great caution in encouraging patients to find supposedly cathartic ways of expressing aggression, such as using punchbags.

The psychiatric nurse requires not only a repertoire of methods for managing violence once it has started but also a repertoire of skills for identifying potentially violent patients and for interacting with them in ways which reduce this potential. Hodgkinson (1980) suggests that attention to the nature of a patient's interactions is the appropriate starting point for nursing observation and interventions, clarifying if possible the different values shaping the behaviour of the nurse and patient.

Nursing history

The need to assess aggressive potential constitutes one of the occasions when a nursing history is particularly useful because it allows a measured and structured way of exploration. A nursing history is mandatory if there is any record of past violence. The admitting doctor may need to be reminded of his or her responsibility to establish whether a history of violence exists and for informing and negotiating with nurse managers before admitting the patient. The nursing history gives the patient the opportunity to ventilate past grievances and to describe how he or she dealt with them, thereby giving the nurse the opportunity to identify the patient's coping methods and vulnerability. The nurse's skill in exploring and responding to answers is directed towards being as non-intrusive as possible while gathering information. That is, the nurse avoids a style which the patient could see as cross-examination, and thus unduly intrusive. It is essential to know what the patient finds distressing or provocative, and what he or she finds helpful and calming.

Individually negotiated care plans

Attention to patient autonomy arises from an ethical view such as Emson's, who notes that many medical procedures involve a violation of a 'patient's mental and physical integrity' (Emson, 1986, p. 218). A paternalistic emphasis in medical care is in conflict with the notion of patient autonomy. Excessive authoritarianism and an excessively *laissez-faire* approach are two ends of a continuum whose middle ground is difficult to establish and maintain in a ward setting.

An experimental ward for patients with sociopathic behaviour disorders was successfully run on the principle of encouraging and maintaining patient responsibility and independence (MIND, 1975; Woodside *et al.*, 1976). Individually negotiated care plans build on the foundation of the patient's freely volunteered history, which, it is hoped, has revealed his or her values, preferred ways of acting and the nature of the insight into his or her behaviour. Sugden (1986) quotes an unpublished paper by Woodside *et al.* which describes how violent behaviour was dealt with 'in the most public part of the unit'.

If a violent incident has occurred, whether without warning or despite precautions, it is essential that repetition of the violence is prevented. As soon as possible after the incident the multidisciplinary team will meet to formulate a management plan.

Verbal interaction
AVOIDING THE REINFORCEMENT OF FEAR-INDUCING BEHAVIOUR
Poverty of interaction between patients and nurses means that the notice taken of fear-inducing behaviour may act as positive reinforcement (Broome, Weaver and Kat, 1978, 1979; Pearson, Wilmot and Padi, 1986). If patients are kept in locked wards intensive interaction between them and the nurses ensures that the emphasis is on treatment, not on segregation. A variation of this problem is the need to remain with a patient after he or she has stopped threatening violence. To walk away when a patient has calmed down may act as a punishment, discouraging desirable behaviour.

Interaction techniques include active listening; using body posture to reduce tension; communication of respect for and an attempt to understand a patient's silence; clarifying, reflecting, echoing in order to help sort out confusions. Sugden (1986) also suggests the need to approach a patient at the first signs of distress or anger and to invite him or her to say what the trouble is. Both psychological and physical privacy reduce the intrusiveness of one-to-one interaction. The nurse will tell colleagues where the interaction takes place and how long it will last, so that they can take any precautions thought to be necessary. Strategies for interactions with individual patients will be planned as part of the routine nursing management. They are recorded and discussed with the supervisor of the nurse responsible for the patient, as well as with other members of the MDCT.

HANDLING FEELINGS
Handling feelings refers to the ways in which the psychiatric nurse tunes in to the experience of patients, identifies and helps patients identify what they are feeling and helps patients to find non-damaging ways to express their feelings.

Tuning in
The phrase 'tuning in' is used to express the notion of careful and effective listening: 'accurate observation of verbal and non-verbal cues, active concentration on spoken words, and caution in interpreting the client's meaning' (Schulman, 1974, p. 121).

The purpose, when used in a one-to-one setting, is to enable a person, the client or patient, to talk about what troubles him or her. Its wider implication is that the nurse is constantly and consistently alert, listening throughout a span of duty. Individualized patient care organized as in primary nursing ensures that a nurse is responsible for a small group of patients and not obliged to maintain vigilance for a whole ward.

Identifying feelings

The phrase 'identifying feelings' does not mean the same as identifying with a patient, a process which risks removing the distinction between the helper and the person being helped, and which jeopardizes the helper's ability to help. To identify with a patient can be especially risky if he or she is potentially violent, as the nurse's identification with him or her may prevent self-evaluation by either person. However, the nurse may have to spend long periods of time with an aggressive patient going over the same ground before the patient is ready to consider alternative forms of behaviour. It is a difficult negotiation which achieves a compromise between acceding to a patient's every wish for interaction, and frustrating him or her when in distress.

Team approach
EMERGENCY TEAM

An example of an emergency team is one where four members of staff from different areas of a hospital – say, the duty clinical nurse manager, the duty doctor, a first-level nurse and a second-level nurse or a senior student or a helper – carry bleeps so that they can be summond by a member of staff requiring help in an emergency. In other settings, wards have an alarm system and a method for gathering together their own staff in an emergency. One computer-controlled radio-alarm system combines touch-sensitive personal alarms; room alarms, sensors and indicators; bleeps which summon other staff to the site of the alarm; a computer with a keyboard, a monitor which displays the current status of the system in the form of a map, and a printer which automatically records the details of all alarms.

Pharmacological intervention

The way in which medication is offered may intensify the aggression it is designed to control. Some aggressive patients are happy to use neuroleptic medication as they feel they need it. A trusting relationship between them and the staff prevents an adversarial or authoritarian response by nurses who may be reluctant to give medication 'on demand'. Compromise is facilitated by the use of elixirs rather than tablets so that nurses can be sure that patients actually take the medicine they ask for.

Training

All members of staff in the hospital require, each year, a specific period of training in the prevention and management of violence, whether initial or refresher training. The health authority will decide on the minimum required, but examples might be ten hours, or two days, a year. The content will vary from demonstrations to role-play to supervised practice. It is the responsibility of the hospital managers to set up and maintain such training, together with a group of selected staff who carry out a training function. It is the responsibility of each charge nurse to ensure that he or she and the nursing staff from the ward or department receive the necessary training.

Administrative issues

Statistics of violence should distinguish between multiple episodes by few people and single episodes by different people. Failure to do so can seriously bias the results of studies of a hospital population. Moreover, studies of the incidence of violence often do not specify where on the continuum of fear-inducing behaviours the episodes being examined are located. A hospital needs a management structure within which data are collected and examined, responsibilities are clearly defined and allocated, and policies and procedures implemented and evaluated by consultation and with reference to documented evidence (Stegne, 1978).

GUIDELINES: PREVENTING VIOLENCE

Action	Rationale
1 Staff are trained to use a variety of techniques with which to nurse patients who are, or may become, violent.	Research shows that nurses tend not to use a repertoire of skills but rely on a restricted range.
2 The hospital policy on the prevention and management of violence states clearly the nature of any restraint techniques to be used.	(a) So that nurses can be trained in their use. (b) So that nurses can select appropriately.

3 Charge nurses are responsible for ensuring that the upkeep of the ward's fixtures and fittings remains of a high standard.

(a) In order to maintain morale.
(b) To discourage damage to an apparently neglected environment.

4 Charge nurses are responsible for ensuring that any broken furniture is sent immediately for repair.

Broken furniture in the ward demonstrates lack of attention to the therapeutic environment.

5 Charge nurses are responsible for ensuring that the mix of patients in their wards is such that, so far as possible, violence is unlikely to be provoked.

Failure to plan and discriminate between types of patients potentiates any risk of violence.

6 On admission the admitting doctor, if possible, elicits from the patient or those accompanying him or her any record of violence.

In order to arrange the most suitable environment in which to nurse the patient.

7 The admitting doctor communicates to the nurse in charge of the admitting ward whether a record of violence exists.

It is essential that the nurse in charge feels confident about the patient's safety in the ward.

8 A nursing history is obtained from each patient with a history of violence.

(a) So that the patient can talk about, among other things, anxieties and conflicts, or air any grievances.
(b) In order to identify precipitants and other risk factors.

9 Nurses avoid reinforcing fear-inducing behaviour by maintaining close interaction with patients along with individually negotiated care plans.

So that patients do not have to use violence to initiate interaction.

10 The charge nurse is responsible for ensuring that the organizational system of nursing in the ward allocates each patient a nurse who is primarily responsible for his or her nursing care together with two other designated nurses who perform a supporting role.

So that the patient will be able to work consistently with the same nurses from day to day.

11 A safety care plan is implemented for every patient with a history of violence until the nursing team is satisfied that violence is no longer a risk.

The objective being that the patient will refrain from serious violence in and outside the ward for periods of time whose length will depend on the risk involved.

12 The charge nurse is responsible for implementing the procedure for supervision (see Chapter 44).

(a) So that nurses' work with violent patients for whose nursing care they are responsible is monitored continuously.
(b) To help nurses deal with the stress involved in nursing violent patients.
(c) To ensure that nurses receive the training necessary to nurse violent patients.

13 All nurses are responsible for familiarizing themselves with the policies, procedures and methods for preventing and managing violence.

So that they can notify their managers when they feel that they require training or practice in specific areas.

14 Primary and associate nurses are responsible for ensuring that patients receive medication which is prescribed.

(a) So that effects can be properly monitored.
(b) So that a schedule may be negotiated whereby the patient requests medication if he or she doubts whether control over impulses to violent behaviour can be maintained.

15 Each nurse who is eligible for membership of the emergency team receives the appropriate demonstration and training before being assigned to the team.

    (a) The composition of the team changes each shift.
    (b) Self-confidence and the necessary skills are required for nurses to function cohesively in the team in an emergency.

16 Once assigned to the team a nurse remains on the hospital premises for the duration of the shift, including the breaks, for which time off in lieu can be claimed on another occasion.

To be in the bleep and response range at all times.

17 The central nursing office maintains the rota of wards and departments responsible for providing members of the emergency team.

To co-ordinate with the clinical nurse manager and duty doctor rotas.

18 Charge nurses are responsible for negotiating in advance with each other the composition of the emergency team for a given week.

So that the necessary mix of first-level mental nurses in the team is maintained.

19 Once a nurse has been assigned to the emergency team he or she negotiates any changes with the clinical nurse manager on duty for the shift in question.

Unauthorized changes may compromise the skill mix and therefore the safety of the team.

20 Nurses and members of other professions attend the same in-service training courses.

So that all staff fulfil their duty to respond in an emergency.

21 All staff fulfil their responsibilities in relation to the documentation of violent incidents.

Well-kept statistics and trends will lead to more effective use of resources.

22 Primary and associate nurses as well as charge nurses initiate if necessary and contribute to multidisciplinary discussions of violent incidents.

    (a) In order to carry out a team discussion of each violent incident, its causes and results.
    (b) To provide an opportunity for learning.

23 Charge nurses arrange with their multidisciplinary clinical teams liaison with hospital systems for monitoring violence and its management.

To ensure free flow of information within and outside a ward or department.

REFERENCE MATERIAL
References

Bandura, A. (1973) *Aggression: A Social Learning Analysis*, Prentice-Hall, Englewood Cliffs, NJ.

Bowden, P. *et al.* (1978) Violence, *Nursing Mirror*, Vol. 146, no. 24, pp. 13–23.

Broome, A.K., Weaver, S.M. and Kat, B.J.B. (1978) Some patterns of disturbed behaviour in a closed ward environment, *Journal of Advanced Nursing*, Vol. 3, pp. 51–63.

Broome, A.K., Weaver, S.M. and Kat, B.J.B. (1979) Long-term behaviour problems in psychiatric hospitals, *Nursing Times*, Vol. 75, no. 12, pp. 493–5.

Crammer, J.L. (1984) The special characteristics of suicide in hospital in-patients, *British Journal of Psychiatry*, Vol. 145, pp. 460–76.

Curtis, J.M. (1985) Considerations in diagnosis and management of violent behaviour, *Psychological Reports*, Vol. 57, pp. 815–23.

Emson, H.E. (1986) Violence and the doctor: 'ethics', *Medicine, Science and the Law*, Vol. 26, no. 3, pp. 218–25.

Fottrell, E. (1980) A study of violent behaviour among paients in psychiatric hospitals, *British Journal of Psychiatry*, Vol. 136, pp. 216–21.

Fromm, E. (1977[1973]) *The Anatomy of Human Destructiveness*, Penguin, Harmondsworth.

Hodgkinson, P.E. (1980) Psychological approaches to violence, *Nursing Times*, Vol. 76, no. 32, pp. 1399–1401.

MIND (1975) *Guidelines for the Care of Patients who Exhibit Violent Behaviour in Mental and Mental Subnormality Hospitals*, National Association for Mental Health, London.

Pearson, M., Wilmot, E. and Padi, M. (1986) A study of violent behaviour among in-patients in a psychiatric hospital, *British Journal of Psychiatry*, Vol. 149, pp. 232–5.

Rossi, A.M. *et al.* (1986) Characteristics of patients who engage in assaultive or other fear-inducing behaviours, *Journal of Nervous and Mental Disease*, Vol. 174, no. 3, pp. 154–60.

Schulman, E.D. (1974) *Intervention in Human Services*, Mosby, St Louis, Mo.

Scott, P.D. (1977) Assessing dangerousness in criminals, *British Journal of Psychiatry*, Vol. 131, pp. 127–42.

Siann, G. (1985) *Accounting for Aggression: Perspectives on Aggression and Violence*, Allen & Unwin, London.

Stegne, L. (1978) A positive approach to negative behaviour, *Canadian Nurse*, Vol. 74, no. 6, pp. 44–8.

Storr, A. (1970) *Human Aggression*, Penguin, Harmondsworth.

Sugden, J. (1986) Coping with violence, *Senior Nurse*, Vol. 4, no. 2, pp. 20–1.

Tanke, E.D. and Yesavage, J.A. (1985) Characteristics of assaultive patients who do and do not provide visible cues of potential, *American Journal of Psychiatry*, Vol. 142, no. 12, pp. 1409–13.

Weller, M.P.I. (1986) Medical concepts in psychopathology and violence, *Medicine, Science and the Law*, Vol. 26, no. 2, pp. 131–43.

Whitman, R.M., Armao, B.B. and Dent, O.B. (1976) Assault on the therapist, *American Journal of Psychiatry*, Vol. 133, no. 4, pp. 426–9.

Woodside, M. *et al.* (1976) Experiment in managing sociopathic behaviour disorders, *British Medical Journal*, Vol. 2, pp. 1056–9.

Further reading

Basque, L.O. and Merhige, J. (1980) Nurses' experiences with dangerous behaviour: implications for training, *Journal of Continuing Education in Nursing*, Vol. 11, no. 5, pp. 47–51.

Berry, P., Leonhardt, W.B. and Stuhm, G. (1982) Differential reinforcement: practical applications to reduce aggressive and disruptive behaviour, *Canadian Journal of Psychiatric Nursing*, Vol. 23, no. 3, pp. 16–18.

Boettcher, E.G. (1983) Preventing violent behaviour: an integrated theoretical model for nursing, *Perspectives in Psychiatric Care*, Vol. 21, no. 2, pp. 54–8.

Cocozza, J.J. and Steadman, H.J. (1978) Prediction in psychiatry: an example of misplaced confidence in experts, *Social Problems*, Vol. 25, no. 3, pp. 265–76.

Convey, J. (1986) A record of violence, *Nursing Times*, Vol. 82, no. 46, pp. 36–8.

Di Fabio, S. and Ackerhalt, E.J. (1978) Teaching the use of restraint through roleplay, *Perspectives in Psychiatric Care*, Vol. 16, nos. 5–6, pp. 218–22.

Eysenck, H.J. (1979) The origins of violence, *Journal of Medical Ethics*, Vol. 5, pp. 105–7.

Garritson, S.H. (1987) Characteristics of restrictiveness, *Journal of Psychosocial Nursing and Mental Health Services*, Vol. 25, no. 1, pp. 11–19.

Gluck, M. (1981) Learning a therapeutic verbal response to anger, *Journal of Psychiatric Nursing*, Vol. 19, no. 3, pp. 22–8.

Gostin, L. (1978) Industrial action: is the target management or patients?, *Nursing Mirror*, Vol. 147, no. 15, pp. 15–17.

Hersen, M. and Bellack, A.S. (1985) *Handbook of Clinical Behaviour Therapy with Adults*, Plenum, New York.

Karshmer, J.F. (1978) The application of social learning theory to aggression, *Perspectives in Psychiatric Care*, Vol. 16, nos. 5–6, pp. 223–7.

Krakowski, M., Volavka, J. and Brizer, D. (1986) Psychopathology and violence: a review of literature, *Comprehensive Psychiatry*, Vol. 27, no. 2, pp. 131–48.

Lanza, M.L. (1985) How nurses react to assault, *Journal of Psychosocial Nursing and Mental Health Services*, Vol. 23, no. 6, pp. 6–11.

Lanza, M.L. (1986) Approaches to studying patient assault, *Western Journal of Nursing Research*, Vol. 8, no. 3, pp. 321–8.

Maier, G.J. *et al.* (1987) A model for understanding and managing cycles of aggression among psychiatric in-patients, *Hospital and Community Psychiatry*, Vol. 38, no. 5, p. 520–4.

Maynard, C.K. (1979) Dealing with anger: guidelines for nursing intervention, *Journal of Psychosocial Nursing and Mental Health Services*, Vol. 17, no. 6, pp. 36–41.

Monahan, J. (1978) Prediction research and the emergency commitment of dangerous mentally ill persons: a reconsideration, *American Journal of Psychiatry*, Vol. 135, no. 2, pp. 198–201.

Montandon, C. and Harding, T. (1984) The reliability of dangerousness assessments: a decision making exercise, *British Journal of Psychiatry*, Vol. 144, pp. 149–55.

Munns, D.C. (1985) A validation of the defining characteristics of the nursing diagnosis 'potential for violence', *Nursing Clinics of North America*, Vol. 20, no. 4, pp. 711–23.

Niskala, H. (1986) Competencies and skills required by

nurses working in forensic areas, *Western Journal of Nursing Research*, Vol. 8, no. 4, pp. 400–13.

Owens, R.G. and Ashcroft, J.B. (1985) *Violence: A Guide for the Caring Professions*, Croom Helm, Beckenham.

Poyner, B. and Warne, C. (1986) *Violence to Staff: A Basis for Assessment and Prevention*, HMSO, London.

Rix, G. (1985) Compassion is better than conflict, *Nursing Times*, Vol. 81, no. 38, pp. 53–5.

Rix, G. (1987) Staff sickness and its relationship to violent incidents on a regional secure psychiatric unit, *Journal of Advanced Nursing*, Vol. 12, pp. 223–8.

Rotter, J.B. (1954) *Social Learning and Clinical Psychology*, Prentice-Hall, Englewood Cliffs, NJ.

Russell, C. and Russell, W.M.S. (1979) The natural history of violence, *Journal of Medical Ethics*, Vol. 5, pp. 108–17.

Sclafani, M. (1986) Violence and behaviour control, *Journal of Psychosocial Nursing and Mental Health Services*, Vol. 24, no. 11, pp. 8–13.

Smith, J.E. (1986) Handling aggression, *The Professional Nurse*, Vol. 1, no. 6, pp. 91–4.

Stewart, A.T. (1978) Handling the aggressive patient, *Perspectives in Psychiatric Nursing Care*, Vol. 16, nos. 5–6, pp. 228–32.

[Unsigned article] (1977) Dangerous patients and prisoners, *British Medical Journal*, Vol. 2, pp. 782–3.

14

Managing Violence

DISCUSSION

Managing violence implies also the management of aggression, because not all fear-inducing behaviour is violence. Although it is not clear whether the aggressive or fear-inducing patient is more or less likely to be violent the techniques for managing aggression fit with the techniques for managing violence. Following Sclafani (1986, pp. 11–12) we can identify five stages in what he calls a 'crisis management protocol':

1 therapeutic environment programming;
2 verbal intervention;
3 team approach;
4 pharmacologic intervention;
5 mechanical restraints.

Therapeutic environment programming

Sclafani (1986) notes, as does Emson (1986), the shift in the USA and Canada away from intrusive and paternalistic methods of managing patient care. However, in the UK physical restraint techniques involving arm locks and other one-to-one fighting techniques are accepted as part of standard practice in the special hospitals and are being more widely used in secure units and elsewhere in psychiatric hospitals. A problem as the techniques become more widely known is that the means of countering them become known as well. Sclafani stresses the need for a quality assurance system to monitor practices and techniques for managing violence (see Chapter 13) (Lenefsky, de Palma and Locicero, 1978). 'In one-to-one situations you cannot subdue – you can only *win* – and to *win* you may have to inflict injury' (Donnelly, 1977, p. 24). The inflicting of injury and the possibility of causing abrasions carry an as yet undetermined risk from people who are HIV-positive or who are carrying hepatitis B antigen. If the single staff member's defence fails, there may be little further protection from the violent patient. For this reason, the techniques of restraint set out in this chapter rely on

using a number of nurses to subdue patients without using the inflicting of pain as a means of controlling behaviour.

ASSESSMENT OF THE POTENTIALLY VIOLENT PATIENT

Assessment of the patient is vital. Weller (1986) suggests that the evidence of abnormal brain functioning in violent patients supports the use of neuroleptic medication to control violent behaviour. Not all hallucinated or deluded patients are aggressive or violent: not all aggressive or violent patients are hallucinated or deluded. Some writers, however, argue that violent people are psychotic for a period of time, however brief.

A detailed baseline assessment of aggressive behaviour and the factors underlying it will be carried out. The accuracy of this assessment will depend in part on the qualities of the nurse–patient interaction. Agitation, fear, feeling of threat, personality, confusion and disorientation, hallucinations, perplexity – will all be possibilities considered by the nurse when assessing a patient.

Observations of and inferences about a potential threat depend on the nurse's ability to make a rapid assessment of the principal factors of the patient's mental state and of his or her subjective experience. The nurse needs to establish whether behaviour is the result of, say, an organic confusional state, possibly involving drugs, or of a delusional state, of fear, agitation or feelings of threat, or of a particular situation, or of the patient's personality or a combination of factors. The inferences from the nurse's observations will lead to the specific plan of management. If triggers of violence for individual patients can be identified it may be possible to construct a care plan which aims to remove or modify their effect. Examples of triggers are alcohol, drugs, grievance, provocation, metabolic disturbance (such as diabetes) and toxic conditions (such as infection).

A behavioural approach provides an understandable basis for helping patients to learn different behaviour in response to staff efforts at reinforcing non-aggressive behaviour. Behavioural approaches in which staff reinforce non-violent, non-threatening behaviour may provide opportunities for patients to learn different behaviours. With patience and careful attention to detail, it is possible to shape behaviour that is incompatible with violence, for example by sitting down when an apparently aggressive patient sits down. Shaping requires the nurse to reinforce all adaptive behaviour by the patient, no matter how minimal.

Treatment agreements have been found to be helpful with violent patients. Details will be found in Chapter 33, 'Treatment agreements'.

CRITICAL INCIDENT DEBRIEFINGS

Debriefing is an essential component of the therapeutic environment. All staff will be used to taking part in debriefings from violent incidents in which they were directly or indirectly involved. Evidence is growing which demonstrates the adverse short- and long-term effects of repeated exposure to psychological trauma such as violence, and the benefits of talking about, reliving, the experience with other victims and with facilitators. Debriefing is carried out by staff for the staff as well as by staff with the patient. Preferably the nurse who is primarily responsible for the patient's nursing care will be closely involved.

TRAINING

Training is discussed in Chapter 13.

Verbal intervention

The first aim of verbal intervention is to enable the patient to desist from his or her fear-inducing behaviour. It is essential that nurses are confident in their judgement about when to intervene verbally, when to withdraw and when to approach a violent patient only with a prepared team of colleagues. (Hence the ten hours of training suggested in Chapter 13.) The assessment of the patient will give an idea about which response is safest. The second aim of verbal intervention is to enable the patient to talk in such a way that further violence becomes gradually more unlikely. This calls again for careful judgement on the nurse's part. It is necessary to be cautious when a very angry person is encouraged to talk about his or her anger. Talking about it may have the effect of arousing rather than diminishing it. Cathartic interventions have to be negotiated and agreed between patient and nurse, and are not suitable for the patient who is already expressing anger.

Self-management when faced with a violent, aggressive or otherwise fear-inducing patient involves the attempt to set limits on the patient's behaviour as well as the nurse's own. The nurse will not retaliate if the patient is swearing or otherwise abusive. If the patient threatens violence the nurse may, depending on his or her knowledge of the patient, withdraw, or intervene verbally (Anders, 1977; Schulman, 1974). The nurse may say something like: 'I'm prepared to listen to you and hear your grievances and to help you, if I can, sort out a way of dealing with them. You do not need to threaten me, and I will not allow you to hurt me'; or 'I can see that you are very angry and I would like to help if I can. But I am afraid you will hurt someone with that cue stick.'

On no account does the nurse make promises or threats – whether or not they can be carried out. The nurse can promise to do his or her best to help the patient. The aim of these interventions is to demonstrate that the nurse takes the patient and what he or she says seriously, so that it is essential not to be dismissive of the reasons for the patient's threatening behaviour.

Team approach

When violence is unexpected, individual nurses are advised to be cautious about approaching the patient. In such circumstances it is advisable to summon help immediately. When violence has been anticipated, even though the first approach to a violent patient may be that of verbal intervention by a single nurse, it will be in the context of a planned strategy by the nursing team as a whole. The strategy may be implemented as a result of prior discussion about how to manage this particular incident. It may be implemented in an emergency, as the team responds to finding one nurse confronted by a violent patient. The strategy and this response will be conditioned by repeated training and debriefings from other violent incidents, including those involving the same patient, so that learning by nurses takes place.

Pharmacologic intervention

Since neuroleptic medication is always to be considered as a means of managing violence even if the patient does not usually carry the label of psychotic, accurate assessment will facilitate such consideration.

Restraint

It is a team decision whether to restrain a patient or not. For example, if a patient is alone in a room destroying property there may be a case for waiting to see if he or she desists voluntarily. If there is any doubt about the safety of people, restraint is the approach of choice. Only if there are at least six members of staff available should restraint be carried out (RCN (1984) guidelines: one person per limb and two for the body).

REASONABLE FORCE

In 1976 there was some disquiet that new DHSS guidelines on violence refrained from clearly defining what was reasonable force when restraining patients (DHSS, 1976). It is not possible or necessarily advisable to give a statutory definition of reasonable force. Rather nurses are protected by section 141 of the Mental Health Act 1983 and by provisions of the Criminal Law Act 1967. Section 141 protects nurses from prosecution by patients, and is intended to allow them to carry out duties necessary to 'maintain good order in the running of the hospital'.

The nurse is protected also from prosecution for assault by means of the provision which allows reasonable force to be used to prevent a crime. Assault, being a crime, may be resisted by the nurse using reasonable force. The common law, consisting of judicial precedent from previous cases concerned with assaults by nurses and patients, is constantly modified with each new judgement. Martin (1979) suggests that the following courses of action are recommended in view of the law as it stands.

1 Run away from an armed patient if he or she cannot be immobilized.
2 Retaliate physically only if there is no other means of protecting yourself from serious harm.
3 Immobilize and disarm a patient rather than fight him or her.
4 Overpower a patient rather than inflict injury.

Suggestions 3 and 4 reflect the notion that there is safety in numbers. Hence the emphasis in these procedures on teamwork and on the use of an emergency team.

If restraint is carried out, it must be decided whether or not to medicate a patient. Clear leadership and sound judgement are required for the right decisions to be thought out on the evidence available.

Documentation

Incident forms are completed after each violent incident, and the staff casualty book completed immediately if any nurse has been injured. The incident forms include the following details:

1 date, time and place;
2 patient's name, age, sex and diagnosis;
3 history of violence;
4 action taken;
5 injuries resulting from the violence;
6 precipitants;
7 consequences of staff intervention.

In the nursing record the nurses involved in the incident write a detailed account as soon as possible. In future admissions the information given about violent behaviour will allow safer assessment of a patient's proneness to violence.

Part of the debriefing process involves discussion with the violent patient in order to try to identify what led to it, whether he or she could have acted differently, how he or she feels now.

Specific techniques for dealing with attacks and restraining patients will not be described in this chapter because it is not possible to learn the necessary skills from the printed page. This chapter supplements training material such as videotapes, demonstrations by qualified trainers, role-play and supervised practice. Each hospital's training programme in restraint must be kept under review and approved by the health authority, acting on legal advice and the views of ethical advisory committees.

GUIDELINES: MANAGING VIOLENCE

Action	Rationale
1 If you go to talk to a potentially violent patient, tell colleagues where you are going and how long you intend to be.	So that other staff will maintain a check on your safety.
2 As soon as you assess that one or more patients are already or are about to be violent, summon help.	(a) To anticipate and forestall violence. (b) To ensure safety.
3 If there is any concern that the patient is dangerous, wait until a team of at least seven staff in addition to you has been assembled.	(a) So that there are six people to restrain the patient if necessary; (b) and two to look after the other patients.

4 If possible ask any other patients to leave while keeping a close eye on the violence.

    (a) To avoid injury to them.
    (b) To avoid provocation.

5 Check whether the patient has a weapon.

    (a) It may be concealed.
    (b) Weapons increase the danger.
    (c) To ensure safety.
    (d) To reduce the chance of serious violence.
    (e) To reduce the chance of injury if violence does occur.

6 Stay at least an arm and a half's distance from the violent patient.

    (a) To avoid entering his or her personal space. Threatening people are easily threatened.
    (b) To be out of fist's reach.

7 Ensure that you have an exit.

In case you have to withdraw.

8 Avoid cornering an angry or disturbed patient.

    (a) Unless restraint is intended,
    (b) and there are enough staff to carry it out.

9 Avoid standing at the top of stairs, by a window, by a door, against glass.

Because you may be pushed through a door or glass, or downstairs, or cornered.

10 Adopt a non-aggressive and relaxed stance:
    (i) Feet apart to maintain balance.
    (ii) Hands by side, fingers lightly curled, clearly holding no weapon, not in pockets, not on hips.

    (a) To maintain safety.
    (b) To reduce the chance of violence.
    (c) To reduce the chance of injury if there is violence.
    (d) In order not to threaten the violent person.

11 Adopt an attentive facial expression.

    (a) Smiling could be interpreted as mockery.
    (b) Frowning could be interpreted as anger.

12 Breathe evenly.

In order not to hyperventilate or breathe too shallowly thereby increasing your own anxiety.

13 Refrain from raising your hands or pointing.

Raised hands may be interpreted as threatening.

14 Avoid sudden movements, move deliberately, slowly if possible.

Sudden movement could be threatening.

15 Lower the pitch and tone of your voice.

    (a) To avoid irritating the patient.
    (b) To give the impression of being relaxed and emotionally neutral.

16 Speak quietly but loudly enough to be heard.

To avoid exciting the violent person.

17 Address the patient by name.

    (a) To help orient him or her.
    (b) To demonstrate respect.

18 Name yourself.

To orient the patient.

19 Remind the patient of the place and time.

To orient him or her.

20 Make suggestions rather than give instructions to the violent person.

(a) Very high arousal will prevent any but the most simple communication from being understood.
(b) It could be dangerous to act on an assumption that the patient has understood what is said.
(c) So that by thinking first, you do your best to see how it is for the violent person.

21 Avoid staring while refraining from appearing shifty.

Persistent eye-contact may be interpreted by the patient as aggressive.

22 Observe the patient's breathing and pitch and tone of voice, bearing in mind that the apparently calm patient may be extremely dangerous.

In order to assess how angry or distressed or both the patient is.

23 Observe the patient for signs of autonomic activity:
   (i) dry mouth;
   (ii) dilated pupils;
   (iii) sweating;
   (iv) rapid breathing;
   (v) rapid pulse (look at carotid).

(a) These will indicate the possibility of a fight or flight reaction.
(b) So that you are prepared to act.
(c) In order that you reflect on what the violent person is feeling to ensure that your own response is accurate.

24 Observe the patient's movements.

In case of a sudden attack.

25 Make a neutral inquiry, for example: 'Tell me what has been happening.'

To give the person a chance to describe his or her subjective experience, thereby making assessment easier.

26 Acknowledge the patient's answers.

To demonstrate interest and respect.

27 Attempt to identify and acknowledge feelings communicated in the answer.

If the patient feels understood he or she may desist from the violence.

28 Make no promises or threats.

You have no guarantee you can carry them out.

29 Avoid arguing.

In order not to provoke the patient.

30 Avoid, if possible, a big dramatic scene.

(a) A highly aroused person may be further pressured if he or she is surrounded by people, noise, competing voices and instructions.
(b) The drama may contribute to the patient's undesirable behaviour.

31 If it is apparent that a patient's behaviour is so dangerous as possibly to need restraint, the emergency team is summoned.

To assemble organized help and management resources.

32 The nurse in charge of the ward directs the procedure.

So that instructions are clearly given by one person and immediately followed.

33 If there are fewer than eight members of staff present, the duty clinical nurse manager will summon help from elsewhere.

(a) Six people are needed to restrain a patient.
(b) At least two nurses, one of whom is a RMN, must be available to look after the patients in the ward.

34   Away from the clinical area the nurse in charge briefly outlines the situation that has led to the emergency.

Preparation is done away from the clinical area so that the nursing team appears united and decisive when it is time to act.

35   The nurse in charge outlines generally what is to be done.

(a)   So that the team knows who the patient is;
(b)   who the ward staff are;
(c)   who has been brought in to help.
(d)   In order to understand the risks.

36   Members of staff remove personal jewellery, badges and pens.

To prevent injury to the patient and to themselves.

37   The nurse in charge assigns to six nurses the task of immobilizing the patient by taking control of his or her limbs after ascertaining that they have been trained in and have practised the techniques of restraint and immobilization.

So that each nurse understands his or her role in relation to the other staff.

38   Each nurse is responsible individually or jointly for immobilizing a specific part of the patient's body.

(a)   So that a method will be selected which meets the requirements of the present emergency.
(b)   So that each nurse knows from which side to approach the patient.

39   The nurse in charge nominates a nurse to fetch any equipment needed, such as mattresses, pillows, blankets, sheets.

(a)   A mattress or pillow may be used as protection against a knife.
(b)   Blankets or sheets may be used to immobilize the patient.
(c)   Pillows may be needed to protect the patient if he or she is on the floor.

40   The nurse in charge maintains contact with the nurses observing the patient.

In order to know where the patient is.

41   The nurse in charge instructs the team members, stating:
(i)   timings;
(ii)   how the patient will be approached;
(iii)   where the team members will position themselves;
(iv)   what the patient is likely to do;
(v)   any other risks which may be present, for example an infected patient.

So that each nurse knows what he or she will do and where to be.

42   The nurse in charge confirms with the doctor and the clinical nurse manager what their roles will be.

So that support and help will be available if needed.

43   The nurse in charge confirms with the remaining nurses in the ward what their role will be.

So that the other patients in the ward will be safely looked after.

44   The nurse in charge says what his or her words of command will be.

So that team members know when to act.

45   The nurse in charge confirms that the members of the team understand their role.

The resulting co-ordination will increase confidence in one another.

46 The nurse in charge asks for any questions from team members.

To confirm finally that the action to be taken is understood by all.

47 The team approaches the patient, led by the nurse in charge.

To make it clear that the patient now does not have a choice about the need to control his or her behaviour.

48 The nurse in charge asks the patient to desist from the dangerous or violent behaviour.

To offer the patient a last chance to take control of his or her behaviour.

49 If the patient will not desist from his or her violent behaviour the nurse in charge gives the prearranged command and the team moves quickly to either side and immobilizes the patient as planned. Depending where the patient is, this might be on the floor, in a chair or on a bed.

The patient is immobilized wherever he or she happens to be because of the risk of injury involved in attempting to move the patient to another location at the same time as restraining him or her.

50 The nurse in charge remains by the patient's head, restraining it if necessary, and talking continuously to him or her.

The effect of one person talking quietly can help to reduce fear and anger, especially in perplexed patients.

51 The team remains in position, the nurse in charge continues to talk to the patient until it is confirmed that he or she is calm enough to be released. This may take some time, and patience is required.

Psychotic patients are especially vulnerable to being suddenly released after being immobilized and may become violent again.

52 If necessary the team quickly and gently lifts the patient using a recognized technique and transfers him or her to the patient's personal accommodation.

(a) In order to prevent a struggle and ensuing injury.
(b) In order to provide privacy for the patient. The privacy may help any loss of face.

53 One or two nurses who know the patient undertake unbroken supervision.

To observe the effects of any medication that has been given.

54 The team returns to the ward office to meet together with the duty clinical nurse manager and the doctor.
  Each member of staff will evaluate his or her own role and will evaluate the work of the team as a whole. Any points for improvement are noted by the nurse in charge.

In order to debrief from the incident.

55 The nurse in charge completes the documentation required by the hospital managers. Examples will include:
  (i)   violent incident form;
  (ii) staff casualty book;
  (iii) patient injury form.

Even when no injury is apparent this will be recorded.

(a) Accurate figures are required of the occurrence of types of violence to facilitate comparison and research.
(b) A record is made of any injury to a nurse so that a claim may be made if necessary at a future date for criminal injuries compensation.
(c) A record is required which states that the patient has been examined for injury at the time of the incident, in case of any complaint or claim later by the patient.

56 The nurse in charge writes an account of the procedure in the patient's nursing record.

To ensure that if necessary the incident can be evaluated after the lapse of some time.

57 The doctor writes in the medical record an account of the patient's mental state before, during and after the incident.

To facilitate a management review by the multidisciplinary team.

58   The patient is examined physically if there is any possibility of injury having occurred.

To record any physical injury to the patient, no matter how slight.

REFERENCE MATERIAL
References

Anders, R.L. (1977) When a patient becomes violent, *American Journal of Nursing*, Vol. 77, pp. 1144–8.

Criminal Law Act 1967, HMSO, London.

DHSS (1976) HC(76)11, *Management of Violent and Potentially Violent Hospital Patients*, DHSS, London.

Donnelly, G. (1977) Violence: Nurse versus patient, *Nursing Mirror*, Vol. 45, no. 20, p. 24.

Emson, H.E. (1986) Violence and the doctor: 'ethics', *Medicine, Science and the Law*, Vol. 26, no. 3, pp. 218–25.

Lenefsky, B., de Palma, T. and Locicero, D. (1978) Management of violent behaviours, *Perspectives in Psychiatric Care*, Vol. 16, nos. 5–6, pp. 212–17.

Martin, A. (1979) Assault, *Nursing Times*, Vol. 75, no. 6, p. 250.

Mental Health Act 1983, HMSO, London.

Royal College of Nursing (1984) *Violence – Policy Guidelines*, RCN, London.

Schulman, E.D. (1974) *Intervention in Human Services*, Mosby, St Louis, Mo.

Sclafani, M. (1986) Violence and behaviour control, *Journal of Psychosocial Nursing and Mental Health Services*, Vol. 24, no. 11, pp. 8–13.

Weller, M.P.I. (1986) Medical concepts in psychopathology and violence, *Medicine, Science and the Law*, Vol. 26, no. 2, pp. 131–43.

Further reading

Brizer, D. *et al.* (1987) A rating scale for reporting violence on psychiatric wards, *Hospital and Community Psychiatry*, Vol. 38, no. 7, pp. 769–70.

Cobb, J.P. and Gossop, M.R. (1976) Locked doors in the management of disturbed psychiatric patients, *Journal of Advanced Nursing*, Vol. 1, pp. 469–80.

Cust, K. (1986) Assault: just part of the job? *Canadian Nurse*, Vol. 82, no. 6, pp. 19–20.

Di Fabio, S. (1978) Teaching the use of restraint through role play, *Perspectives in Psychiatric Nursing Care*, Vol. 16, nos. 5–6, pp. 218–22.

Fein, B.A., Gareri, E. and Hansen, P. (1981) Teaching staff to cope with patient violence, *Journal of Continuing Education in Nursing*, Vol. 12, no. 3, pp. 7–11.

Hoge, S.K. and Gutheil, T.G. (1987) The prosecution of psychiatric patients for assaults on staff: a preliminary empirical study, *Hospital and Community Psychiatry*, Vol. 38, no. 1, pp. 44–9.

Jones, M.K. (1985) Patient violence: report of 200 incidents, *Journal of Psychosocial Nursing and Mental Health Services*, Vol. 23, no. 6, pp. 12–17.

Katz, L., Weber, F. and Dodge, P. (1981) Patient restraint and safety vests: minimizing the hazards, *Dimensions in Health Service*, Vol. 58, no. 5, pp. 10–11.

Lanza, M.L. (1984) Factors affecting blame placement for patient assault on nurses, *Issues in Mental Health Nursing*, Vol. 6, pp. 143–61.

Lion, J.R. (1987) Training for battle: thoughts on managing aggressive patients, *Hospital and Community Psychiatry*, Vol. 38, no. 8, pp. 883–4.

Lion, J.R., Levenberg, L.B. and Strange, R.E. (1972) Restraining the violent patient, *Journal of Psychiatric Nursing*, Vol. 10, no. 2, pp. 9–11.

MIND (1975) *Guidelines for the Care of Patients who Exhibit Violent Behaviour in Mental and Mental Subnormality Hospitals*, National Association for Mental Health, London.

Moran, J.F. (1984) Teaching the management of violent behaviour to nursing staff: a health care model, in J.T. Turner (ed.) *Violence in the Medical Care Setting: A Survival Guide*, Aspen Systems Corporation, Rockville, MD.

Neizo, B.A. and Lanza, M.L. (1984) Post violence dialogue: change through language restructuring, *Issues in Mental Health Nursing*, Vol. 6, pp. 245–54.

Owens, R.G. and Ashcroft, J.B. (1985) *Violence: A Guide for the Caring Professions*, Croom Helm, Beckenham.

Packham, H. *et al.* (1978) Violence, *Nursing Mirror*, Vol. 146, no. 25, pp. 17–27.

Slack, P. (1983) Facing up to aggression, *Nursing Times*, Vol. 79, no. 20, pp. 10–11.

Stegne, L. (1978) A positive approach to negative behaviour, *Canadian Nurse*, Vol. 74, no. 6, pp. 44–8.

Sugden, J. (1986) Coping with violence, *Senior Nurse*, Vol. 4, no. 2, pp. 20–1.

Turner, J.T. (ed.) (1984) *Violence in the Medical Care Setting: A Survival Guide*, Aspen Systems Corporation, Rockville, MD.

[Unattributed news item] (1975) 'Reasonable force', *Nursing Times*, Vol. 71, no. 7, p. 245.

15

Deliberate Self-Harm

DEFINITIONS

There is no unitary explanation for suicide, nor is there agreement on a definition. Moreover, at least seven different groupings must be considered, as shown in Figure 15.1:

1 those who complete suicide;
2 those who attempt suicide;
3 an overlap group of those who attempt and complete suicide;
4 inpatients;
5 inpatients who complete suicide;
6 inpatients who attempt suicide;
7 an overlap group of inpatients who attempt and complete suicide.

The result of this complexity is that, on the one hand, a blurring of distinction may mean that staff are immobilized by the threats of a coercive patient. On the other hand, excessive reliance on categories and labels means that it is possible that staff do not recognize the proximity to death of a chronically distressed patient at the end of his or her tether.

To reduce ambiguity, this chapter will be restricted to the terms 'suicide', 'attempted suicide', 'suicidal', and 'inpatients'. The definitions in this chapter are taken from the World Health Organization's (WHO) International Classification of Diseases, ninth edition (WHO, 1977) and from the report of a WHO working group. The reason for this is that causes of death in the UK are analysed by WHO classification. A procedure based on the WHO definitions follows Durkheim's (1951) recommendation to deal only in comparable facts: to use established groupings so that any subsequent research can be compared with existing findings.

However, to establish an operational definition does not necessarily clarify management of individual

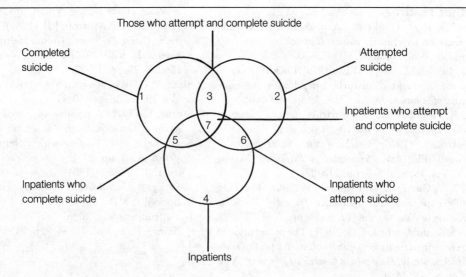

Figure 15.1 Those who attempt and complete suicide

patients. No definition of suicide is satisfactory because of the need to describe intent to die. Few people would argue that to swallow a handful of aspirin tablets in the midst of a quarrel is qualitatively the same kind of action as asphyxiation with a car exhaust after many months of intractable and incurable pain. Yet if both such actions end in death they are called suicide.

For the purposes of nursing the suicidal patient, suicide is death due to an intentional act of self-injury or self-poisoning. Attempted suicide is a non-fatal act of self-injury or self-poisoning, which in the case of drug poisoning means that the recommended dose has been deliberately exceeded.

The term 'suicidal' will be used to refer to any person thought to be at risk of self-injury or self-poisoning. The term 'inpatient' will be used to refer to a person admitted to 'an institution for the care of the sick and wounded or for those who require medical treatment', as in the *Shorter Oxford English Dictionary*.

Differentiation between attempted and completed suicide

The reason for retaining a global definition of the term 'suicidal' is that to have one procedure designed for the person at risk of completed suicide and another designed for the person at risk of attempted suicide runs the risk of missing the overlap group described earlier. The nursing procedure described in this chapter includes an assessment tool used to discriminate between levels of suicidal risk; risk implying the danger of death as the result of self-injurious behaviour. The word 'suicidal' does not in itself imply any specific degree of risk for that individual. Once the risk is measured and stated, a decision as to management can follow.

DISCUSSION

The rate of suicide for hospital inpatients is at least three times greater than for the population at large. Most classifications of suicide do not discriminate between inpatients and others, so that there are few pointers to whether the risk of suicide is increased or reduced by being in hospital, or to the factors which can be used specifically to predict the risk to individuals resident in hospital.

The population or grouping of those people who complete suicide overlaps with the population of those who attempt suicide. That is, although it is likely that up to half of those who eventually complete suicide have previously attempted it, the two populations remain socially, clinically and demographically distinct groups. Inpatients form a further population which overlaps with the other two. They are a complex group of people at risk, as shown in Figure 15.1.

Causes of suicide and contributory factors

SOCIAL AND ENVIRONMENTAL FACTORS

From Durkheim (1951) onwards writers have hypothesized the social and interpersonal nature of suicide and attempted suicide. Durkheim believed that the nature of a society determined its types and rates of suicide. Douglas (1967) criticized Durkheim's failure to define the nature of the social forces hypothesized to influence suicide, and called for more accurate description and measurement before attempts at explanation. Much of the research in the UK describes and measures suicidal phenomena, attempting to find patterns from which hypotheses can be constructed.

Some writers have speculated that covert hostility by family, friends or hospital staff increases the risk of suicide for some people. The part played in completed and attempted suicide by social forces and interpersonal relationships is by no means quantified or clear, but interpersonal conflict is present for many who attempt or complete suicide. A high suicide rate exists in prisons. Broken homes have been found to be a significant factor in both attempted and completed suicide. Social isolation, whether in the form of residential mobility or divorce, separation or widowhood, is associated with attempted and completed suicide. Although between 1975 and 1980 increases in unemployment, alcohol consumption and suicide occurred in England and Wales, strict causal connections between these phenomena have not been demonstrated (Barraclough *et al.*, 1974; Flood and Seager, 1968; McClure, 1984; Pallis *et al.*, 1982).

CHARACTERISTICS OF INPATIENT SUICIDE

Factors associated with inpatient suicide have been identified. Many patients kill themselves towards the beginning and end of admission and soon after discharge. Up to half the inpatients who kill themselves do so while on leave. Many patients who kill themselves appear to be improving at the time of their suicide. The juxtaposition of two other findings causes concern. That is, up to two-thirds of completed suicides give advance warning, and up to three-fifths of suicides come as a surprise to staff. What this could imply is a deficit in listening to patients, as well as in predicting their eventual suicide.

The occurrence of suicides at a time of disruption or change in wards has been documented. Further attention to this association of suicide with the ward environment has been demonstrated by a number of hypotheses which require testing. One is that suicides occur when ward routine and staff confidence are disturbed.

Another is that a patient is more likely to kill him- or herself if he or she fails to make a relationship with staff or fellow patients. A third hypothesis is that diffusion of responsibility in a ward team leads to decision-making by less skilled members, thus putting patients at risk. A fourth is that a team in the early stages of formation is less skilful in its assessment of suicidal patients than a long-established team.

PSYCHOPATHOLOGY AND SUICIDE
The association of mental illness and suicidal behaviour leads to considerable argument. It will have been noticed that the definition of inpatient given earlier made no reference to illness; a requirement for medical treatment implies nothing about disease. For this reason care should be taken not to confuse a history of previous psychiatric treatment with a history of mental illness. Previous psychiatric treatment in both patients' and patients' families is significantly associated with attempted and completed suicide. The phenomena which have been identified as being associated with suicide tend not only to cross disease boundaries but to be associated with social, developmental and personality factors. A statement about suicidal risk may be made independently of or in addition to a diagnosis of disease process.

DEPENDENCE
Conflict with friends, relatives and staff has been found to be associated with issues of a person's dependence on and independence of significant others, oscillation between the two occurring in ways that put considerable strain on relationships.

DEPRESSION
Clinical findings in a number of studies indicate that depressive phenomena are commonly present in both attempted and completed suicide. It may be less useful to try to classify types of depression than to use a continuum model such as that described by Hill (1968). Phenomena from the 'mild' end of the continuum are as likely to be associated with self-injury as phenomena from the 'severe' end. Depression rating scales may be useful for measuring changes in patients' complaints and other phenomena over time.

HOPELESSNESS
Hopelessness and despair are common clinical findings in suicidal persons. Research with the Beck Depression Inventory has demonstrated that hopelessness correlates significantly with suicidal intent (Beck *et al.*, 1979).

IMPULSIVENESS
Although many suicides are carefully planned, there are a number of people whose inability to tolerate distress and frustration is displayed in impulsive behaviour. Impulsiveness increases the risk of self-injury.

INSOMNIA
Sleep disturbance and early-morning waking have been associated with both attempted and completed suicide.

PSYCHOMOTOR RETARDATION
There is no evidence that retardation protects depressed patients from suicide. Some findings indicate that shortly before suicide some people become very calm.

PSYCHOSIS
Psychotic patients may attempt serious self-injury in response to hallucinations and delusions. The more lethal and sometimes bizarre methods tend to be preferred. Examples are jumping from a height, self-incineration, shooting, drowning and hanging. Psychotic patients can represent maximum suicidal risk while denying suicidal intent.

SCHIZOPHRENIA
The suicide rate in patients with a diagnosis of schizophrenia or schizo-affective disorder appears to be higher in the early stages of the illness and at times when improvement is occurring. For inpatients this is near the start of the first admission to hospital, and shortly before or after discharge from hospital.

SUBSTANCE ABUSE
Heavy drinking is associated with both attempted and completed suicide. Up to 60 per cent of men and up to 45 per cent of women take alcohol before overdosing. Alcohol addiction combined with depressive phenomena and severe social disorganization is associated with suicide attempts. In its late stages, chronic alcoholism carries a high risk of suicide. Suicide and opiate abuse are significantly correlated, but rates of suicide for all addicts are difficult to infer because of the unreliability of estimates of the number of addicts.

Diurnal variation
It has been demonstrated that the majority of suicides occur between 0600 and 1200.

The risk of suicide
MEASURING SUICIDE RISK
The importance of attending to the social environment as well as to the individual patient when calculating suicide risk is emphasized by a continuing increase in the rate of suicide for inpatients. This increase has occurred independently of the downward fluctuation in the suicide rate as a whole (Copas and Robin, 1982;

Extremely high	High	Moderately high	Moderately low
Hanging	Paracetamol	Natural gas	Delicate cutting
Self-incineration	Tricyclics	Benzodiazepines with alcohol	Benzodiazepines without alcohol
Jumping from a height	Anticholinergics	Phenothiazines	
Jumping under a train	Lithium	Aspirin	
Asphyxiation: Carbon monoxide Strangulation Suffocation	Anticonvulsants	Coarse cutting	
Drowning	Opiates	Exposure to cold	
Car crash	Corrosives		
Insulin	Weed killer		
Gunshot			

Figure 15.2 Risk of completed suicide of different methods

Perris, Beskow and Jacobson, 1980; Report of a Working Group, 1982).

Reliance on intuition or common sense or clinical experience is not enough when measuring suicidal risk. In recent years there has been a rapid increase in the number of rating scales being used to try to predict suicide. Care must be taken to use scales developed specifically for the kinds of patient proposed for rating. Additionally, 'the clinical assessment of a person's proclivity to suicide can never be reduced to a mere scoring of a few items on any single scale' (Pallis, Gribbons and Pierce 1984, p. 147).

CLASSIFYING SUICIDE RISK
The classification of suicide risk in this procedure follows that used by Pallis (Pallis et al., 1982). There are five categories: extremely high, high, moderately high, moderately low and low. Levels of supervision are ranged against levels of risk. It is emphasized that the levels and intervals of supervision prescribed for each type of risk are independent of and additional to any other plan for individualized nursing care. The patient's safety is the foundation upon which negotiated treatment objectives are constructed.

ASSESSMENT OF SUICIDE RISK
Assessment of suicide risk involves six steps. These steps will not necessarily follow the order set out here because a suicidal crisis may require an immediate plan of intervention based on clinical impressions and a global assessment of:

1 the suicide risk of any method already used (as shown in Figure 15.2);
2 self-rating by the patient;
3 personal interaction between the nurse and patient;
4 global assessment by the nurse of the suicide risk;
5 discussion between the staff based so far as possible on the material assembled in the previous steps;
6 classification of the suicide risk.

Self-rating by the patient
Examples of useful scales are the Hopelessness Scale (Beck, 1974), the Leeds Specific Depression Scale (Snaith et al., 1971) or the Irritability–Depression–Anxiety Scale (Snaith et al., 1978).

Personal interaction between nurse and patient
Interactions are documented as laid out in the procedures for carrying out the nursing process (see Chapters 1 and 23).

Discussion between staff
The results of the different types of assessment are compared and a decision made about the final risk classification. If the various scales identify different levels of risk, the team decides which aspect to emphasize. For example, an extremely high risk method used in the past may be considered better evidence of overall

risk than a low self-rating on the Hopelessness Scale. The decision is made individually how to rate each patient's risk.

Global assessment and classification of suicide risk

Figure 15.3 shows the Global Assessment of Functioning Scale (DSM-III (rev), 1987). The codes may be divided into five sections, corresponding to low (71–90), moderately low (51–70), moderately high (31–50), high (11–30), and extremely high (1–10) risk of self-harm. These may be used as guidelines for nurses who wish to estimate a risk level for self-harm by the patient being assessed. This estimate may be compared with the findings of the rest of the ward team in order to arrive at the final risk classification.

Planning

Planning for the suicidal patient involves two additional steps to those detailed in the procedure for planning (see Chapter 2). They are, first, the specification of the level of supervision required for the patient and, second, the initiation of a suicide alert form if the risk is extremely high or moderately high.

Figure 15.4 shows a method of matching risks to levels of supervision and types of recording. Figure 15.5 is an example of a nursing care plan, and a suicide alert form is shown in Figure 15.6.

Global Assessment of Functioning Scale (GAF Scale)

Consider psychological, social, and occupational functioning on a hypothetical continuum of mental health-illness. Do not include impairment in functioning due to physical (or environmental) limitations.

Note: Use intermediate codes when appropriate, e.g. 45, 68, 72.

Code

90 | **Absent or minimal symptoms** (e.g., mild anxiety before an exam), **good functioning in all areas, interested and involved in a wide range of activities, socially effective, generally satisfied with life, no**
81 | **more than everyday problems or concerns** (e.g., an occasional argument with family members).

80 | **If symptoms are present, they are transient and expectable reactions to psychosocial stressors** (e.g., difficulty concentrating after family argument); **no more than slight impairment in social, occupational, or**
71 | **school functioning** (e.g., temporarily falling behind in school work).

70 | **Some mild symptoms** (e.g., depressed mood and mild insomnia) **OR some difficulty in social, occupational, or school functioning** (e.g., occasional truancy, or theft within the household), **but generally**
61 | **functioning pretty well, has some meaningful interpersonal relationships.**

60 | **Moderate symptoms** (e.g., flat affect and circumstantial speech, occasional panic attacks) **OR moderate**
51 | **difficulty in social, occupational, or school functioning** (e.g., few friends, conflicts with co-workers).

50 | **Serious symptoms** (e.g., suicidal ideation, severe obsessional rituals, frequent shoplifting) **OR any serious**
41 | **impairment in social, occupational, or school functioning** (e.g., no friends, unable to keep a job).

40 | **Some impairment in reality testing or communication** (e.g., speech is at times illogical, obscure, or irrelevant) **OR major impairment in several areas, such as work or school, family relations, judgement, thinking, or mood** (e.g., depressed man avoids friends, neglects family, and is unable to work; child
31 | frequently beats up younger children, is defiant at home, and is failing at school).

30 | **Behaviour is considerably influenced by delusions or hallucinations OR serious impairment in communication or judgement** (e.g., sometimes incoherent, acts grossly inappropriately, suicidal preoccupation) **OR inability to function in almost all areas** (e.g., stays in bed all day; no job, home, or
21 | friends).

20 | **Some danger of hurting self or others** (e.g., suicide attempts without clear expectation of death, frequently violent, manic excitement) **OR occasionally fails to maintain minimal personal hygiene** (e.g., smears
11 | feces) **OR gross impairment in communication** (e.g., largely incoherent or mute).

10 | **Persistent danger of severely hurting self or others** (e.g., recurrent violence) **OR persistent inability to**
1 | **maintain minimal personal hygiene OR serious suicidal act with clear expectation of death.**

Figure 15.3 Global assessment of functioning scale (GAF Scale). Reprinted with permission from the *Diagnostic and Statistical Manual of Mental Disorders, Third Edition, Revised.* Copyright 1987 American Psychiatric Association.

Risk classification	Level of supervision	Initiated by	Intervals of supervision	Duration	Carried out by	Type of recording	Discontinued by
Extremely high	Maximum supervision	First level nurse or registered medical practitioner	One-to-one contact every minute of 24 hours	30 mins + 15 mins for reporting	First level nurse	Suicide alert form, nurses' notes each shift, day and night reports	First level nurse and registered medical practitioner
High	Full supervision	First level nurse or registered medical practitioner	One-to-one contact every minute the patient is awake. Fifteen-minute checks while the patient is asleep	45 mins + 15 mins for reporting	First level nurse	Suicide alert form, nurses' notes each shift, day and night reports	First level nurse and registered medical practitioner
Moderately high	Close supervision	First level nurse or registered medical practitioner	Fifteen-minute checks while patient is awake. Thirty-minute checks while the patient is asleep at night	Not applicable	First level, second level or senior student nurse	Suicide alert form, nurses' notes each shift, day and night reports	First level nurse and registered medical practitioner
Moderately low	Intermittent supervision	First level nurse or registered medical practitioner	Thirty-minute checks while the patient is awake. Thirty-minute checks while the patient is asleep at night	Not applicable	First level, second level or student nurse	Nurses' notes each shift	First level nurse and registered medical practitioner
Low	Periodic supervision	Patient's allocated nurse	Hourly checks while the patient is awake. Thirty-minute checks while the patient is asleep at night	Not applicable	First level, second level or student nurse	Nurses' notes each day	Never discontinued

Figure 15.4 Risk classification and supervision chart

Primary and associate nurses: Chris   Burgess
                    Joan Laurence, Ann Rogers, Ray Sullivan

Patient: Steven Wilson

Date: 19 February 19—

Problem: Over the last four days Steven has become more preoccupied with thoughts of burning himself both on and off the
          ward.

Risk: Moderately high

Level of supervision: Close

Objective: Steven will remain free from serious self-injury both on and off the ward for the next 24 hours.

Patient action: Steven will:
    1. Approach his nurses whenever he feels like burning himself.
    2. Hand in his matches and lighter to one of the nurses.
    3. Keep a record of when he wants to burn himself, what he feels, and what is going on round him at the
       time.

Nursing intervention: Steven's nurses will:
    1. Initiate a suicide alert form.
    2. Initiate close supervision.
    3. Ensure that each shift Steven has a named nurse to approach if he feels like burning himself.
    4. Ensure that Steven can obtain a light for his cigarettes when he wants a smoke.
    5. Give Steven a diary for him to record his thoughts when he feels like burning himself.

Signed: Steven Wilson
         Chris Burgess, Joan Laurence, Ann Rogers, Ray Sullivan
         Frank Brown, charge nurse

Review: 1700, 20 February 19—

Figure 15.5   Example of nursing care plan

GUIDELINES: REDUCING RISK OF DELIBERATE SELF-HARM

Action	**Rationale**
1 Invite the patient to describe his or her present situation.	To obtain information about: (a) the patient's previous level of coping compared with the present; (b) what has led up to the present upset; (c) to give the patient a sense that his or her view of events is valued.
2 Confirm with the patient that you both agree on your understanding of the present situation.	To ensure that you have not missed essential information.

Patient_____   Hospital No. _____

Nurse_____   Doctor_____

Date_____   Time_____

INITIATING/CHANGING TO/MAXIMUM/
FULL/CLOSE SUPERVISION

Please ring the action and level of
supervision for this shift

Time taken over	Time handed over	Name and signature of nurse with notes as appropriate

Instructions for the use of suicide risk alert

1. **Suicide risk alert** is to be initiated by a registered medical practitioner or a registered mental nurse, but preferably jointly, when a patient is thought to be so at risk of suicide that close, full or maximum supervision is thought to be necessary. Please ensure that you are familiar with the hospital's *Policy on the Care of Suicidal Patients* before you use this form.
2. The **Suicide risk alert** form is to be used in addition to plans and progress notes in the medical and nursing records.
3. The brief notes on the **Suicide risk alert** form may be amplified in the nursing and medical notes. The abbreviations SNN and SMN would mean respectively: See Nurses' Notes and See Medical Notes.
4. The **Suicide risk alert** form is to be finally filed in the nursing notes.
5. While in use it is to be drawn to the attention of the day and night nursing staff in the ward by the charge nurse. The consultant or his deputy is to inform the rest of the ward team as appropriate.
6. The person prescribing the level of supervision required is to be either a registered medical practitioner or a registered mental nurse, but preferably they will prescribe jointly. If there is disagreement, the higher level of supervision will be carried out until the issue is decided, if necessary, by the executive group.
7. In the case of periodic supervision the senior registered mental nurse on duty may designate any nurse to carry it out.
8. In the case of close supervision the senior registered mental nurse on duty may designate a trained or senior student nurse to carry it out.
9. If in the nurses' view the nursing resources in the ward do not cover the provision of the agreed level of supervision the clinical nurse manager will be consulted. Should this not result in a solution, the Director of Nursing Services/In-patient Services Manager will be informed and asked to provide a solution, before the executive group is asked to decide the matter.
10. The nurse responsible for carrying out the required supervision will be designated by the senior registered mental nurse on duty from the trained and senior student nurses on duty for that shift.
11. Periods of supervision are recorded with the time started [Taken over] and the time finished [Handed over].
12. A new form is started at the beginning of each day and of each night shift by the senior registered mental nurse on duty for that shift.
13. Discontinuation of the **Suicide risk alert** may be ordered only by a registered medical practitioner *and* a registered mental nurse, *jointly*, after discussion with as wide a membership of the ward team as appropriate.

Figure 15.6 Example of suicide risk alert form (with permission Bethlem Royal and Maudsley Hospital)

3 Obtain a full history of any previous suicide attempts.

Previous history of suicidal behaviour is a proven feature of completed suicide in inpatients.

4 Using the chart in Figure 15.2, assess the risk of any method of self-injury already used by the patient.

The more lethal the method the higher the risk.

5 Obtain a full history of any family suicide or psychiatric treatment.

Family history of suicide or psychiatric treatment is associated with both attempted and completed suicide.

6 Ask the patient to complete the Hopelessness Scale.

Hopelessness is a significant predictor of suicidal behaviour.

7 Ask the patient to complete a tested specific depression scale.

Depressive phenomena often accompany suicidal behaviour and are responsive to treatment.

8 Start a graph with the time in weeks on the horizontal axis and the hopelessness and depression ratings on the vertical axis.

So that changes over time can be measured and compared, giving an accurate picture of the patient's progress. The graph can be used to monitor response to treatments such as medication, cognitive therapy, ECT, as well as responses to environmental and social stresses.

9 Start two sleep charts: one to be kept by the patient, the other by the nurses.

Insomnia is associated with suicidal behaviour. Patients' subjective assessment of their insomnia often differs widely from that of nurses.

10 Set at least thirty minutes aside each shift for interaction with the patient. That is, joining with the patient in an activity of his or her choice.

The low self-esteem of suicidal patients is linked with a great sensitivity to actions that can be perceived as rejection. For example, perceiving that a nurse spends more time with more sociable patients.

11 Inform the patient at least a shift in advance of your inability to keep an appointment.

As in 10 above.

12 Be punctual in beginning and finishing time with the patient.

It is hypothesized that a calm adherence to routine contributes to an atmosphere of staff confidence in what they are doing.

13 Record all interactions with the patient in the progress notes.

Good written communication between staff is essential for safeguarding the patient.

14 Using the scale in Figure 15.3 record your global assessment of the potential suicide risk of the patient.

A combination of different methods for rating suicidal risk is more reliable than any single method.

15 Inform other members of the nursing and multidisciplinary clinical teams of the results of your assessment of the patient.

So that decision-making can be carried out on the basis of information from those closest to the patient.

16 Discuss with the team what the classification of suicide risk for the patient will be.

Participation in decision-making increases motivation to implement the decisions.

17 Record in the nurses' notes the classification of risk decided by the team.

Written communication is more reliably preserved than oral communication.

18 Always discuss the patient's fitness for leave with the patient, the patient's nurse, the nurse in charge of the ward, the patient's doctor and the patient's relative or friend who will take responsibility for the patient.

Many suicides occur while patients are on leave from hospital. At times of staff shortage decisions may be made by persons with insufficient skills or experience.

19 Tell the patient who his or her primary and associated nurse will be.

So that the patient can predict who will be on duty, and so can have a sense of something in the future on which to rely.

20 Discuss with the patient the team's classification of his or her suicide risk.

(a) To negotiate consent.
(b) So that the patient has a sense of being a co-worker on his or her needs and problems.

21 Explain the level of supervision to be implemented, together with the suicide alert form if necessary.

Supervision implies interaction with the patient whereas observation does not. Observation is likely to reinforce alienation and a sense of rejection.

22 Write a care plan which incorporates, if necessary, the suicide alert form.

The suicide alert is not a substitute for the nursing care plan.

23 Agree with the patient review dates for each objective.

(a) In order to be able to evaluate the plan.
(b) To provide a sense of the future.

24 Provide the patient with the means of obtaining a copy of the nursing care plan.

So that the patient takes responsibility for the planning aspect of his or her nursing care.

25 Agree with the patient and relatives to enter in the property record gifts or supplies brought in for his or her use.

(a) Monitoring of the patient's access to potentially dangerous items is continued after the admission property check.
(b) Continued monitoring prevents unnecessary debate and argument about any need to search patients' property. (See procedure for conducting searches, Chapter 26.)

26 Agree with the patient that he or she entrusts personal monies, cheque book and guarantee, credit and cashcards to the hospital safe.

The procedure involved in retrieving personal property allows you to discuss with the patient his or her reasons for having money. For example, to buy a train ticket to Eastbourne *en route* for Beachy Head. Many patients kill themselves while on leave without permission.

27 Discuss with the patient's relatives the nurse's monitoring of the patient's money.

(a) To gain their help in protecting the patient.
(b) To provide a safety net if the patient leaves the ward with money.
(c) To elicit potentially destructive responses and so define a specific area of intervention whether by a social worker or by a family therapist.

28 Arrange with the patient's relatives the circumstances in which they are prepared to take over responsibility for the patient's safety when he or she is off the ward.

(a) Because staff are handing over responsibility for the patient's life, it is essential that both parties are clear that this is so, and that relatives can decline if they wish.
(b) If the patient subsequently insists on leaving alone, it will help to have already involved relatives who may be asked to help in a process to detain the patient under the Mental Health Act 1983.

29 Arrange for any drugs which are to be taken out of the ward to be dispensed by the pharmacy in small amounts.

(a) To ensure that the correct drugs are given.
(b) To ensure that the amounts dispensed are less than a lethal dose.

30 Ask the patient to return unused drugs.

To prevent hoarding.

31 Agree with the patient that he or she refrains from alcohol or other unprescribed substances.

(a) Alcohol potentiates risk-taking behaviour.
(b) Up to 60 per cent of men and 45 per cent of women are found to have taken alcohol before overdosing.

32 If you discover that a patient may have taken an overdose, inform the nurse in charge immediately.

So that he or she is in a position to co-ordinate what may become a medical emergency.

33 If you are the nurse in charge, inform the duty clinical nurse manager and the patient's doctor or duty doctor immediately.

In order to anticipate any rapid development of an emergency.

34 Measure and record vital signs.

To establish a baseline record.

35 If possible, elicit from the patient:
   (i) what has been taken;
   (ii) how much;
   (iii) when;
   (iv) if he or she has vomited;
   (v) if there any symptoms now.

(a) In order to decide immediate management.
(b) For example, whether to perform gastric lavage, administer antidotes, or observe and wait.

36 Complete an incident report form, the patient's casualty book, and write a full account in the nurses' notes.

To provide the basis for later evaluation.

37 Decide with the ward team or the clinical nurse manager and the duty doctor what the suicide risk classification will be.

So that appropriate supervision can be implemented.

38 If the risk is extremely high, high or moderately high, initiate a suicide alert form.

So that the resources required to carry out the necessary supervision can be implemented.

39 The nurse in charge nominates the nurses to be responsible for carrying out supervision of the patient.

As soon as the suicide alert form is initiated, supervision of the patient is handed and taken over between the responsible nurses face to face without interruption.

40 If the ward nursing resources are too limited to allow relief of supervising nurses at least every hour, help may be requested from the duty clinical nurse manager.

The risk classification is designed to enable the nurse in charge to determine accurately the resources needed by a suicidal patient.

41 Keep the clinical nurse manager in the picture.

So that, for instance, an admission could be diverted to another ward if necessary.

42 The charge nurse is responsible for ensuring that regular teaching and supervision takes place concerning suicidal patients.

(a) In order to familiarize nurses with the principles behind the procedures.
(b) So that nurses can practise the procedures in a safe setting before applying them to a patient.

43 Reserve space in meetings for nurses to discuss their work with suicidal patients.

(a) The suicidal patient needs intensive input by nurses, who can become isolated from the rest of the ward team.
(b) Discussion offers the opportunity for group problem-solving as well as for identification of common concerns among the team.

44 The charge nurse arranges immediate attention to the maintenance and repair of the ward fabric. The following items need frequent checking:
 (i) windows (frames, blocks, catches, panes);
 (ii) locks;
 (iii) gas, electricity and water supplies.

(a) A patient can put together a lethal method of self-injury within a few minutes.
(b) Tampering by patients intent on self-injury may go unnoticed.
(c) Poor maintenance and housekeeping facilitate (a) and (b).

45 Check routinely and unobtrusively each shift, and as often as you check on a suicidal patient, any door that can be jammed, exposed pipework, cleaning materials.

(a) Poor design in psychiatric wards must be compensated by extra vigilance.
(b) There is little point in inadvertently instructing patients on the danger areas in a ward.

46 Avoid using anxiolytics and hypnotics except as titrated specifically against mood, behaviour or sleep charts, kept by the patient and the nurses.

(a) The suicidal patient may look anxious, complain of anxiety and be restless. He or she may be impatient of the length of time needed to achieve therapeutic levels of an appropriate antidepressant and the subsequent time before subjective improvement can be experienced.
(b) Anxiolytics may effect transient reduction in distress but impair motivation for longer-term strategies of treatment, for example cognitive therapy.
(c) Anxiolytics and hypnotics are liable to abuse, especially in conjunction with alcohol.

47 Review all care plans at the time stated in the plan.

(a) So that outcomes occur against controlled objectives.
(b) Strategies that are not working need to be identified quickly.

48 Discuss the risk classification with the patient at least every twenty-four hours.

(a) So that the suicide alert form can be changed, initiated or discontinued, thus using nursing resources as economically as possible.
(b) So that the nursing team retains a cohesive approach to the suicidal patient.

49 Review all outcomes, if possible, with the patient.

The patient's problems do not exist independently of the patient, who is the co-worker in any strategy to deal with them.

50 Obtain the agreement of the patient to keep him- or herself safe if given leave from the ward.

Agreements have been found to be useful in helping patients to desist from self-injury.

51 See the procedure for negotiating treatment agreements, Chapter 33.

52 Agree with the patient a specific time limit to any leave out.

In order to help him or her weather any trouble while out on leave.

53 Discuss with the patient, his or her relatives and friends their plans for leave out.

You have the opportunity to assess the likely atmosphere of the patient's leave, and to document detailed plans in the nurses' notes.

54 Give the patient, relatives and friends the names of the nurses on duty over the period of leave, as well as the hospital telephone number.

So that they have a route for help if the patient feels unable to manage while away from the ward.

55 Ask the patient to ring or return to the ward or both if he or she begins to feel unable to manage out of the ward.

To safeguard the patient.

56 Ensure that on discharge the patient returns to as favourable surroundings as could be achieved during the admission.

Many suicides of inpatients occur soon after discharge.

57 Ensure that the patient's first follow-up appointment has been booked properly and an appointment card given to relatives if necessary.

As for 31 above.

58 If the team agrees, offer the patient a named member of the ward nursing staff to return to see during the first stages of discharge.

As for 31 and 32 above.

59 Make any referral to the community psychiatric nursing services before discharge in liaison with the ward team, general practitioner and local social services.

(a) So that the patient can meet the new person in familiar surroundings.
(b) Changes in personnel are thought to contribute to an increased risk of self-injurious behaviour.

60 Operate a bring-forward system so that inquiries can be started early if the patient does not show up for an appointment.

Poor communication may result in early deterioration not being quickly noticed.

REFERENCE MATERIAL
References

Barraclough, B., Bunch, J., Nelson, B. and Sainsbury, P. (1974) A hundred cases of suicide: clinical aspects, *British Journal of Psychiatry*, Vol. 125, pp. 355–73.

Beck, A.T. *et al.* (1974) *Cognitive Therapy of Depression*, Guilford, New York.

Copas, J.B. and Robin, A. (1982) Suicide in psychiatric in-patients, *British Journal of Psychiatry*, Vol. 141, pp. 503–11.

Douglas, J.D. (1967) *The Social Meanings of Suicide*, Princeton University Press.

DSM-III (rev) (1987) Diagnostic and Statistical Manual of Mental Disorders, 3rd edn, revised, DSM-III-R, American Psychiatric Association, Washington DC.

Durkheim, E. (1951) *Suicide: A Study in Sociology*, Free Press, Glencoe.

Flood, R.A. and Seager, C.P. (1968) A retrospective examination of psychiatric case records of patients who subsequently committed suicide, *British Journal of Psychiatry*, Vol. 114, pp. 443–50.

Hill, D. (1968) Depression: disease, reaction or posture, *American Journal of Psychiatry*, Vol. 125, no. 4, pp. 37–49.

Kearns, N.P. *et al.* (1982) A comparison of depression rating scales, *British Journal of Psychiatry*, Vol. 141, pp. 45–9.

McClure, G.M.G. (1984) Trends in suicide rate for England and Wales 1975–1980, *British Journal of Psychiatry*, Vol. 114, pp. 119–26.

Pallis, D.J. *et al.* (1982) Estimating suicide risk among attempted suicides: I The development of new clinical scales, *British Journal of Psychiatry*, Vol. 144, pp. 37–44.

Pallis, D.J., Gibbons, J.S. and Pierce, D.W. (1984) Estimating suicide risk among attempted suicides: II Efficiency of predictive scales after the attempt, *British Journal of Psychiatry*, Vol. 144, pp. 139–48.

Perris, C., Beskow, J. and Jacobson, L. (1980) Some remarks on the incidence of successful suicide in psychiatric care, *Social Psychiatry,* Vol. 15, pp. 161–6.

Report of a Working Group (1982) *Changing Patterns in Suicide Behaviour*, WHO, Copenhagen.

Snaith, R.P. *et al.* (1971) Assessment of the severity of primary depressive illness, *Psychological Medicine*, Vol. 1, pp. 143–9.

Snaith, R.P. *et al.* (1978) A clinical scale for the self-assessment of irritability, *British Journal of Psychiatry*, Vol. 32, pp. 164–71.

WHO (1977) *Manual of the International Statistical Classification of Diseases, Injuries and Causes of Death, Volumes One and Two*, World Health Organization, Geneva.

Further reading

Andreason, N.C. and Noyes, R. (1975) Suicide attempts by self-immolation, *American Journal of Psychiatry*, Vol. 132, no. 5, pp. 554–6.

Ashton, J.R. and Donnan, S.P.B. (1979) Suicide by burning: a current epidemic, *British Medical Journal*, Vol. 2, pp. 769–70.

Barbee, E.L. (1978) Lethality assessment: whose role?, *Issues in Mental Health Nursing*, Vol. 1, pp. 67–84.

Beck, A.T., Kovacs, M. and Weissman, A. (1979) Assessment of suicidal intention: the Scale for Suicidal Ideation, *Journal of Consulting and Clinical Psychology*, Vol. 47, pp. 343–52.

Beck, R.W., Morris, J.B. and Beck, A.T. (1974) Cross-validation of the suicidal intent scale, *Psychological Reports*, Vol. 34, pp. 445–6.

Berger, M.M. and Rosenbaum, M. (1967) Notes on help-rejecting complainers, *International Journal of Group Psychotherapy*, Vol. 17, pp. 357–70.

Breier, A. and Astrachan, B.M. (1984) Characterization of schizophrenic patients who commit suicide, *American Journal of Psychiatry*, Vol. 141, no. 2, pp. 206–9.

Busteed, E.L. and Johnstone, C. (1983) The development of suicide precautions for an inpatient psychiatric unit, *Journal of Psychosocial Nursing and Mental Health Services*, Vol. 21, no. 5, pp. 15–19.

Central Statistical Office (1980) *Guide to Official Statistics*, HMSO, London.

Coser, R.L. (1979) *Training in Ambiguity*, Free Press, New York.

Crammer, J.L. (1984) The special characteristics of suicide in hospital in-patients, *British Journal of Psychiatry*, Vol. 145, pp. 460–76.

Crammer, J.L. *et al.* (1984) Symposium on suicide in hospital, *British Journal of Psychiatry*, Vol. 145, pp. 460–76.

Crammer, J.L. (1985) Suicide: don't wait for the publicity, *Bulletin of the Royal College of Psychiatrists*, Vol. 9, p. 103.

Delbridge, P.M. (1974) Identifying the suicidal person in the community, *Canadian Nurse*, Vol. 70, no. 11, pp. 14–17.

Diller, J. (1979) The psychological autopsy in equivocal deaths, *Perspectives in Psychiatric Care*, Vol. 17, no. 4, pp. 156–61.

Dyer, J.A.T. and Kreitman, N. (1984) Hopelessness, depression and suicidal intent in parasuicide, *British Journal of Psychiatry*, Vol. 144, pp. 127–33.

Evans, D.L. (1982) Explaining suicide among the young: an analytical review of the literature, *Journal of Psychosocial Nursing and Mental Health Services*, Vol. 20, no. 8, pp. 9–16.

Farmer, R. and Rohde, J. (1980) Effect of availability and acceptability of lethal instruments on suicide mortality, *Acta Psychiatrica Scandinavica*, Vol. 62, pp. 436–46.

Finch, J. (1983) Whose life is it anyway?, *Nursing Mirror*, Vol. 157, no. 10, p. 38.

Finch, J. (1983) Attempted suicide, *Nursing Mirror*, Vol. 157, no. 12, p. 30.

Finley, B. and Mynatt, S. (1981) Faculty intervention into suicidal crisis, *Nurse Educator*, Vol. 6, no. 2, pp. 12–16.

Fitzpatrick, J.J. (1983) Suicidology and suicide prevention: historical perspectives from the nursing literature, *Journal of Psychosocial Nursing and Mental Health Services*, Vol. 21, no. 5, pp. 20–7.

Getz, W.L. *et al.* (1983) *Brief Counselling with Suicidal Persons*, Heath, Lexington, Mass.

Guze, S.B. and Robins, E. (1970) Suicide and primary affective disorders, *British Journal of Psychiatry*, Vol. 117, pp. 437–8.

Hamel-Bissell, B.P. (1985) Suicidal casework: assessing nurses' reactions, *Journal of Psychosocial Nursing and Mental Health Services*, Vol. 23, no. 10, pp. 20–23.

Harris, R.A. (1966) Factors related to continued suicidal behaviour in dyadic relationships, *Nursing Research*, Vol. 15, no. 1, pp. 72–5.

Hessö, R. (1977) Suicide in Norwegian, Finnish and Swedish psychiatric hospitals, *Archiv fur Psychiatrie und Nervenkrankheifen*, Vol. 224, pp. 119–27.

Hoff, L.A. and Resing, M. (1982) Was this suicide preventable?, *American Journal of Nursing*, Vol. 82, pp. 1106–11.

Horoshak, I. (1977) How to spot and handle high-risk patients, *RN*, Vol. 40, no. 9, pp. 58–63.

Hoyt, W. (1979) The psychological autopsy in equivocal deaths, *Perspectives in Psychiatric Care*, Vol. 17, no. 4, pp. 156–61.

Jacobson, R., Jackson, M., and Berelowitz, M. (1986)

Self-incineration: a controlled comparison of in-patient suicide attempts, *Psychological Medicine*, Vol. 16, pp. 107–16.

Joel, L.A. and Collins, D.L. (1978) *Psychiatric Nursing*, McGraw-Hill, New York.

Knight, L. (1980) Suicide, *Mindout*, Vol. 44, pp. 14–16.

Kumler, F.R. (1964) Communication between suicide attemptors and significant others: an exploratory study, *Nursing Research*, Vol. 13, no. 3, pp. 268–70.

Lawrence, E. (ed.) (1986) *CSO Annual Abstract of Statistics* (1986 edn), HMSO, London.

Lester, D. (1980) The validity of national suicide rates, *British Journal of Psychiatry*, Vol. 136, pp. 107–8.

Lester, D. and Beck, A.T. (1974) Suicidal intent, medical lethality of the suicide intent, and components of depression, *Journal of Clinical Psychology*, Vol. 31, pp. 11–12.

Litman, R.E. (1964) Immobilization response to suicidal behaviour, *Archives of General Psychiatry*, Vol. 11, pp. 282–5.

Maddison, D. and Mackey, K.H. (1966) Suicide: the clinical problem, *British Journal of Psychiatry*, Vol. 112, pp. 693–703.

Mayer, D.Y. (1971) A psychotherapeutic approach to the suicidal patient, *British Journal of Psychiatry*, Vol. 119, pp. 629–33.

Miles, C.P. (1977) Conditions predisposing to suicide: a review, *Journal of Nervous and Mental Disease*, Vol. 164, no. 4, pp. 231–46.

Miller, M. (ed.) (1982) *Suicide Intervention by Nurses*, Springer, New York.

Morse, S.J. (1973) The after-pleasure of suicide, *British Journal of Medical Psychology*, Vol. 46, pp. 227–38.

Myers, D.H. and Neal, C.D. (1978) Suicide in psychiatric patients, *British Journal of Psychiatry*, Vol. 133, pp. 38–44.

Orsolits, M. and Morphy, M. (1982) A depression algorithm for psychiatric emergencies, *Journal of Psychiatric Treatment and Evaluation*, Vol. 4, pp. 137–45.

Ovenstone, I.M.K. (1973) A psychiatric approach to the diagnosis of suicide and its effect on the Edinburgh statistics, *British Journal of Psychiatry*, Vol. 123, pp. 15–21.

Ovenstone, I.M.K. and Kreitman, N. (1974) Two syndromes of suicide, *British Journal of Psychiatry*, Vol. 124, pp. 336–45.

Pallis, D.J. and Sainsbury, P. (1976) The value of assessing intent in attempted suicide, *Psychological Medicine*, Vol. 6, pp. 487–92.

Pao, P.-N. *et al.* (1969) Symposium on impulsive self-mutilation, *British Journal of Medical Psychology*, Vol. 42, pp. 195–229.

Pierce, D.W. (1981) The predictive validity of a suicide intent scale: a five-year follow-up, *British Journal of Psychiatry*, Vol. 139, pp. 391–6.

Post, J.M. and Oteri, E.M. (1983) Sign-out rounds, *Journal of Psychosocial Nursing and Mental Health Services*, Vol. 21, no. 9, pp. 11–17.

Pownall, M. (1986) No place to die, *Nursing Times*, Vol. 82, no. 37, pp. 16–18.

Prentice, G. (1977) Evaluating suicide potential, *Nurse Practitioner*, Vol. 2, no. 5, pp. 30–1.

Report (1984) *Report of the Health Service Commissioner*, HMSO, London.

Resnick, J.H. and Kendra, J.M. (1973) Predictive value of the 'Scale for Assessing Suicide Risk' (SASR) with hospitalized psychiatric patients, *Journal of Clinical Psychology*, Vol. 29, pp. 187–90.

Rosen, A. (1954) Detection of suicidal patients: an example of some limitations in the prediction of infrequent events, *Journal of Consulting Psychology*, Vol. 18, no. 6, pp. 397–403.

Roy, A. (1982) Suicide in chronic schizophrenia, *British Journal of Psychiatry*, Vol. 141, pp. 171–7.

Rudestam, K.E. (1971) Stockholm and Los Angeles: a cross-cultural study of the communication of suicidal intent, *Journal of Consulting and Clinical Psychology*, Vol. 36, no. 1, pp. 82–90.

Sartorius, R. (1983) Coercive suicide prevention: a libertarian perspective, *Suicide and Life Threatening Behaviour*, Vol. 13, no. 4, pp. 293–303.

Seager, C.P. and Flood, R.A. (1965) Suicide in Bristol, *British Journal of Psychiatry*, Vol. 111, pp. 919–32.

Shields, E.A. (1946) Depression, then suicide, *American Journal of Nursing*, Vol. 46, pp. 677–9.

Shneidman, E.S. (1976) *Suicidology: Contemporary Developments*, Grune & Stratton, New York.

Sims, A. and O'Brien, K. (1979) Autokabalesis: an account of mentally ill people who jump from buildings, *Medicine, Science and the Law*, Vol. 19, no. 3, pp. 195–8.

Stein, G.S. (1982) Dangerous episodes occurring around the time of discharge of four chronic schizophrenics, *British Journal of Psychiatry*, Vol. 141, pp. 586–9.

Temoohe, A., Pugh, T.F. and MacMahon, B. (1964) Suicide rates among current and former mental institution patients, *Journal of Nervous and Mental Disease*, Vol. 138, pp. 124–30.

Tishler, C.L., Lent, W.J. and McKenry, P.C. (1980) Assessment of suicide potential in adolescents, *Journal of Emergency Nursing*, Vol. 6, no. 2, pp. 24–6.

Topalis, M. and Aguiler, D.C. (1978) *Psychiatric Nursing*, Mosby, St Louis, Mo.

Tuskan, J.J. and Thase, M.E. (1983) Suicides in jails and prisons, *Journal of Psychosocial Nursing and Mental Health Services*, Vol. 21, no. 5, pp. 29–33.

Twiname, B.G. (1981) No-suicide contract for nurses, *Journal of Psychosocial Nursing and Mental Health Services*, Vol. 19, no. 7, pp. 11–12.

Wetzel, R.D. (1987) The changing relationships between age and suicide rates: cohort effect, period effect or both?, *Psychiatric Developments*, Vol. 3, pp. 179–218.

Whiteworth, R.A. (1982) The ethics of suicide intervention: seen as a nursing problem, *Psychiatric Nursing*, Vol. 23, no. 1, pp. 12–14.

Wilson, H.S. and Kneisl, C.R. (1983) *Psychiatric Nursing*, Addison-Wesley, Menlo Park, Calif.

Yale, L.P. (1934) Nurses and suicide prevention, *American Journal of Nursing*, Vol. 34, no. 9, pp. 882–6.

16

Patients' Sexual Activities

DISCUSSION

The traditional role of the psychiatric nurse involved policing the activities of patients, counting cutlery, locking up sharp objects, locking ward kitchens, inspecting their rooms, segregating men and women. While nurses now aspire to base their practice on rational conclusions derived from research, the profession exists in a society where people's beliefs and attitudes about sex may result more from confusion and prejudice than from reason (Kelleher, 1987).

Manchester, Eastland and Sugden (1985) suggest along with Stuart and Sundeen (1983) that their education may have taught nurses about normal sexual behaviour and the importance of discussing it openly, but this teaching does not necessarily square with their personal experience of and beliefs about sexuality.

A problem with nurses' mixed feelings and thoughts about sex is that they may lead to distortions in judgements and so reduce the quality of their decision-making. Furthermore, because society's attitudes towards sex and its regulation are far from clear, nurses occupy a difficult position, being expected to enforce rules on the one hand and, on the other, to display tolerance and understanding. This is illustrated in a case history candidly described by therapists at the Cassel Hospital. An incident occurred in which a child of five said that she had been touched by a youngster, who asked her in turn to touch his penis. As discussion of the incident went on over the next few days, the account by staff developed into one where the youngster had sexually assaulted the little girl. Her parents and some of the staff called for the boy to be charged by the police. When the youngster was eventually listened to, he denied any sexual contact with the little girl, and staff concluded he was telling the truth (James and Wilson, 1987). Although James and Wilson discuss the case in relation to the structure of a therapeutic community, their perspec-

tives illuminate and are relevant to general psychiatric settings.

In another example from a therapeutic community, Rapoport (1960) describes how a patient helped another to discuss openly in the community meeting a homosexual attachment that he feared developing with a third patient in the ward.

The nurse's relationship with a patient affords privileged access to many areas which a person usually has the right to keep private, and which the patient shares with the nurse on the basis of an understanding regarding confidentiality, veracity and consent. In the case of homosexual men and women, the social stigma that still influences judgement of their capacity to fulfil professional and public responsibilities means that nurses have a big responsibility for exercising discretion in their handling of information obtained in the course of their work. The rights of homosexual men under twenty-one, mentally retarded people, prisoners and disabled people to sexual freedom are heavily circumscribed. The law relating to their sexual rights is most unlikely to be changed in the near future. Privileged access to such people who become psychiatric patients involves complex ethical and professional issues for nurses.

The issues involved

The issues may be specified. Should sexual intercourse between patients be allowed on hospital premises? Does it make any difference if the patients do it in private? Should there be rules for dealing with masturbation or other exposure of the genitals in public? Should any rules depend on whether sexual intercourse takes place between patients; or between patients and visitors; whether between heterosexual or homosexual partners? Would a nurse's attitude towards sexual activity by patients be any different if a patient was known to be HIV antibody positive?

Emotional and sexual relationships

It is emphasized that it is impossible to pronounce a rule by which nurses will work. Certain kinds of emotional relationships are unavoidable in hospital given that most people have a need for close and confiding involvement with others. In their lives outside hospital this may or may not be in the context of sexual relations. The development and use by nurses of emotional relationships are regarded as the basis of the nurse's therapeutic function. Other kinds of relationship are more problematic. Just as nurses are particularly wary of possible sexual links with patients, so they need to be wary of such liaisons between patients. Emotional ties, whether sexual or not, between patients may be dangerous for a number of reasons, including:

1 disruption to a previously established partnership;
2 a temporary solution to distressing problems, whose failure may result in self-injurious behaviour;
3 a temporary alleviation of responses such as depressed mood, whose failure to lift permanently may also lead to self-injurious behaviour.

It may be argued that emotional needs are often the antecedents to sexual relationships, but the consequences may be emotional problems as well as pregnancy, disease or injury. People in predicaments search for solutions to them. An apparently satisfying emotional relationship may be experienced as such a solution, however temporary. There is a danger that an excessive dependence may develop as a result of the relief experienced, and which prolongs the relationship beyond a time when other solutions may be more appropriate.

Nurses will view more cautiously relationships newly formed by patients under their care as opposed to previously established relationships. An established relationship, whether between heterosexual or homosexual partners, has implications for the planning of nursing care that are quite different from those of a relationship which occurs as a result of admission to hospital.

Sexual approaches by patients towards nurses

The nursing literature implies that the majority of patient–nurse sexual approaches are made by male patients to female nurses. Although in the UK it is a criminal offence for a male nurse to have a sexual relationship with a female patient, the issue is rarely discussed in the nursing literature. It is, nevertheless, central to the practice of psychotherapy and to the professional conduct of doctors. It has been suggested that patients who make sexual approaches to nurses may do so because of doubts about their own sexuality; or as a means of expressing resentment and hostility; or

to attempt to form a relationship (Assey and Herbet, 1983). A patient who touches or otherwise behaves sexually towards a nurse is not one who has a working relationship with a professional helper. The nurse therefore requires intensive supervision to ensure that he or she can form a professional relationship with the patient, bounded by clearly defined limits, and directed to negotiated specific objectives.

Assey and Herbet (1983) note ways in which nurses may unwittingly provoke sexual approaches by their non-verbal behaviour and the clothes they wear, as well as by the quality of their conversation with patients. They recommend the acquisition of self-awareness and self-monitoring skills, supervision and role-play as strategies to prevent or manage seductive behaviours.

Sexual acts by patients in hospital

The nurse's duty of care to patients requires that account is taken of the patient's capacity for sound judgement, and the question whether the patient's mental state is such as to promote behaviour in ways that he or she later regrets. Nurses also have a duty to attempt to understand what patients who perform usually private sexual acts in public may be trying to say. That is, as Assey and Herbet (1983) suggest, sexual behaviour may be communicating a non-sexual message. Once this message is understood and put into words, the need for actions may disappear. On the other hand, Stewart (1979) suggests that complaints of financial and housing problems often obscure sexual difficulties, and recommends that careful attention is paid to the context as well as the content of what patients say. He points out that long-term residents are limited in sexual opportunities. He recommends that, for staff training, self-awareness inventories may be used, such as can be found in Lego's (1984) handbook.

Hospital managers are responsible for consulting with staff in order to produce policies to guide nurses in charge of wards in determining what sexual behaviour may be acceptable, as well as what standard of dress by nurses is acceptable. If a hospital policy states that sexual intercourse is unacceptable in any area of the hospital, the charge nurse has the right to ask patients to desist. If visitors and patients were then to engage in sexual intercourse, the visitor, by doing so, would define her- or himself as unacceptable and could be asked to leave. Refusal to do so would further define the visitor as a trespasser (Finch, 1983). It is essential that nurses are guided by their own hospital policies and that they receive the necessary support to carry them out, and to manage wards in such a way that situations do not develop to points where extreme measures must be taken. At the centre is the principle of professional clinical supervision of all nurse–patient relationships.

GUIDELINES: MONITORING PATIENTS' SEXUAL ACTIVITIES

Action

Rationale

1 The nurse in charge of the ward ensures that regular supervision is available concerning sex and how to assess patients' needs and problems.

(a) So that patients' problems may be correctly identified.
(b) So that appropriate interventions to assist patients meet their needs and resolve problems can be implemented.

2 The nurse in charge of the ward ensures that nurses comply with hospital policies regarding dress and appearance.

In order that provocative clothes are not worn at work.

3 If the necessary skills do not exist in the ward, the charge nurse ensures that at least one of the permanent first-level nurses attends educational and training seminars in the subject.

In order that he or she will return to the ward or department and provide training and supervision for the other staff.

4 Nurses conduct or attend self-awareness workshops for staff.

In order to feel more at ease when discussing sex with patients and with each other.

5 Primary nurses liaise with other members of the multidisciplinary clinical team in assessing patients' sexuality and in planning interventions.

(a) In order to anticipate and prevent if possible untoward sexual liaisons between patients while they are the responsibility of the team.
(b) In order to protect vulnerable patients.

6 First-level nurses are responsible for ensuring that their supervisees understand hospital policy regarding sexual activities between patients by, for example:
  (i) role-playing nurse–patient interactions concerning patients' sexual behaviour;
  (ii) emphasizing the need for a co-ordinated approach between members of the team;
  (iii) emphasizing the role of the clinical nurse manager in helping nurses deal with problems;
  (iv) encouraging student nurses to make use of educational settings to learn about and discuss the nursing care of patients with problematic sexual behaviour.

To ensure that clinical and interpersonal support is available for supervisees to learn and practise the relevant nursing care skills.

7 Primary nurses ensure that their patients are able to negotiate visits to their partners as soon as is practicable after admission.

So that the admission to hospital does not necessarily cut them off from their partner and from all sexual expression.

8 The charge nurse ensures that patients and their visitors are made aware of hospital policies regarding sexual activities by patients while in hospital.

In order that sexual needs and activities may be discussed with nurses, and plans negotiated to help patients meet their needs in acceptable ways.

9 The charge nurse ensures that each patient has the opportunity for privacy and for visits in private with their partners, balancing the needs of the patient against the potential problems of promiscuous behaviour and exploitation by psychotic or personality-disordered others.

In order that patients' needs for intimacy and closeness with their partners or friends (that is, affiliative needs) are not necessarily confused with sexual needs.

10 The nurse in charge is responsible for ensuring that nursing observation and supervision of all patients remains at least at the minimum stated in Chapter 20. This means arranging the necessary supervision while nurses are in meetings.

(a) So that patients are not left without nursing supervision.
(b) In order that nurses can take responsibility for patients who are not competent to exercise choice and who may become victims as a result.

11 Nurses observe social conventions whereby men and women have private areas even in mixed wards.

(a) The social convention of such discretion between the sexes is a deeply rooted one.
(b) To ignore it is likely to cause distress.

12 A nurse who doubts his or her ability to cope with a sexual approach from a patient will use supervision to anticipate and discuss ways of dealing with such approaches, for example by role-playing suitable verbal responses.

In order that a sexual approach does not become a crisis for the nurse or patient.

13 The procedures for documenting and carrying out the nursing process are used to record accurately all nursing observations of and interactions with patients.

(a) So that a patient's sexual behaviour is seen in the context of the nursing assessment as a whole.
(b) To ensure accurate communication of facts as well as of opinions.

REFERENCE MATERIAL
References
Assey, J.L. and Herbet, J.M. (1983) Who is the seductive patient?, *American Journal of Nursing*, Vol. 83, pp. 530–2.
Finch, J. (1983) Unwanted visitors, *Nursing Mirror*, Vol. 157, no. 4, p. 25.
James, O. and Wilson, A. (1987) A sexually charged clinical problem, in R. Kennedy, A. Heymans and L. Tischler (eds.) *The Family as In-Patient*, Free Association Books, London.
Kelleher, A. (1987) *Sex Within Reason*, Cape, London.
Lego, S. (ed.) (1984) *The American Handbook of Psychiatric Nursing*, Lippincott, Philadelphia.
Manchester, J., Eastland, M. and Sugden, J. (1985) Sexuality, *Nursing*, Vol. 2, no. 35, pp. 1026–8.
Rapoport, R.N. (1960) *Community as Doctor*, Tavistock, London.
Stewart, W.F.R. (1979) *Sexual Aspects of Social Work*, Woodhead-Faulkner, Cambridge.
Stuart, G.W. and Sundeen, S.J. (eds.) (1983) *The Principles and Practice of Psychiatric Nursing*, Mosby, St Louis, Mo.

Further reading
ANA (1978) Resolution on mental health status of gay persons, *Journal of Psychiatric Nursing*, Vol. 16, no. 12, p. 25.
Anderson, M.L. (1980) Talking about sex – with less anxiety, *Journal of Psychiatric Nursing*, Vol. 18, no. 6, pp. 10–15.
Bartscher, P.W. (1983) Human sexuality and implications for nursing intervention: a format for teaching, *Journal of Nursing Education*, Vol. 22, no. 3, pp. 123–7.
Birchall, J. (1984) Unspoken anxieties, *Nursing Times*, Vol. 80, no. 50, pp. 29–30.
Birchall, J. (1984) In a private place, *Nursing Times*, Vol. 80, no. 50, pp. 31–4.
Brossart, J. (1979) The gay patient: what you should be doing, *RN*, Vol. 42, no. 4, pp. 50–2.

Byers, J. (1983) Sexuality and the aged, *Geriatric Nursing*, Vol. 4, no. 5, pp. 293–7.

Crown, S. (1985) Psychosocial aspects of homosexuality, *Journal of Medical Ethics*, Vol. 6, pp. 130–2.

Curtin, L. (1983) Sex in the hospital, *Nursing Management*, Vol. 14, no. 6, pp. 9–10.

Damrosch, S.P. (1982) Nursing students' attitudes toward sexually active older persons, *Nursing Research*, Vol. 31, pp. 252–8.

Davies, M. (1984) Coping with sexuality: unspoken anxieties, *Nursing Times*, Vol. 80, no. 50, pp. 29–30.

DeMoya, D. and DeMoya, A. (1979) Sex Q and A: frank answers to your most delicate patient counselling questions, *RN*, Vol. 42, no. 9, pp. 129–30.

Falk, G. and Falk, U.A. (1980) Sexuality and the aged, *Nursing Outlook*, Vol. 28, no. 1, pp. 51–5.

Golub, S. (1975) When your patient's problem involves sex, *RN*, Vol. 38, no. 3, pp. 27–31.

Gott, M. (1980) Quite comfortable, *Nursing Times*, Vol. 76, no. 14, p. 582.

Hampton, P.J. (1979) Coping with the male patient's sexuality, *Nursing Forum*, Vol. 18, no. 3, pp. 304–10.

Hicks, C. (1980) Taking the lid off: sexuality and the nurse, *Nursing Times*, Vol. 76, no. 39, pp. 1681–2.

Irish, A.C. (1983) Straight talk about gay patients, *American Journal of Nursing*, Vol. 83, pp. 1168–70.

Krozy, R. (1978) Becoming comfortable with sexual assessment, *American Journal of Nursing*, Vol. 78, p. 1036.

Lawrence, J.C. (1975) Homosexuals, hospitalization and the nurse, *Nursing Forum*, Vol. 14, no. 3, pp. 305–17.

Leonard, C. (1981) Talking through a taboo, *Nursing Mirror*, Vol. 153, no. 5, pp. 19–20.

Lion, E.M. (ed.) (1982) *Human Sexuality in Nursing Process*, Wiley, New York.

Llewellyn, S. and Fielding, G. (1983) Sex: more than the facts, *Nursing Mirror*, Vol. 156, no. 11, pp. 38–9.

Miller, M.H. and Flynn, B.C. (eds.) (1977) *Current Perspectives in Nursing: Social Issues and Trends*, Mosby, St Louis, Mo.

Miller, S. (1984) Recognizing the sexual health care needs of hospitalized patients, *Canadian Nurse*, Vol. 80, no. 3, pp. 43–6, 49.

Oakley, A. (1982) *Sex, Gender and Society*, Temple Smith, London.

Pogoncheff, E. (1979) The gay patient: what not to do, *RN*, Vol. 42, no. 4, pp. 46–50.

Randell, J. (1977) Transsexualism and its management, *Nursing Mirror*, Vol. 144, no. 12, pp. 45–7.

Ryan, D., Watson, N. and Moffat, L. (1982) Skill training and heterosexual social difficulties, *Canadian Journal of Psychiatric Nursing*, Vol. 23, no. 3, pp. 13–15.

Schuster, E., Unsain, K. and Goodwin, M.H. (1982) Nursing practice in human sexuality, *Nursing Clinics of North America*, Vol. 17, no. 3, pp. 345–9.

Shilts, R. (1987) *The Band Played On*, Penguin, Harmondsworth.

Silverberg, R.A. (1984) Being gay: helping clients to cope, *Journal of Psychosocial Nursing and Mental Health Services*, Vol. 22, no. 2, pp. 18–25.

Tauer, K.M. (1983) Promoting effective decision-making in sexually active adolescents, *Nursing Clinics of North America*, Vol. 18, no. 2, pp. 275–92.

Webb, C. (1985) *Sexuality, Nursing and Health*, Wiley, Chichester.

Webb, C. (1986) *Feminist Practice in Women's Health Care*, Wiley, Chichester.

Webb, C. (1987) Nurses' knowledge and attitudes about sexuality: report of a study, *Nurse Education Today*, Vol. 7, pp. 209–14.

Whitley, M.P. (1978) Seduction and the hospitalized person, *Journal of Nursing Education*, Vol. 16, no. 6, pp. 34–9.

Zalar, M.K. (1982) Role preparation for nurses in human sexual functioning, *Nursing Clinics of North America*, Vol. 17, no. 3, pp. 351–63.

Part Three

Administrative Aspects of Patient Care

17

Admitting Patients

DISCUSSION

Admission to hospital can be seen both as a cause of stress and as an expression of an inability to tolerate stress further. On admission, patients are faced with two interacting tasks: to deal with whatever has brought them into hospital; and to deal with the admission itself. In a review of the literature on stress and hospitalization, Ahmadi (1985) noted deficiencies in 'definitions, conceptualization and theorizing' about patient satisfaction and hospital stress. Her study demonstrated racial differences in the stress experienced by hospitalized patients, related to items concerned with nurse–patient interaction. She suggests that an alienation exists between nurses and patients. Wilson-Barnett (Wilson-Barnett and Carrigy, 1978) reviewed findings which show that patients often remain anxious for some days after admission to hospital. Volicer (Volicer and Bohannon, 1975) has developed a hospital stress rating scale in order to elicit patients' perceptions of the hospitalization experience.

The studies mentioned deal with patients admitted to general hospitals. In the absence of research, it is suggested that the issues mentioned are intensified for patients admitted to psychiatric hospitals. Käppeli (1986) suggests that systematic individualized nursing care depends on the nurse's ability to gather and record information from the patient. An admission procedure has as its target obtaining, communicating, discussing and documenting essential information in order to produce an immediate plan of care acceptable, so far as possible, both to the patient and the nursing staff.

Giving information to the patient

Giving information to the patient, orienting him or her to the ward, is as important as collecting information. It follows that the admission procedure is unlikely to be completed in a set time, certainly not in a few minutes, and may need a day or two. Relatives and friends who accompany patients need to express their own anxieties at the time of a person's admission. A nurse who walks away with the designated patient can seem to relatives to be taking little account of them. If the nurse spends time with the relatives, he or she will need to follow up the initial contact, because under stress they are unlikely fully to take in explanations. In these circumstances, booklets for patients and their relatives and friends are useful.

Special cases

DISTURBED PATIENTS

Emergency admissions of disturbed patients may occur under a section of the Mental Health Act. The admitting nurse will ensure that the necessary documentation has been completed, that the process of informing the patient's nearest relative is under way, and that the patient has a means of claiming his or her rights as detailed in the leaflet given to patients who are detained under the Act. Merely giving the leaflet to the patient is not sufficient.

VERY DISTURBED PATIENTS

Very disturbed patients may be admitted informally. Nurses will ensure that psychotic patients or those who are intoxicated are carefully assessed and screened for potential safety problems, and will monitor carefully how they are tolerating the admission process.

PATIENTS PRESENTING HAZARDS

It is recommended that, if possible, the form for recording the pre-admission assessment of patients who present hazards is completed, in order that any special precautions may be implemented as necessary. Examples of hazards include violence, suicide, infection such as HIV or hepatitis B, physical disability or frailty, mental retardation or impairment.

Documents and equipment

To fulfil the bureaucratic requirements of admission a formidable set of assorted documents and equipment is needed, which the admitting nurse assembles before approaching the patient. To someone who is already anxious, the comings and goings of a nurse in search of items needed to conduct the procedure can begin the process of alienation referred to above.

An example of a checklist of such items follows.

CHECKLIST

Patient record file
Nursing process documentation
Two missing persons forms
Weight chart
Other record charts as needed
Pass form
Ward admission record
Locker and wardrobe keys
Inpatient certificate
Certificate and benefit record
Ward cash record
Receipt and deposit book
Property retained book
Night safe cash deposit book and envelopes (if the admission is out of office hours)
Specimen signature card
Sphygmomanometer
Stethoscope
Urine specimen pot.

After assembling the checklisted items, the nurse is faced with four main tasks:

1 gathering information from the patient;
2 communicating information to the patient;
3 sifting, reporting, discussing and recording the information;
4 negotiating a care plan.

The broad principles behind these tasks are reasonably easy to identify:

1 to ensure the patient's safety;
2 to establish a working relationship;
3 to outline the informal agreement implied in each admission whereby the patient accepts certain constraints in order that the hospital may continue to run smoothly according to its policies and procedures.

The emphasis on each task during the procedure will vary with the needs of the individual patient, and be worked out between the patient with his or her friends or relatives if available, and the admitting nurse with his or her senior nursing colleagues and the medical staff.

Institutional constraints

Sociological and anthropological views of psychiatric hospitals have seen admission as a ritual whereby the stigma of deviance is affixed to individuals by removing their property from them, giving them numbers and labelling them with diagnoses. According to this view the patient then behaves in ways that both result from and conform to the label (Spitzer and Denzin, 1968). Staff perceive the deviant behaviour without perceiving the vicious circle which produces and amplifies it. Deviant behaviour is likely to be reinforced by insensitive application of institutional constraints to patients.

However, the smooth running of the hospital does involve constraints on individuals, whether patients or staff. Fire precautions require that the occupants of a building can be accounted for in case of fire. Food supplies must be based on accurate tallies of potential consumers. Linen and laundry services are based on predictions of actual use. Patients who present varying degrees of risk are housed together. It is suggested that if, on admission, the nurse is explicit about the constraints on a patient's freedom to do as he or she wishes, while at the same time attempting to clarify what is on offer from the institution, he or she stands a better chance of tackling problems of non-compliance.

GUIDELINES: ADMITTING A PATIENT

Action

1 As soon as the patient arrives in the ward, introduce him or her to the nurse who will be assigned primary responsibility for his or her nursing care, and inform the doctor of the patient's arrival.

Rationale

(a) In order that the patient's first contact with the ward or department is structured round an individualized approach.
(b) So that it is clear that the nursing care is effectively organized and puts the patient's interests first.

2   Having negotiated times with the doctor, arrange with another nurse what time you will check the patient's property.

(a)   In order that he or she will assist with the property check according to hospital policy.

(b)   In order that he or she will continue supervision of the patient while the admitting nurse completes the documentation.

3   Book a quiet area in the ward to conduct the admission procedure.

To ensure privacy and freedom from interruptions.

4   Arrange for tea or coffee to be brought to this area for the patient, those accompanying him or her and the admitting nurse.

To provide a sense of unhurried welcome.

5   The admitting nurse introduces him- or herself to the patient.

Common courtesy.

6   Introduce other staff and patients in the immediate vicinity.

Common courtesy.

7   Show the patient the sleeping area and personal storage facilities.

In order to explain where he or she will be living and how he or she will store his or her property.

8   Explain that he or she will be given keys to his or her locker and wardrobe.

To preview aspects of the admission procedure.

9   Depending on the patient's state of mind, show him or her round the ward.

In order to demonstrate fire exits and alarm systems.

10   Accompany the patient to the quiet area booked earlier.

In order to explain how the next period of time will be spent.

11   Check the time.

In order to let the patient know when you will be finishing this part of the procedure.

12   Explain, if necessary, who the patient's consultant is.

A new patient is sometimes allocated to a consultant on arrival in the ward.

13   Name the registrar or ward doctor and state where his or her office is located.

So that the patient knows how and where to find him or her.

14   Explain how the nursing is organized in the ward.

So that the patient knows who the nurses will be and who is in charge of the ward.

15   Identify the nurses' duty rotas, the ward timetable and the nurse–patient allocation.

So that the patient knows where to find them.

16   State the visiting hours.

So that relatives and friends can be told.

17   Give relevant phone numbers: e.g. ward payphone, hospital number, ward extension.

So that relatives and friends can freely get in touch both with the patient and with staff.

18   Explain hospital policies concerning sharps, valuables, money, electrical equipment and medication.

(a)   So that relatives or friends can take unsuitable items home if necessary.
(b)   So that relatives can arrange, for instance, to bring in disposable razors.
(c)   So that any personal medications can be shown to the doctor for prescribing or discontinuing, before being taken home by the relatives or sent to the pharmacy.

19   Pause at intervals and ask if the patient has any questions.

(a)   It is likely that the patient has concerns that are not covered by routine procedures.
(b)   To find out how he or she is coping with the procedure.
(c)   In order to determine how to conduct the next stage.

20   Explain that information is needed from the patient.

To make it clear that the admission process is interactive.

21   Complete the administrative documents required by the hospital medical records and under the provisions of the Mental Health Act 1983.

(a)   Following the Körner Reports (DHSS, 1982; 1984), hospitals are required to maintain standardized information for nationwide collation.
(b)   If the admitting nurse completes it, the patient will not need to have repetitious interviews to gain the same information.
(c)   So that the patient can claim his or her rights, particularly for an appeal against detention.

22   Elicit from the patient in his or her own words the reason for admission.

(a)   It is likely that this will differ from that given by medical staff or friends and relatives.
(b)   It is important that the patient's own views are recorded.

23   Elicit from the patient in his or her own words what kind of help is wanted.

(a)   In order to establish what the patient's complaints are.
(b)   In order to establish why the patient thinks he or she is in hospital.
(c)   In order to establish what the patient's assets and strengths are at this time.

24   Decide whether the patient is likely to be at risk of accidental or deliberate self-harm.

The nurse's duty of care to the patient involves ensuring his or her safety and the safety of other patients and staff.

25   Elicit from the patient what he or she thinks are priorities and needs in addition to safety factors.

In order to identify personal and cultural values which will influence the patient's perception of his or her predicament.

26   Ask the patient again if he or she has any questions.

To help you decide whether you can move to the next stage.

27   Fill out a medical certificate, recording on the nursing front sheet that this has been done.

(a)   To ensure that the patient will receive any benefits due as soon as possible.
(b)   So that the patient can make necessary arrangements with his or her employers without delay.

28   Complete two missing persons forms and record on the nursing front sheet that this has been done. If a missing persons form as such is not used, ensure that the information that would be required in the event of the police being asked to search for a patient has been recorded on admission.

Patients' mental states may change suddenly, and it is difficult to fill out missing persons forms accurately from memory.

29 Explain to the patient that he or she will have a safety care plan.

(a) In order to achieve agreement with the patient if possible.
(b) To make it clear that safety of the patient is the main concern.

30 Explain what a safety care plan entails.

In order to try to achieve agreement.

31 Give the patient a copy of his or her safety care plan.

The safety care plan is not negotiable.

32 Explain the arrangements for taking into safekeeping medication, razors, blades and other potentially dangerous items.

(a) Disposable razors can be broken and the blades exposed.
(b) Electric razor points are near wash basins and so electric shock is a risk.
(c) Razor blades may be used either for direct self-injury, or for preparation of other means: e.g. cutting up a clothes dryer to make a rope for hanging oneself.

33 Explain that you will check the patient's property.

(a) So that valuables may be deposited into safe custody.
(b) To ensure that medicines are sent to pharmacy before being prescribed for new dispensing, and for administering by ward staff.
(c) To ensure the safety of individual items of property.

34 Issue a wardrobe and locker key, recording the patient's name, the date and the numbers of the keys and the furniture.

It is essential that patients have personal and private storage facilities.

35 Ask the patient whether he or she would like to combine the property-checking procedure with packing things away in the locker and wardrobe.

To try to make the checking procedure less intrusive.

36 If the second nurse has not by now joined you, go with the patient to collect him or her.

So that the checking of the patient's property will be witnessed.

37 Go to the patient's sleeping area and follow the procedures for checking monies, valuables, clothing and other property.

So that the procedures are conducted in private.

38 Take into safekeeping any potentially dangerous items.

(a) To safeguard the patient.
(b) To safeguard other patients and staff.

39 Label them with embossing tape or with a similar relatively permanent form of label.

Property deposited into safe custody must be clearly identified.

40 Store the razors in a locked cupboard, in a well-ventilated container separate from those of other patients.

Storage of razors in a single area creates the risk of contamination and cross-infection, particularly of pathogens such as those causing hepatitis.

41 Ensure that any hospital razors use a locking device, are disinfected between patients and have new blades for each patient.

This is an intrusive procedure. The patient will be requiring his razor daily. The patient who is presented with a dirty razor and a dull blade is likely to be encouraged to acquire and hoard his own razors so that assessment of the suicide risk becomes more difficult.

42 Measure and record on the nursing front sheet the patient's temperature, pulse and blood pressure.

(a) To provide baselines in case of any changes later.
(b) To evaluate any changes from previous recordings.

43 Measure and record on the nursing front sheet the patient's weight.

Weight is an important somatic indicator of states of mind, and is not easily predictable or easy to judge clinically.

44 Carry out and record the results of analysis of the patient's urine, having first established whether there is thought to be any risk of infection from pathogens such as the human immunodeficiency virus (HIV) or hepatitis B.

Some somatic illnesses which are accompanied by psychiatric symptoms are characterized by abnormal findings in urinalysis.

45 If any specimen of urine is sent for biochemical examination in the hospital pathology department, ensure that it is placed in the correct bag, correctly sealed and labelled.

(a) To prevent accidental spillage in transport.
(b) So that other hospital staff will take the correct precautions when handling the specimen, should it be considered infectious.

46 Confirm with the patient that he or she feels comfortable with the admission procedure so far.

(a) This stage of the procedure has been intrusive and is being drawn to a close.
(b) In order to spend a few minutes helping the patient to settle down before leaving him or her.

47 Finish at the time you said you would.

In order to demonstrate reliability and attention to detail.

48 Explain that you are going to write up some notes and state a time when you will next see the patient.

(a) Common courtesy.
(b) To provide a sense of continuity for the patient.
(c) So that the patient knows where to find you if he or she has any questions.

49 Leave the patient with the nurse with whom you arranged for supervision to be taken over.

(a) On admission it is essential that patients have as full and as rapid nursing assessment as possible.
(b) To ensure the safety of the patient.

50 Set out your findings in accordance with the headings on the nursing front sheet.

(a) To provide the baseline information for subsequent assessment.
(b) So that essential information such as name and address of the next of kin is recorded.
(c) So that the nature of any hazards is clearly stated. Examples of hazards include violence, suicide, infection such as HIV or hepatitis B, physical disability or frailty, mental retardation or impairment.

51 Make any additional notes on the nursing assessment form.

The front sheet will not provide room for all the information gained during the admission procedure.

52 Summarize what the patient has said verbatim if possible.

It is preferable to record the patient's own words than to record the nurse's opinions of them.

53 Discuss your notes with the senior registered nurse on duty.

(a) In order that safety aspects may be fully evaluated.
(b) In order that the nurse in charge of the shift can make a full report to the nurse in charge of the next shift on duty.

54	Discuss the patient's permission to go out unaccompanied with the senior registered nurse on duty.	In order to arrive at the safest decision given the state of the patient and of the ward or department as a whole.
55	Discuss your notes and the patient's permission to go out unaccompanied with his or her doctor.	So that the ward team works as a team.
56	If appropriate, arrange with the doctor to see the patient with him or her.	To do so can be helpful in case of disagreement with the patient about aspects of management such as the safety care plan or the permission to go out unaccompanied.
57	Ask the doctor to complete all documentation that will be required by the nursing staff and, if necessary, record that the request has been made.	So that the nurses on duty out of office hours will be informed about the medical contribution to the assessment and planning so far.
58	Start an entry in the day report ready for completion by the nurse in charge on the evening shift.	So that there is no possibility of the patient's being forgotten when the reports are written.
59	Finish any other documentation using the checklist above as an *aide-mémoire*.	In order to hand over efficiently to nurses coming on duty later.
60	Return to the patient at the time you said you would.	To ensure that he or she has the opportunity to ask questions and receive necessary information.

REFERENCE MATERIAL

References

Ahmadi, K.S. (1985) The experience of being hospitalized: stress, social support and satisfaction, *International Journal of Nursing Studies*, Vol. 22, pp. 137–48.

DHSS (1982) *Steering Group on Health Services Information First Report*, HMSO, London.

DHSS (1984) *Steering Group on Health Services Information Reports 2–6*, HMSO, London.

Käppeli, S. (1986) Nurses' management of patients' self-care, *Nursing Times*, Vol. 82, no. 11, pp. 40–3.

Spitzer, S.P. and Denzin, N.K. (1968) *The Mental Patient: Studies in the Sociology of Deviance*, McGraw-Hill, New York.

Volicer, B.J. and Bohannon, M.W. (1975) A hospital stress rating scale, *Nursing Research*, Vol. 24, no. 5, pp. 352–9.

Wilson-Barnett, J. and Carrigy, A. (1978) Factors influencing patients' emotional reactions to hospitalization, *Journal of Advanced Nursing*, Vol. 3, pp. 221–9.

Further reading

Aspinall, M.J. (1975) Development of a patient-completed admission questionnaire and its comparison with the nursing interview, *Nursing Research*, Vol. 24, no. 5, pp. 377–81.

Bean, P. (1980) *Compulsory Admissions to Mental Hospitals*, Wiley, Chichester.

Betemps, E. (1981) Management of the withdrawal syndrome of barbiturates and other central nervous system depressants, *Journal of Psychosocial Nursing and Mental Health Services*, Vol. 19, no. 9, pp. 31–4.

Boylan, A. (1982) Nursing at the crossroads: assessment of the patient's physical condition, *Nursing Times*, Vol. 78, no. 35, pp. 1485–6.

Chalmers, H. (1977) First impressions stick, *Nursing Mirror*, Vol. 145, no. 1, pp. i–iv.

Cohn, L. *et al.* (1982) The hospitalized alcoholic, *American Journal of Nursing*, Vol. 82, pp. 1862–77.

Coupar, A. and Conway, C. (1986) Hospital admission for depression, *Journal of Advanced Nursing*, Vol. 11, pp. 697–704.

Dowell, L. (1985) The rights of admission, *Nursing Mirror*, Vol. 160, no. 1, p. 33.

Franklin, B.L. (1974) *Patient Anxiety on Admission to Hospital*, RCN, London.

Fultz, J.M. *et al.* (1980) When a narcotic addict is hospitalized, *American Journal of Nursing*, Vol. 80, pp. 478–81.

James, S.D. (1982) *The Hospital Shop Window*, Institute of

Health Services Administrators, London.

Kennard, D. (1974) The newly admitted psychiatric patient as seen by self and others, *British Journal of Medical Psychology*, Vol. 47, pp. 27–41.

Lego, S. (ed.) (1984) *The American Handbook of Psychiatric Nursing*, Lippincott, Philadelphia.

Local Government Training Board (1984) *Admission of the Mentally Disordered to Hospital or Guardianship: A Guide for Social Workers*, Local Government Training Board.

Loweree, F., Freng, S. and Barnes, B.C. (1984) Admitting an intoxicated patient, *American Journal of Nursing*, Vol. 84, pp. 617–18.

Platt, C. (1986) Social class, underprivileged areas and psychiatric disorder in the city of Stoke-on-Trent, *Journal of Advanced Nursing*, Vol. 11, pp. 309–14.

Porter, A. (1977) Patient needs on admission, *American Journal of Nursing*, Vol. 77, pp. 112–13.

Price, B. (1983) Just a few forms to fill in, *Nursing Times*, Vol. 79, no. 44, pp. 26–8.

Price, B. (1983) Role playing the admission procedure, *Nursing Times*, Vol. 79, no. 44, pp. 28–9.

Price, B. (1986) In sickness, health or in-between, *Nursing Times*, Vol. 82, no. 16, pp. 32–4.

Price, B. (1987) First impressions: patient assessment paradigms, in *Clinical Excellence in Nursing International Networking*, Department of Nursing Studies, University of Edinburgh.

Reid, H. (1980) A nurse's objectives for newly arrived patients, *Nursing Times*, Vol. 76, no. 4, pp. 165–6.

Rix, G. (1985) An admission of crisis, *Nursing Times*, Vol. 81, no. 16, pp. 28–9.

Roslaniec, A. and Fitzpatrick, J.J. (1979) Changes in mental status in older adults within four days of hospitalization, *Research in Nursing and Health*, Vol. 2, pp. 177–87.

Silver, K. and Wilcox, P.A. (1986) Admission: the consumer's first impression, *Journal of Nursing Administration*, Vol. 16, no. 9, pp. 14–18.

Smith, D.S. (1985) Admitting, transfer and discharge: capturing savings from system design, *Nursing Management*, Vol. 16, no. 5, pp. 25–33.

Sofaer, B. (1979) The loss of dentures in hospital, *Nursing Times*, Vol. 75, no. 21, pp. 85–8.

Volicer, B.J. (1973) Perceived stress levels of events associated with the experience of hospitalization: development and testing of a measurement tool, *Nursing Research*, Vol. 22, pp. 491–7.

Volicer, B.J. (1974) Patients' perception of stressful events associated with hospitalization, *Nursing Research*, Vol. 23, pp. 235–8.

Webster, R.A. (1986) Sleep in hospital, *Journal of Advanced Nursing*, Vol. 11, pp. 447–57.

Williamson, C. (1984) What's in a name?, *Nursing Times*, Vol. 80, no. 48, pp. 30–2.

Wilson-Barnett, J. (1978) In hospital: patients' feelings and opinions 1, *Nursing Times*, Vol. 74, no. 8, pp. 29–32.

Wilson-Barnett, J. (1978) In hospital: patients' feelings and opinions 2, *Nursing Times*, Vol. 74, no. 9, pp. 33–4.

18

Admitting Patients who are Likely to Cause Hazards

DISCUSSION

For a patient to be safely nursed after admission to hospital, nurses need to possess information about the degree of risk posed by him or her, and whether the risk is to the patient or to others or both. Risks include suicide, violent behaviour including aggressive sexual behaviour, fire-raising, physical disability or frailty, infection such as HIV or hepatitis B antigen, substance abuse and self-injurious behaviour. A ward on the second floor, say, whose access by lift is controlled by a hospital key is not a suitable place for an informal patient confined to a wheelchair, because of the unacceptable constraints placed on the patient's liberty.

The system for negotiating the admission of patients who present hazards is always under pressure. However, research is not helpful in determining how resources should be matched to patients thought to present risks. It seems likely that outcomes of admission or transfer of patients likely to cause hazards are conditional upon organizational factors rather than on characteristics of individual patients. That is, the quality of the negotiation process before admission, of liaison between different disciplines and between health care agencies, of liaison between penal institutions or law-enforcement agencies and admitting hospitals may be measured against the quality of outcome for a given patient (Roscoe, 1988).

The extended form which is provided in this procedure attempts to document as fully as possible from the nursing point of view how joint assessment and negotiation has been carried out before admission. Further discussion of the effects of transferring patients from one institution to another will be found in Chapter 27.

GUIDELINES: ADMITTING A PATIENT LIKELY TO CAUSE HAZARDS

Action

1 The nurse in charge of a ward to which a patient is to be admitted discusses with the admitting doctor any history of hazards presented by the patient.

2 The nurse in charge discusses with the local nurse manager whether the patient can be managed by day and by night.

3 If the proposed admission is from another hospital or institution, the multidisciplinary clinical team (MDCT) undertakes a hazard assessment.

Rationale

An experienced nurse may well give a different weight to aspects of a patient's history which could affect the nursing of him or her.

So that if extra nursing resources are required they can be negotiated before the patient is admitted.

(a) In order to determine the resources required to nurse the patient safely.
(b) To try to predict any risk involved in the admission.

FORM FOR RECORDING THE PRE-ADMISSION ASSESSMENT OF PATIENTS WHO PRESENT HAZARDS

PATIENT'S NAME
CURRENT ADDRESS

TELEPHONE

DATE OF BIRTH
DATE OF ADMISSION

DETAINED/INFORMAL
DATE FROM WHICH DETAINED
SECTION NUMBER

WHERE MANAGED AT PRESENT: COMMUNITY ☐   LOCKED WARD ☐   OPEN WARD ☐   PRISON ☐

CONTACT PERSON: NAME   GRADE   POSITION
ADDRESS
TELEPHONE

PATIENT'S HOME ADDRESS
TELEPHONE

CATCHMENT AREA HOSPITAL

REASON FOR REQUEST FOR ADMISSION

STATE PRECISELY NATURE OF THE HAZARD THE PATIENT PRESENTS

CURRENT CARE PLAN

PROBLEM/NEED	OBJECTIVE	REVIEW DATE

CURRENT MEDICATION

DATE PRESCRIBED	MEDICATION	DOSE	FREQUENCY

HOW THE PATIENT BECAME INVOLVED WITH CURRENT CAREGIVERS

Figure 18.1   Example of a hazard assessment form

| VISITING NURSE'S ASSESSMENT |

HISTORY OF HAZARD PRESENTED

KNOWN PRECIPITANTS

KNOWN SETTINGS

FORENSIC HISTORY

HISTORY OF SUBSTANCE ABUSE

MEDICAL HISTORY RELEVANT TO HAZARD PRESENTED

PSYCHIATRIC HISTORY RELEVANT TO HAZARD

| FAMILY AND SOCIAL BACKGROUND |

GENOGRAM

INVOLVEMENT OF FRIENDS AND RELATIVES IN CURRENT MANAGEMENT

PATIENT'S VIEW OF NURSING NEEDS

SUMMARY OF CURRENT NURSING CARE

Figure 18.1   (continued)

INTERVIEW WITH PATIENT

INTERVIEWED WITH

DEMEANOUR AND ATTITUDE OF THE PATIENT TO THE INTERVIEW

SUMMARY

VERBATIM NOTES OF FORM AND CONTENT OF PATIENT'S CONVERSATION

INTERVIEWER'S CONCLUSIONS

ANY AGREEMENT MADE WITH PATIENT?

Figure 18.1   (continued)

RECOMMENDATION OF NURSE CONDUCTING THE ASSESSMENT

NAME OF ASSESSING NURSE [   ] GRADE [   ] DATE [   ] SIGNATURE [   ]

DISCUSSION WITH MULTIDISCIPLINARY TEAM

NAME OF NURSE [   ] GRADE [   ] DATE [   ] SIGNATURE [   ]

DISCUSSION WITH SENIOR NURSE MANAGER(S)

DECISION: ADMIT [   ] PLANNED DATE [   ] NOT ADMIT [   ]

REFERRERS INFORMED? YES/NO [   ] PATIENT INFORMED? YES/NO [   ]

SPECIAL ARRANGEMENTS TO BE MADE BEFORE ADMISSION

NAME OF NURSE [   ] GRADE [   ] DATE [   ] SIGNATURE [   ]

Figure 18.1 (continued)

4 A senior first-level nurse conducts a nursing assessment by visiting the patient along with another member of the MDCT.

In order that any recommendation to admit is made by a person with the necessary authority to do so.

5 The assessing nurse interviews the patient alone or together with his or her colleague from the MDCT, as agreed between them.

Co-operation between team members is essential to preserve open communication upon which to base difficult decisions.

6 The assessing nurse meets with the nurses of the transferring ward or unit and reads the nursing record.

In order to get a clear idea of the therapy so far offered and its results.

7 The two assessors report in writing to the MDCT and to the nurse manager of the admitting ward or unit, using the hazard assessment form, shown in Figure 18.1.

The standardized form acts as a checklist for essential information, a means of organizing it in a familiar way, and displaying it for examination by all team members.

8 The first page of the form provides a summary of administrative details.

(a) Details of detention under the Mental Health Act are essential to protect the patient's civil liberties as well as to ensure the legal restraint of a dangerous person.
(b) If the admitting hospital is not the same as the catchment area hospital it is likely that liaison will be necessary for planning any psychiatric aftercare as well as social services provision.
(c) A summary of the care being currently provided will help in the estimate of future requirements for nursing resources.

9 The second and third pages summarize the visiting nurse's assessment.

(a) The history and known precipitants for any hazard are essential for planning management strategies. A history of substance abuse or forensic involvement or both will indicate the likelihood of lapses of impulse control by the patient.
(b) A genogram is useful because it indicates the cohesion or otherwise of a person's family, along with significant deaths, separations and illnesses. These all provide evidence of environmental and genetic influences which can be used as the basis for prediction.
(c) The report of the interview and of the patient's own views will provide significant evidence for the assessment of safety.

10 The final page concludes the assessment by the nurse with his or her recommendations.

The recommendations made soon after the interviews with the patient and his or her current caregivers will give a sense, it is hoped, of what interaction with this particular person is like, even if, later, the recommendations are changed.

11 The assessment will provide information in such a way that it can be evaluated by any member of the team.

A summary of the discussion by the MDCT may be given by a nurse other than the nurse who conducted the assessment.

12 A summary of the discussion with the senior nurse managers is usually made by the nurse in charge of the ward or unit.

Because the nurse in charge of the ward or unit is accountable for the health and safety of the people who work there, as well as for the safety of the patients.

13 The decision whether to admit or not, and the summary of special arrangements to be made before admission are recorded by the nurse in charge of the ward or unit.

The nurse in charge is accountable, with the rest of the MDCT, for the decision, but can later delegate some of the special arrangements. If so, the person to whom they are delegated will need a record of what is to be done, as well as evidence of the authority delegated.

14 A copy of the hazard assessment form is available for all nurses in the ward or unit as well as for the person who will be the patient's primary nurse.

(a) So that all the nursing team will participate in the necessary planning.

(b) So that the primary nurse can make preparations such as beginning liaison with other disciplines, making appointments with family members and friends, and possibly visiting the patient before admission.

REFERENCE MATERIAL
Reference

Roscoe, J.J. (1988) *The Context of Professional Decisions: Clinical, Social, Psychological and Organisational Influences on the Transfer of Patients from Secure Accommodation to NHS Hospitals*, PhD Thesis, University of London.

Further reading

Cocozza, J.J. and Steadman, H.J. (1978) Prediction in psychiatry: an example of misplaced confidence in experts, *Social Problems*, Vol. 25, no. 3, pp. 265–76.

Curtis, J.M. (1985) Considerations in diagnosis and management of violent behaviour, *Psychological Reports*, Vol. 57, pp. 815–23.

Farrington, D.P. and Gunn, J. (eds.)(1985) *Aggression and Dangerousness*, Wiley, Chichester.

Gostin, L. (1978) Industrial action: is the target management or patients?, *Nursing Mirror*, Vol. 147, no. 15, pp. 15–17.

Hyman, S.E. (ed.) (1984) *Manual of Psychiatric Emergencies*, Little Brown, Boston, Mass.

Krakowski, M., Volavka, J. and Brizer, D. (1986) Psychopathology and violence: a review of literature, *Comprehensive Psychiatry*, Vol. 27, no. 2, pp. 131–48.

Kroll, J. and Mackenzie, T.B. (1983) When psychiatrists are liable: risk management and violent patients, *Hospital and Community Psychiatry*, Vol. 34, no. 1, pp. 29–37.

Loo, A. (1984) Assessing mentally disordered offenders, *Nursing Times*, Vol. 80, no. 18, pp. 44–6.

McKillop, W. (1987) Weapon screening, *Hospital and Community Psychiatry*, Vol. 38, no. 2, pp. 202–3.

Monahan, J. (1978) Prediction research and the emergency commitment of dangerous mentally ill persons: a reconsideration, *American Journal of Psychiatry*, Vol. 135, no. 2, pp. 198–201.

Montandon, C. and Harding, T. (1984) The reliability of dangerousness assessments: a decision making exercise, *British Journal of Psychiatry*, Vol. 144, pp. 149–55.

Munns, D.C. (1985) A validation of the defining characteristics of the nursing diagnosis 'potential for violence', *Nursing Clinics of North America*, Vol. 20, no. 4, pp. 711–23.

Scott, P.D. (1977) Assessing dangerousness in criminals, *British Journal of Psychiatry*, Vol. 131, pp. 127–42.

Soreff, S.M. (1981) *Management of the Psychiatric Emergency*, Wiley, New York.

[Unsigned article] (1977) Dangerous patients and prisoners, *British Medical Journal*, Vol. 2, pp. 782–3.

19

Patients' Property

DISCUSSION

This manual does not attempt to cover detailed procedures for the handling of patients' property. Different hospitals will have different nomenclatures for the relevant offices, finance officers, property record books and accounts systems. Brief guidelines are included here in order to give a general outline of the principles involved in safekeeping patients' property.

Care and diligence

The legal responsibilities of nurses were outlined in 1963 by the Association of Chief Financial Officers in the Hospital Service in England and Wales. They have not changed. Where a patient hands over his or her property for safe custody, the 'standard of care and diligence employed' by a nurse will be the same as that which a 'careful and diligent nurse would exercise in the care and custody of his or her own property of a similar description and character' (Research Committee, 1978, p. 2). The following decisions must be made for each patient:

1 Is the patient's capacity to be a careful and diligent guardian of his or her money likely to be affected by his or her mental state?
2 Are the items capable of being stored in such a way as to prevent theft?
3 Will the patient consent to a third party taking charge of his or her monies?

Role of the charge nurse

The charge nurse is the key person in administering hospital policies regarding patients' money and other property. He or she or a designated deputy retains custody of the ward safe keys. He or she is responsible for designating who will check bookkeeping and accounts in accordance with hospital policy. The charge nurse will administer an organizational system where first-level nurses direct the care of all patients so that those thought to be incapable of looking after their own valuables have their interests safeguarded in accordance with hospital policy. Finally, the quality of the charge nurse's liaison with other disciplines will determine the effectiveness of any help offered to a patient with the management of his or her property and money.

GUIDELINES: SAFE-KEEPING A PATIENT'S PROPERTY

Action	Rationale
1 Transfer immediately to proper storage facilities any property or valuables handed over by patients.	In order to prevent theft or loss after the patient has entrusted articles to the nurse.
2 Ensure that the patient understands his or her responsibilities in relation to his or her property.	In order to prevent theft or loss of any property or valuables retained by the patient.
3 Refrain from handing over to third parties the property of patients without the patient's consent.	To prevent theft or loss.

4   Record all transactions involving patients' property or valuables in the presence of the patient and another witnessing nurse.

(a) To demonstrate 'care and diligence'.
(b) In case of any subsequent theft or loss.

5   Find out whether the patient's mental state is likely to affect his or her diligence in looking after property, money and valuables.

To decide whether statutory measures such as the Court of Protection, guardianship or power of attorney will need to be negotiated in order to safeguard the patient's interests.

6   Examine and transfer immediately to proper storage facilities the contents of patients' clothing or other items brought by the patient on admission to hospital.

(a) To ensure that no dangerous or valuable articles are left unaccounted for.
(b) To ensure that the patient has the necessary private facilities in which to store his or her personal property.

7   Where such facilities are provided for the patient's use, the nurse supplies him or her with a key to them on admission.

So that the patient can exercise due care and diligence in the care of his or her property.

8   Record with a witness when a patient refuses consent for property to be taken into safe custody.

So that it is clear who is responsible for the safe-keeping of the property.

9   Take advice from a hospital manager if such property is thought to be dangerous to other people. (See Chapter 26.)

In order to decide what action to take to ensure the safety of all patients and staff.

10 Take advice from a hospital manager if such a property is thought to jeopardize confidentiality.

(a) Cameras and tape recorders endanger the confidentiality of patients other than the patient owning them.
(b) The patient who records him- or herself may regret having done so in the future.

11 Treat the following articles as patients' monies:
   (i)   cash;
   (ii)   cash cards;
   (iii) cheque books;
   (iv)   cheque guarantee cards;
   (v)   charge cards;
   (vi)   credit cards, including store accounts;
   (vii) building society pass books;
   (viii) savings account books, including savings certificates;
   (ix)   pension books;
   (x)   benefit order books.

They represent actual or potential possession by the patient of cash.

12 The nurse ensures the safe custody of everything: a special example is that of order books.

Pension books and benefit order books represent sources of income that are likely to be affected by admission to hospital.

13 Record the name of the person responsible for a pension or order book.

To ensure that the patient receives the sums due at the times specified in the pension or order book.

14 Notify the hospital welfare officer of the patient's admission immediately.

Even a short delay in letting the welfare officer know of an admission can result in long delays before patients receive benefits or allowances due to them.

15 Issue witnessed receipts whenever monies, valuables or other property are received from a patient.	So that any subsequent loss or theft can be effectively investigated.
16 Obtain witnessed receipts from patients whenever monies, valuables or other property are restored or issued to them.	To prevent fraud.
17 Maintain accounts for each patient, showing balances and all payments in or out, each entry being signed by two nurses and dated.	(a) To prevent fraud. (b) To facilitate audit.
18 Regularly check records of accounts in accordance with hospital policy.	(a) To ensure that storage is effective. (b) To maintain records to an acceptable standard between audits.
19 Record details of all property retained by patients on admission or transfer to the ward.	So that any theft or loss may be effectively investigated.
20 Even if no property is retained or received from a patient the nurse and a witnessing nurse will complete both the property retained book and the receipt and deposit book with entries saying, 'Nil property', or 'Nil received'.	So that it is clear that a check was made at the time of admission.

REFERENCE MATERIAL
Reference
Research Committee (1978) *Patients' Property, Income and Allowances*, Association of Health Service Treasurers, Cardiff.

Further reading
DHSS (1971) HM(71)90, *Patients' Moneys*, DHSS, London.
Faulkner, B. and Taylor, V.M. (1982) The nurse and patients' property, *Nursing*, Vol. 1, no. 36, pp. 1532–3.
Mental Welfare Commission (1981) *Does the Patient Come First?*, HMSO, Edinburgh.
MIND (1979) *Your Money in Hospital*, National Association for Mental Health, London.
Scottish Hospital Centre (1974) *Handling of Patients' Clothes and Valuables in Long-Stay Hospitals*, Scottish Hospital Centre.

20

Observing and Supervising Patients

DEFINITIONS
Descriptive observation
Descriptive observation answers the question: 'What is happening here?'

Relational observation
Relational observation asks the question: 'What is this for?'

Experimental observation
Experimental observation answers the question: 'What happens if the situation changes?' (Rosenthal and Rosnow, 1975).

DISCUSSION
Aims of observation and supervision
The aim of observation is to assess patients. The aim of supervision is to keep safe those patients thought to be at risk.

Types of observation
Following Rosenthal and Rosnow (1975), three kinds of observation are distinguished here – descriptive, relational and experimental.

DESCRIPTIVE OBSERVATION
Descriptive observation answers the question, 'What is happening here?' It involves defining behaviour in specific and discrete rather than global ways. That is, identifying and measuring specific activities rather than using words like 'hostile', 'inappropriate', 'disturbed', 'manipulative'.

RELATIONAL OBSERVATION
Relational observation is geared towards identifying what precedes actions, and what the consequences of actions are. Functional analysis has much in common with relational observation, and is a problem-solving method which fits with the nursing process. It asks the question, 'What is this for?', thereby relating the things which affect the behaviour being observed to the effects of the behaviour. By focusing on the unique activities of individuals, functional analysis avoids lumping people into groups such as 'obsessionals', 'dements', 'schizophrenics', or 'inadequate personalities'. Functional analysis and relational observation can be used to support any theoretical viewpoint (Owens and Ashcroft, 1982). The scheme which is commonly used to describe the functional analysis is the ABC paradigm: Antecedent events, Behaviour and Consequences (Yule and Carr, 1987).

EXPERIMENTAL OBSERVATION
Descriptive and relational observations pinpoint the behaviour which become the targets to be looked at more closely. Experimental observation answers the question, 'What happens if the situation changes?' For a functional analysis to be effective it may be necessary for the observer to vary the environment of the person being observed, thereby seeing whether situational changes are associated with changes in behaviour. The function of problem behaviours becomes clearer when aspects of the environment which influence them are identified. For instance, Yule notes the research which demonstrates that some kinds of disruptive behaviour have the function of allowing escape from difficult situations (Yule and Carr, 1987). If aspects of a patient's environment are changed systematically, making one change at a time, an accurate assessment of the functions of behaviours is more easily made. Such systematic assessment is called experimental observation. Examples of naturally occurring events which can be used for experimental observation include alterations in medication, weekend leave, visits and changes in the staff duty rota.

Observation skills

Observers' behaviour ranges on a continuum from passive surveillance to active manipulation of patients' environment. The two main strands of observation technique are the psychological and physiological factors which affect perception; and the communication skills which enable the nurse to be receptive to behavioural cues of patients (Janzen, 1980). Observation also involves the accumulation of a variety of different kinds of evidence whose nature is as carefully as possible discriminated in the process of recording.

In recent years attempts have been made to identify and classify observation skills, again using the principle of naming specific behaviours rather than global descriptions (Boice, 1983). A selection follows.

1 Perceptual skills:
  (a) selective attention;
  (b) screening;
  (c) recall;
  (d) recognition.
2 Interaction skills:
  (a) noting and responding to non-verbal cues;
  (b) noting and responding to ambiguous verbal cues;
  (c) communicating attention;
  (d) active listening;
  (e) empathizing;
  (f) questioning;
  (g) adjusting the environment both physically and psychologically;
  (h) participating in groups.
3 Reasoning skills:
  (a) making inferences;
  (b) drawing conclusions;
  (c) discussing.
4 Writing skills:
  (a) summarizing;
  (b) narrative presentation of data;
  (c) graphic presentation of data.
5 Case presentation:
  (a) organizing information;
  (b) defining problems;
  (c) making plans;
  (d) reporting.

Interaction between the observed and the observers

Weick (1985) describes a problem familiar to psychiatric nurses: 'People have strong needs not to examine their lives, and observers threaten this avoidance' (p. 587). He describes research which shows that people's reactions to being observed range from attacks on the observers to efforts to impress observers favourably by, for example, kindness to others or boasting.

Weick therefore describes what he calls the 'socially competent observer'. That is, someone who can maintain friendly and sustained contact with the people he or she is observing. Such an observer is able to assess the effects of his or her behaviour on others; can discuss these effects with the people observed; can use the discussion as experimental material for comparing behaviours before and afterwards; can devise ways of being more or less conspicuous as an observer (pp. 584–7). He notes that liking generally precedes trust. In support of Weick, at least one definition of a therapeutic milieu is a place which 'facilitates observation of self and other' (Szjanberg, 1985).

Reliability

Gregory (1966, 1970) has defined the physiological and psychological issues which are involved in the act of perception. He emphasizes how far from being a total awareness of our surroundings our perceptions are; and how many of our behaviours result from perceptions of which we are not conscious. Because perception and, therefore, observation can only ever be selective, observation must be controlled in order that an account is made which remains stable over time. This does not imply that the behaviour is observed until it stabilizes, rather it is observed until the observer is satisfied that his or her account is accurate.

A number of methods exist for ensuring the reliability of observation and records of observations. They include (Weick, 1985):
1 Continuous recording: using, for example, checklists and running logs.
2 Event recording: counting the numbers of times a behaviour occurs over a predetermined length of time.
3 Duration recording: measuring the total amount of time during which a behaviour occurs over a predetermined period.
4 Interval recording: estimating the frequency of a behaviour by recording how often it occurs in a predetermined period, say an hour which has been divided into intervals of, for example, forty seconds' observation, followed by twenty seconds' recording.
5 Time sampling: counting the occurrences of a behaviour at predetermined intervals, say at every ten minutes over four hours.

Attribution

Attribution theory attempts to explain the causes of behaviour. Jones and Nisbett (1987) examine the relationship between observers and actors. They warn that, in general, observers are tempted, on the basis of quite limited contact, to attribute qualities or traits to the people whom they observe. These attributions tend not only to become more stable over time, rather like self-fulfilling prophecies, but to receive confirmation from other observers. Worsley (1980, p. 170) found that patients who found favour with nurses were those who 'facilitat[ed] the nurse's performance of her role'. Worsley suggests that nurses often simply ignore behaviours that do not fit with their stereotypes of men and women. In Jones and Nisbett's terms, observers thereby construct for themselves apparently consistent explanations of puzzling phenomena. Awareness of the pitfalls of attribution is necessary to protect patients' rights and civil liberties.

Supervision

So far it has been argued that observation techniques run a continuum of interaction between nurses and patients. Even where interaction with a patient is minimal the nurse retains responsibility for his or her safety. The purpose of this chapter is to define a hierarchy of supervision which allows the nurse to judge how active and controlling his or her observation of patients must be to be compatible with the safety of both patients and staff.

Supervision is divided into five levels, each comprising different types of observation. The nurse is always active in supervising patients' safety even when the risk is apparently low. Moran (1979) criticized one-to-one supervision as wasteful of nursing resources and as encouraging dysfunctional dependence by patients. As an alternative, she proposed a checklist whereby all patients in a ward are checked every thirty minutes.

However, this chapter proposes that five levels of supervision allow nurses to make plans for use of resources and for predicting and dealing with interpersonal problems between them and the patients being supervised.

Because nurses actually carry out observation, it is necessary that they take a lead in the multidisciplinary clinical team's definition of the level of supervision for patients. There is evidence that where doctors prescribe supervision, nurses are unlikely to carry out their instructions (Aidroos, 1986). It must be clear who has the authority to initiate and discontinue different levels of supervision; who may carry out supervision; how often the need for supervision is reviewed; how often and what kind of records are written; what the role is of families and friends of patients (Goldberg, 1987).

Risk classification

The classification of risk used in this chapter, and shown in Figure 15.4 (p. 103), was originally devised for suicidal patients. However, it may be applied to patients who present any kind of risk, the nature of which will be defined in the nursing care plan, which states the risk and the level of supervision to be used.

The chart in Figure 15.4 states that the lowest categorization of risk is 'Low'. There is not a category labelled 'No risk'. It is essential that the safety aspect of this is understood by nurses. That is, no patient is left unsupervised. In particular, at the beginning and end of each shift, the well-being and whereabouts of every patient on the current bed-state or register are accounted for by both the outgoing and incoming nurses.

GUIDELINES: OBSERVING AND SUPERVISING A PATIENT

Action

1 Any level of supervision is initiated by a registered nurse or a registered medical practitioner, but preferably jointly.

2 If there is disagreement between the registered nurse and the doctor about the level of supervision to be carried out the higher level is implemented until the issue is decided by consultation with other members of the team or senior colleagues or both.

Rationale

(a) Some research has shown that unless nurses are involved in determining the level of supervision, it may not be carried out.
(b) Joint decisions characterize effective teamwork.

So that the safety of the patient is given priority while any disagreement is resolved.

3 If a registered mental nurse initiates or increases the level of supervision, he or she will arrange for the patient to have a mental state assessment by a psychiatrist as soon as possible.

In order that contingency plans may be made in case more restrictive management and possibly legal detention become necessary.

4 Orders for supervision are written and signed in the patient's medical and nursing records.

(a) So that all members of the MDCT are made aware of the patient's requirements for supervision.
(b) To record that the decision to implement supervision has been correctly taken.

5 The senior registered nurse on duty in a given shift designates nurses to supervise patients as follows:
 (i)   maximum supervision – RMN;
 (ii) full supervision – RMN;
 (iii) close supervision – RMN, EN(M), senior student nurse;
 (iv) intermittent supervision – RMN, EN(M), senior student nurse;
 (v)   periodic supervision – RMN, EN(M), senior student nurse.

The senior registered nurse on duty is deemed to be the nurse in charge of the ward and therefore responsible for the safety of patients and staff.

6 Depending on the system of nurse–patient allocation, nurses who usually work most closely with the patient being supervised are designated to carry out supervision.

Nurses who know the patient are more likely to be able to maintain the role of friendly and diligent observers.

7 The longest that a nurse will be required to carry out maximum supervision at one time will be thirty minutes, followed by fifteen minutes for handing over supervision, discussion and writing of observations, making a total of forty-five minutes.

(a) Because maximum supervision is stressful nurses are not expected to maintain vigilance for longer than half an hour.
(b) Reporting is defined as being part of the supervision process.

8 The longest that a nurse will be required to carry out full supervision will be forty-five minutes, followed by fifteen minutes for handing over supervision, discussion and writing of observations, making a total of one hour.

(a) Because full supervision is stressful nurses are not expected to maintain vigilance for longer than three-quarters of an hour.
(b) Reporting is defined as being part of the supervision process.

9 If in the nurses' view the nursing resources in the ward do not cover the provision of the level of supervision, the nurse manager will be consulted.

So that arrangements can be made to provide the necessary resources. For example, redeployment of staff, restriction on admissions, transfer of the patient.

10 If this consultation does not resolve the problem, senior managers are consulted until a decision is made.

So that satisfactory arrangements are made as soon as possible in order to preserve the safety of patients and staff.

11 The senior registered nurse on duty and the nurse manager make temporary arrangements for supervision of the patient while consultation takes place.

So that disagreement between staff does not jeopardize the patient's safety.

12 Periods of supervision are recorded with the time started (the time one nurse takes over from another) and the time finished (the time one nurse hands over to another).

So that the MDCT can draw inferences and conclusions about the effects of supervision.

13 Records of supervision are kept as follows:
  (i)   maximum, full and close supervision: every shift – (if used) suicide alert form, nurses' notes by supervising nurses; twelve-hourly – day and night reports;
  (ii) intermittent supervision: each shift – nurses' notes by supervising nurses;
  (iii) periodic supervision: each day – nurses' notes by supervising nurses.

Reporting is integral to observation and supervision. The closer the supervision the more detailed the records need to be.

14 Discontinuation or reduction of any level of supervision above intermittent may be ordered only by a registered mental nurse and a registered medical practitioner, jointly, after discussion with as wide a membership of the ward team as appropriate.

The decision to discontinue or reduce supervision carries some risk which needs to be assessed and accepted by team members.

15 A nurse may be asked to give maximum or full supervision to a patient up to three times during a shift.

Because supervision is stressful nurses are not expected to maintain vigilance for longer than a total of one and a half hours (maximum supervision) or two and a quarter hours (full supervision), plus a total of three-quarters of an hour for reporting and discussion.

16 No nurse is left alone to give maximum supervision to a patient who is thought to be at risk of violence to others.

(a) So that the nurse is not placed in danger.
(b) So that the patient's behaviour can be effectively controlled if necessary.

17 The senior registered nurse on duty, together with representatives of the MDCT, decides where the patient will be supervised, preparing a special room if necessary.

So that a safe environment can be provided for both patients and staff.

18 The senior registered nurse on duty, in consultation with the nurses supervising a patient, arranges the environment.

So that supervision can be safely carried out.

19 Each nurse will conduct periods of supervision according to the patient's current care plan, negotiated if possible with the patient, and based on detailed knowledge of the patient's history.

Because patients vary in their responses to prolonged observation and supervision; for example, by hostility to physical nearness of the observer; or, on the other hand, by hostility to distant surveillance, it is necessary for a decision to be made on the spot, based on the evidence available.

20 The nurse taking over maximum or full supervision meets with the nurse handing over in the presence of the patient to discuss how supervision is going.

So that the patient's views can be considered in decisions to maintain, increase or reduce levels of supervision.

21 The nurse who is supervising a patient discusses with him or her how the time will be occupied.

(a) The outcome of this discussion provides a useful assessment of the patient's current risk.
(b) It may be possible to move towards an agreement with the patient that he or she will refrain from self-injury or harm to others. Such an agreement could be made at the beginning of each supervision interval.

22 In the case of patients receiving maximum, full or close supervision, the senior registered nurse on duty consults at least once with the line manager and another member of the MDCT.

(a) To confirm that the existing nursing resources are enough to supervise all patients at the level thought to be necessary.
(b) To review the need for a given level of supervision.

23 The senior registered nurse on duty or the patient's allocated nurse explains to relatives and friends that a nurse will be present during visits when a patient is receiving maximum and full supervision and that the patient has been asked not to leave the ward without the agreement of the MDCT.

Because supervision of disturbed patients has been defined as the responsibility of registered nurses, it is not possible for the designated nurse to absent him- or herself during visits.

24 If relatives or friends insist on private visits or on taking the patient out of the ward, the senior registered nurse on duty consults immediately with a nurse manager.

(a) In order to confirm the need to place the patient's interests before those of his or her visitors.
(b) Although the nurse in charge of a ward has the right to request any visitor to leave immediately, the nurse manager is informed in case any difficulties arise as a result of such a request.

25 At the beginning of each shift, each nurse satisfies him- or herself about the safety of the ward environment in general. For example, emergency exits, alarm systems, fire-fighting equipment.

Such a safety check ensures that all nurses are prepared to supervise patients, and to give immediate and effective assistance to other supervising nurses whenever necessary.

26 At the beginning and end of each shift, the senior registered nurse on duty satisfies him- or herself about the whereabouts and well-being of every patient on the current bed-state.

In order to hand over safely and effectively to the incoming nurse in charge of the ward.

REFERENCE MATERIAL
References

Aidroos, N. (1986) Nurses' response to doctors' orders for close observation, *Canadian Journal of Psychiatry*, Vol. 31, pp. 831–3.

Boice, R. (1983) Observational skills, *Psychological Bulletin*, Vol. 93, no. 1, pp. 3–29.

Goldberg, R.J. (1987) Use of constant observation with potentially suicidal patients in general hospitals, *Hospital and Community Psychiatry*, Vol. 38, no. 3, pp. 303–5.

Gregory, R.L. (1966) *Eye and Brain*, Weidenfeld, London.

Gregory, R.L. (1970) *The Intelligent Eye*, Weidenfeld, London.

Janzen, S. (1980) Taxonomy for development of perceptual skills, *Journal of Nurse Education*, Vol. 19, no. 1, pp. 33–40.

Jones, E.E. and Nisbett, R.E. (1987) The actor and the observer: divergent perceptions of the causes of behaviour, in E.E. Jones *et al.* (eds) *Attribution: Perceiving the Causes of Behaviour*, Lawrence Erlbaum Associates, Hillsdale, NJ.

Moran, J.C. (1979) An alternative to constant observation, *Perspectives in Psychiatric Care*, Vol. 17, no. 3, pp. 114–17.

Owens, G. and Ashcroft, J.B. (1982) Functional analysis in applied psychology, *British Journal of Clinical Psychology*, Vol. 21, pp. 181–9.

Rosenthal, R. and Rosnow, R.L. (1975) *Primer of Methods for the Behavioural Sciences*, Wiley, New York.

Szjanberg, N. (1985) Staff counter-transference in the therapeutic milieu: creating an average expectable environment, *British Journal of Medical Psychology*, Vol. 58, pp. 331–6.

Weick, K.E. (1985) Systematic observation methods, in G. Lindzey and E. Aronson (eds.) *Handbook of Social Psychiatry*, Vol. 1, Random House, New York.

Worsley, A. (1980) Exploration of student nurses' stereotypes of patients, *International Journal of Nursing Studies*, Vol. 17, pp. 163–74.

Yule, W. and Carr, J. (eds.) (1987) *Behaviour Modification for People with Mental Handicaps*, Croom Helm, Beckenham.

Further reading

Barbee, E.L. (1978) Lethality assessment: whose role?, *Issues in Mental Health Nursing*, Vol. 1, pp. 67–84.

Beck, C.M., Rawlins, R.P. and Williams, S.R. (1984) *Mental-Health Psychiatric Nursing: A Holistic Life-Cycle Approach*, Mosby, St Louis, Mo.

Blyth, M.M. and Pearlmutter, D.R. (1983) The suicide watch: a re-examination of maximum observation, *Perspectives in Psychiatric Care*, Vol. 21, no. 3, pp. 90–3.

Bonaparte, B. (1979) Ego defensiveness, open–closed mindedness, and nurses' attitudes toward culturally different patients, *Nursing Research*, Vol. 28, no. 3, pp. 166–71.

Boylan, A. (1982) Assessment of the patient's physical condition, *Nursing Times*, Vol. 78, no. 35, pp. 1485–6.

Broome, A. (1977) Observation in a psychiatric hospital, *Nursing Times*, Vol. 73, no. 22, pp. 837–8.

Broome, A.K. and Weaver, S.M. (1978) Nursing in mental hospitals: who cares for the patients?, *Nursing Mirror*, Vol. 146, no. 23, pp. 16–18.

Collister, B. (1985) Communication: tuning into patients' needs, *Nursing Times*, Vol. 81, no. 10, p. 19.

Dwyer, M., Fricker, R. and Johnson, A.L. (1978) Effect of hospitalization on weight of psychiatric patients, *Journal of Advanced Nursing*, Vol. 3, pp. 433–6.

Frenkel, S.I. *et al.* (1980) Does patient contact change racial perceptions?, *American Journal of Nursing*, Vol. 80, pp. 1340–2.

Gladstone, T.U. and McKegney, F.P. (1980) Relationship between patient behaviours and nursing staff attitudes, *Supervisor Nurse*, Vol. 11, no. 6, pp. 32–5.

Goodwin, L. *et al.* (1981) The Nurse Practitioner Rating Form 2: methodological development, *Nursing Research*, Vol. 30, no. 5, pp. 270–6.

Gottheil, E., Exline, R.V. and Winkelmayer, R. (1979) Judging emotions of normal and schizophrenic subjects, *American Journal of Psychiatry*, Vol. 136, no. 8, pp. 1047–54.

Guirguis, E.F. and Durost, H.B. (1978) The role of mechanical restraints in the management of disturbed behaviour, *Canadian Psychiatric Association Journal*, Vol. 23, no. 4, pp. 209–18.

Hardin, S.B. and Halaris, A.L. (1983) Nonverbal communication of patients and high and low empathy nurses, *Journal of Psychosocial Nursing and Mental Health Services*, Vol. 21, no. 1, pp. 14–20.

Hargreaves, W.A. (1968) Systematic nursing observation of psychopathology, *Archives of General Psychiatry*, Vol. 18, pp. 518–31.

Hogstel, M.O. (1987) Teaching students observational skills, *Nursing Outlook*, Vol. 35, no. 3, pp. 89–91.

Johnson, J.P. (1978) Interpersonal process recall: a useful adjunctive to psychotherapy, *Journal of Psychiatric Nursing*, Vol. 16, no. 2, pp. 14–21.

Kemp, J. (1984) Nursing at night, *Journal of Advanced Nursing*, Vol. 9, pp. 217–23.

Kjervik, D.K. and Palta, M. (1978) Sex-role stereotyping in assessments of mental health, *Nursing Research*, Vol. 27, no. 3, pp. 166–71.

Lane, B.J. and Rae, D.I. (1983) The prejudice of language: effects of word choice on impressions formed by nurses, *Nursing Papers*, Vol. 15, no. 1, pp. 21–3.

Leonard, R. (1983) Attending: letting the patient know you are listening, *Journal of Practical Nursing*, Vol. 33, no. 8, pp. 28–9.

McNamee, C. (1978) Communicating, *Canadian Nurse*, Vol. 74, no. 3, pp. 27–9.

Orsolits, M. and Morphy, M. (1982) A depression algorithm for psychiatric emergencies, *Journal of Psychiatric Treatment and Evaluation*, Vol. 4, pp. 137–45.

Phillips, M. *et al.* (1977) Continuous observation, *Canadian Psychiatric Association Journal*, Vol. 22, no. 1, pp. 25–30.

Piaget, J. (1950) *The Psychology of Intelligence*, Routledge & Kegan Paul, London.

Raffel, S. (1979) *Matters of Fact*, Routledge & Kegan Paul, London.

Royal College of Nurses (1985) *Guidelines on Observation*, RCN, London.

Sackett, G.P. (ed.) (1978) *Observing Behaviour*, Vol. 2, University Park Press, Baltimore, Ma.

Snaith, R.P. (1981) Rating scales, *British Journal of Psychiatry*, Vol. 138, pp. 512–14.

Stricklin, M.L.V. (1979) Mental health patient assessment record: interobserver reliability, *Nursing Research*, Vol. 28, no. 1, pp. 11–15.

Tallent, N. (1983) *Psychological Report Writing*, Prentice-Hall, Englewood Cliffs, NJ.

Ward, M.F. (1985) *The Nursing Process in Psychiatry*, Churchill Livingstone, Edinburgh.

Wolfgang, A. (ed.) (1979) *Nonverbal Behaviour: Applications and Cultural Implications*, Academic Press, New York.

21

Welfare and Voluntary Services

DISCUSSION
Patients' income and allowances
The income of patients is certain to be affected by admission to hospital. The responsibility of nurses is to liaise with the patients' affairs officer or welfare officer in order to:
1 ensure that the patient receives the income due to him or her;
2 assist the patient to carry out the necessary actions to maintain his or her income in as stable a position as possible;
3 ensure that the patient applies for benefits due to him or her;
4 ensure that the patient or a duly appointed agent receives benefits due to him or her;
5 ensure that the patient is not caused to receive benefits to which he or she is not entitled and so be liable to repay them.

The first task of the nurse in relation to the patient's welfare is to issue an inpatient certificate on the day of admission for forwarding to the patient's local DHSS office, to enable the process of claiming and adjusting benefits to begin immediately. Any delay in issuing and forwarding this certificate can result in wrong or non-payment of benefit in the short term and, in the long term, jeopardize future claims based on the length of admission – thus causing hardship to the patient, his or her family and any dependants.

INCOME
Types of income will include salary or wages which continue to be paid depending on the policy of the patient's employer and the duration of the illness. Welfare officers in a patient's workplace may liaise with hospital welfare officers with the consent of the patient, to help him or her to make the necessary plans for managing financial responsibilities while in hospital.

The *Supplementary Benefits Handbook* (DHSS, 1984) states:

> A person's normal requirements are subject to reduction while he is a NHS patient in hospital. The amount and timing of any reduction depend on such factors as whether the person has a partner or dependent children and how long the person has been an in-patient. The general aim is to ensure that the hospital in-patient has sufficient resources to cover any continuing commitments such as home rent or the requirements of his partner and children, with a margin for his personal expenses while in hospital.
>
> (DHSS, 1984, p. 63)

That is, the DHSS assesses each patient's needs on an individual basis. Because of the scrutiny of each case, delays in sending the correct forms or mistakes or omissions or both can result in patients waiting for a considerable time before receiving any money, and so suffering hardship and possibly running into debt. It is essential, therefore, that patients receive prompt and adequate advice about claiming benefits while in hospital.

The system includes an important feature whereby patients who go on leave are entitled to increased payments of supplementary benefit for the time spent out of hospital. The nurse who is primarily responsible for a patient's nursing care is in the best position to liaise with the hospital welfare officer and the patient and to maintain the necessary documentation of the patient's periods of leave.

ALLOWANCES
Allowances to which patients may be entitled include pocket money, whether paid by the hospital or as part of a disability pension; payments for work in the hospital; one-off payments by the hospital authority or the DHSS; therapeutic expenses, for example for cooking in the

ward; reward monies, for example for work in the occupational therapy units. The nurse is responsible for liaising with other departments to ensure that the patient receives the allowance to which he or she is entitled.

Quinn (1985) found that nurses in Scotland receive little or no training for assisting patients to claim the benefits to which they are entitled. She recommends that hospitals employ welfare officers, distinct from the social work departments, in order to provide patients with the necessary information and help in claiming benefits, negotiating and liaising with employers, Departments of Employment and Social Security, building societies and landlords.

Some of the responsibilities of the welfare officer inevitably overlap with those of the social worker. The primary nurse liaises with the welfare officer and the social worker to ensure that they have the necessary information with which to assess patients' needs and to advise them. The welfare officer is equipped with detailed knowledge of the specific regulations for the administration of social security legislation but, in a large organization, needs the assistance of the nurses to ensure that patients are referred and their income and allowances monitored so that their welfare is not jeopardized.

Court of Protection

> The Court of Protection is an office of the Lord Chancellor's department which exists for the purpose of protecting and managing the financial affairs and property of people who, because of mental disorder, are unable to manage for themselves.
>
> (Court of Protection, 1986)

It was re-established with the Mental Health Act 1959, and is an office of the Supreme Court. It operates by the principle of examining individual cases in order to judge whether a person (regardless of whether he or she is in hospital or not, and whether he or she is detained or not) is capable of managing his or her property and affairs. Gostin (1983) and Carson (1987) describe the history of the Court and the detailed procedures for making best use of it. Application to the Court of Protection can be made by the nearest relative or any interested party with the help of a solicitor or with the help of the Court itself. Two medical recommendations are required. The Court's services are provided free if necessary, unless the patient's estate can afford to pay expenses in proportion to the patient's income. Applications are made to the:

Court of Protection
Staffordshire House
25 Store Street
London WC1E 7BP

Guardianship

The function of guardianship as enacted in the Mental Health Act 1983 is to provide compulsory supervision of patients' welfare in order to protect the interests of the patient or other people or both.

It is utilized primarily for the long-term treatment of patients living in the community. Application is by the nearest relative or an approved social worker, and medical recommendation is required by two doctors. The guardian, who is usually the local social services department, is given authority for supervision of patients in the community, with power to require the patient to live at a specified place; to attend specified places for treatment; and ensures that a doctor, social worker or other person, such as a community psychiatric nurse, can see the patient at home.

Hospital resettlement officer

The hospital resettlement officer is employed by the local health authority to provide advice and help for unemployed patients wishing to find work or training for employment. Patients often require help with setting up the necessary training and experience in order to return to work, make a complete change in career or obtain work for the first time. The hospital resettlement officer liaises with the disablement resettlement officer based at the local Department of Employment office, and with the hospital occupational therapy and social work departments, by whom referrals are made. The hospital resettlement officer can provide assistance during patients' rehabilitation, helping nurses and patients set realistic targets and timetables.

Hospital voluntary services

From 1948 the Ministry of Health encouraged hospitals to make use of voluntary services. Hospital Leagues of Friends and the Women's Royal Voluntary Service were the main kinds of organization which undertook fund-raising to provide services and equipment for which funding was not available. The Hospital Car Service is another example of such a service, and provides volunteers to supplement patient transport services.

Few voluntary services existed in the 1950s, but they grew again in the 1960s to the point where they needed an organization and a structure. Training for voluntary service co-ordinators began with a pilot project in 1972, organized by King Edward's Hospital Fund and the National Institute for Social Work. Rocha (1968) for the King Edward's Hospital Fund recommended that hospitals set up any post for a voluntary services organizer only after negotiation with trade union and professional organization representatives so that the responsibilities of paid staff and volunteers could be kept distinct.

From 1969 to 1974 a voluntary services information

officer was appointed at King Edward's Hospital Fund, a role that was later divided between the National Association of Voluntary Help Organizers and the Volunteer Centre. Pitkeathley (1983) edited a report on volunteers in mental health services, which reiterated the need for careful liaison with trade unions, and defined volunteering as 'work undertaken on behalf of oneself or of others, outside the immediate family, not directly for wages and by free choice' (p. 4). The voluntary sector is now well established nationally and has international links. It represents an important part of the services available to the health services.

Chapter 5, 'Nurse–patient relationships', emphasizes the privileged nature of the access to patients and the absolute prohibition of any contact with patients other than that which is strictly professional. Close liaison between charge nurses and the voluntary services organizer is necessary to ensure that any volunteers applying to work with patients are carefully scrutinized and their work monitored to ensure that they understand and stay within the boundaries on relationships imposed by their privileged access to patients. It is helpful if each ward has a member of staff, if not the charge nurse, who is nominated to carry out this liaison by means of regular meetings and evaluation of the relationship between ward staff and volunteers.

REFERENCE MATERIAL
References

Carson, D. (ed.) (1987) *Making the Most of the Court of Protection*, King Edward's Hospital Fund, London.

Court of Protection (1986) *Receivers*, Court of Protection, London.

DHSS (1984) *Supplementary Benefits Handbook*, HMSO, London.

Gostin, L. (1983) *The Court of Protection*, National Association for Mental Health, London.

Pitkeathley, J. (ed.) (1983) *Volunteers in Mental Health: The Next Five Years*, Volunteer Centre, Berkhamsted.

Quinn, C. (1985) *Out of Pocket*, SCCL, Glasgow.

Rocha, J. (1968) *Organizers of Voluntary Services in Hospitals*, King Edward's Hospital Fund, London.

Further reading

Avebury, K. (1986) *Volunteers in Mental Health*, Volunteer Centre, Berkhamsted.

Bradshaw, M. and Davis, A. (1986) *Not a Penny to Call my Own*, King Edward's Hospital Fund & Disability Alliance, London.

Dartington, T. (1978) *Volunteers and Psychiatric Aftercare*, Volunteer Centre, Berkhamsted.

DHSS (1971) HM(71)90, *Patients' Moneys*, DHSS, London.

Donabedian, D. (1980) What students should know about the health and welfare systems, *Nursing Outlook*, Vol. 28, no. 2, pp. 122–5.

Gay, P. and Pitkeathley, J. (1982) *Mobilising Voluntary Resources – the Work of the Voluntary Services Coordinator*, King's Fund Centre, London.

Gay, P. and Pitkeathley, J. (1982) *Just Like a Friend: Befriending Discharged Psychiatric Patients*, King Edward's Hospital Fund, London.

Gostin, L. and Rassaby, E. (1980) *Representing the Mentally Ill and Handicapped*, Quartermaine House, Sunbury.

Gostin, L., Rassaby, E. and Buchan, A. (1984) *Mental Health: Tribunal Procedure*, Longman, London.

MIND (1983) *Money in Hospital: The Incomes of People Living in Long Stay Hospitals*, National Association for Mental Health, London.

MIND (1986) *Guidelines for Training Volunteers*, National Association for Mental Health, London.

Ministry of Health (1953) *The Reception and Welfare of In-Patients in Hospitals*, HMSO, London.

Morby, G. (1982) *Know how to Find out your Rights*, Pluto Press, London.

Pitkeathley, J. (1983) *Community Service Volunteers in Hospitals*, King Edward's Hospital Fund, London.

Shearer, A. (1976) *The Poor in Hospital*, Disability Alliance, London.

Skeet, M. and Crout, E. (1977) *Health Needs Help*, Blackwell, Oxford.

22

Reporting Between Shifts

DEFINITION

The report, to be communicated at the start of a shift, is the summary of current information about all the patients in a ward to enable nurses coming on duty safely to take over responsibility should circumstances temporarily prevent access to more detailed information. It routinely happens at changeovers of shifts between night and morning staff, morning and evening staff, and evening and night staff. The time available is usually short, say fifteen minutes, and so the delivery of information must be accurate, brief and clear.

DISCUSSION

Because the report represents the handing over of responsibility it is performed by the nurse in charge of the ward (the senior registered nurse on duty). Those listening are all the nurses coming on duty led by the senior registered nurse for that shift. It can be helpful for the ward doctors to listen to the midday report.

The report is a summary by the nurse in charge. The nurses responsible for individual patient care maintain their own documentation in the nursing record.

The report is an activity distinct from case-oriented teaching sessions, care planning sessions, evaluations of nursing performance, management discussions, case conferences or presentations. Its objective is the accurate transmission of information as free from interference as possible (Gagneaux and Shaver, 1977). Questions, therefore, are asked only for the purpose of clarifying points of information, and discussion is kept for the meetings which have it as their aim. Interruptions rarely clarify what is being transmitted, unless they prompt or consist of factual information which supersedes that being given by the reporting nurse.

Safety

The nurse in charge of the outgoing shift is responsible for ensuring that nurses have conducted a safety check of:
1 all fire exits;
2 all fire equipment;
3 kitchens;
4 bathrooms;
5 sleeping and communal areas;
and that the whereabouts and well-being of all patients on the current bed-state are accounted for.

The nurse in charge of the incoming shift is responsible for ensuring that the incoming nurses conduct their own safety check, and that the complement of the patients corresponds to the information given by the outgoing nurses.

GUIDELINES: REPORTING BETWEEN SHIFTS

Action	Rationale
1 Start the report promptly.	(a) To enable nurses to get off duty on time. (b) To ensure that any meeting which follows the report starts on time.
2 The senior registered nurse on duty in the outgoing shift gives the report.	He or she is accountable for the information delivered to the senior registered nurse on the incoming shift.
3 For reports between the morning and evening staff, and the evening and night staff, the next most senior nurse on duty answers the telephone and deals with other interruptions.	(a) In order to prevent interruptions to the report. (b) This nurse will be competent to deal with most matters that arise without interrupting the nurse in charge.
4 For reports where the outgoing shift consists of only two nurses, the second nurse remains in the patient area of the ward, while the next most senior nurse on the incoming shift deals with the telephone and other interruptions.	Nurses from the outgoing shift remain responsible for patient safety until the incoming shift has the information necessary to take over responsibility safely.
5 Use the following headings to give the report for each patient: (i) safety; (ii) permission to go out unaccompanied; (iii) changes in treatment; (iv) changes in behaviour; (v) review of forthcoming events for the shift.	There may be as little as thirty seconds per patient and information must be organized in patterns that facilitate transmission and reception, and remain constant from ward to ward.
6 State where all information given orally can be found in written form. For example, the ward diary, nursing process documentation (specify which section), medical records.	In order that the incoming nurses can confirm the accuracy of any information which has been transmitted orally.
7 The nurse giving the report is questioned only in order to clarify points of information.	(a) Because of the limited time available. (b) To maintain clarity in the transmission of information.
8 Routinely verify oral information as soon as practicable after the report. For example, laboratory results, prescriptions, incident notifications.	To ensure that any action necessary has been taken.
9 Inform the duty nurse manager as soon as possible after the report if it seems likely there will be difficulties in administering the ward in the light of the report.	So that nursing resources can be redeployed if necessary.
10 Inform the duty nurse manager of any absences of nurses due on duty but not present.	(a) To ensure adequate staffing levels. (b) Administrative action may be necessary regarding the absence.
11 Take immediate action to rectify any deficiencies discovered during the safety checks.	In order that patient safety is not endangered.

12 Immediately the report is finished, the nurse in charge confirms that the complement of patients in the ward corresponds to the information provided by the outgoing shift.

So that unpredictable patients, or patients on heavy doses of medication, or patients with physical problems are not left unobserved or unaccounted for.

REFERENCE MATERIAL
Reference

Gagneaux, V. and Shaver, D.V. (1977) Distractions at nurses' stations during intershift report, *Nursing Research*, Vol. 26, no. 1, pp. 42–6.

Further reading

Damrosch, S.P. and Soeken, K. (1983) Communicating probability in clinical reports: nurses' numerical associations to verbal expressions, *Research in Nursing and Health*, Vol. 6, pp. 85–7.

Hay, M., Drake, N.L. and Lindy, J.D. (1985) The evening shift, *Journal of Psychosocial Nursing and Mental Health Services*, Vol. 23, no. 10, pp. 24–30.

King Edward's Hospital Fund (1983) *A Handbook for Nurse to Nurse Reporting*, KEHF, London.

Lane, B.J. and Rae, D.I. (1983) The prejudice of language: effects of word choice on impressions formed by nurses, *Nursing Papers*, Vol. 15, pp. 21–33.

Mathieson, A. (1984) Wasted opportunities, *Nursing Mirror*, Vol. 158, no. 6, pp. 22–3.

Matthews, A. (1986) Patient-centred handovers, *Nursing Times*, Vol. 82, no. 24, pp. 47–8.

Norberg, A. and Lindsten, I. (1987) The effect of training in human relations on the content of the daily reports between staff in long-term care, in *Excellence in Nursing: International Networking*, Department of Nursing Studies, University of Edinburgh, pp. 214–15.

Parrino, T.A. and Villanueva, A.G. (1986) The principles and practice of morning report, *Journal of the American Medical Association*, Vol. 256, no. 6, pp. 730–3.

Richard, J.A. (1988) Congruence between intershift reports and patients' actual conditions, *Image*, Vol. 20, no. 1, pp. 4–6.

Rowe, M.A. and Perry, A. (1984) Don't sit down nurse – it's time for report, *Nursing Times*, Vol. 80, no. 26, pp. 42–3.

23

Documenting Nursing Care

DEFINITION

Nursing care incorporates observations, interactions, negotiations with the patient and the nursing and multi-disciplinary teams, definitions of problems, plans, evaluations and assessments. These activities accumulate complex records and require a format which will accommodate the heterogeneous data that form the basis of a psychiatric nursing assessment.

DISCUSSION

The nursing process seems to have been first described in Peplau's (1952) *Interpersonal Relations in Nursing*. She described the steps by which the nurse assesses a problem, explores the conditions necessary to resolve it and sets goals to achieve resolution. The stages in the process were seen by Peplau to be performed in the context not only of the nurse–patient relationship, but of the nurse's relationship with the multidisciplinary clinical team (MDCT).

Since 1952 many nursing models other than Peplau's psychodynamic educative model have emerged. Perhaps reflecting the fragmentation of theories and concepts, documentation of clinical nursing practice has tended to become bogged down in a superfluity of paperwork, little of which has been validated by systematic research. However, this is not necessarily a disadvantage. Even a well-established schedule such as the present state examination (PSE) contains the proviso: 'using the PSE schedule will not in itself guarantee useful results. The quality of the output of any system depends on the quality of the input' (Wing, Cooper and Sartorius, 1974, p. 190).

It is possible to maintain the accountability of individual nurses for the standard of their record-keeping within broadly defined guidelines. Basic documentation, in line with the four stages of the nursing process, allows nurses to use a variety of organizational systems and models according to the needs of their unit or ward.

The main principles and functions of documentation remain constant and will be described in this chapter.

Terminology

DHSS guidelines indicate that patient records are termed 'personal health records'. The 'nursing record [can] be combined with the medical [i.e. doctor's record] as in hospitals – or [can] be a professional record in its own right' (DHSS, 1983, p. 3). It has been noted in a doctor's magazine, however, that some general practitioners perceive nurses' notes as representing nurses' intentions to work independently of doctors rather than under their direction (Duncan, 1983). Even where nurses' and other records are not integrated it is important that nurses and other members of the MDCT agree their systems for documentation and communication in order that collaborative teamwork is encouraged rather than adversarial independence.

Confidentiality

Confidentiality is discussed in the chapters on confidentiality and nurse–patient relationships. In relation to this procedure confidentiality requires that the nursing record is kept secure from access by persons other than nursing staff and the MDCT with which they work. There is now an increasing trend towards sharing patients' nursing records with the patients themselves and encouraging them to participate in their own record-keeping. This trend helps to ensure that material written about patients adheres to professional standards and remains relevant to their needs. 'The nursing record demonstrates that professionally acceptable standards of care are being delivered' (King Edward's Hospital Fund, 1983, p. 18).

The functions of documentation

In this chapter the functions of documentation are divided into two kinds. The division is made to empha size the general requirements of any systematically planned activity, and the particular requirements of nursing activity.

The first fourteen actions in the guidelines which follow refer to the principles of documentation. The next eight (15–22) refer to the functions of documentation generally in planning work. The last seven (23–29) refer to specific functions of documentation related to the nursing process.

GUIDELINES: DOCUMENTING NURSING CARE

Action	Rationale
1 Entries in the record are written legibly in blue or black ink.	Use of coloured ink to emphasize entries can lead to habituation and diminished attention to the occurrence of small changes.
2 Each entry is signed in full with the time and date it was made. If the signature is illegible, it is accompanied by block capitals.	(a) To ensure accountability. (b) To facilitate information retrieval. (c) To facilitate audit.
3 A confidential record is kept in the ward or unit of the signatures of nurses who have worked there.	In order that they may be identified if any questions arise from the nursing documentation.
4 No writing is erased or obliterated with correcting fluid.	(a) To ensure a true record of events. (b) To safeguard both patient and nurse in case of litigation.
5 Corrections are made by ruling through with a single line, noting 'error' above the correction, dating and signing the note.	So that the original writing remains legible.
6 Entries by unqualified nurses or helpers are countersigned by a first-level nurse.	The Nurses Rules (S.I. 1983/873) require that nurses qualified in Parts 1, 3, 5 or 8 of the register (first-level nurses) direct the care provided by nurses in training for those parts of the register and by nurses qualified in Parts 2, 4, 6 or 8 of the register (second-level nurses).
7 Abbreviations are not used.	To avoid ambiguity and misunderstanding.
8 Interactions with or observations of patients are recorded as soon as practicable after they have taken place.	To ensure optimal accuracy.
9 Where possible, patients are quoted verbatim.	To distinguish between observation and interpretation.
10 Management decisions and discussions are documented as they happen.	To ensure reliable transmission of information and instructions.
11 The nurse confirms with other members of the team that his or her record is a true one.	To ensure reliable transmission of information and instructions.

12 Description of a patient's actual behaviour is recorded separately from interpretations of the behaviour. For example: 'At 11:15 Sam ran out of the day room, slamming the door'; 'Sam seemed angry about losing at cards with another patient.'

So that it is clear what is an observation and what is an inference by the nurse from observation.

13 Catch-all phrases such as 'slept well' are avoided in favour of precise description. For example: 'Sam took 20 mg of temazepam at 22:15. He went to bed at 23:00 and slept until 07:00.'

(a) Such phrases may be misleading.
(b) They may lead to mistaken decisions about nursing care and management.

14 An entry is made in a patient's nursing record at least once a day and once a night.

To provide evidence that nursing care of patients is both individual and continuous.

15 Nursing interventions are prescribed, implemented and evaluated according to the competencies detailed in the Nurses Rules.

(a) So that work is divided into manageable components.
(b) So that personnel are deployed effectively.

16 Outstanding problems and uncompleted tasks are recorded.

(a) To identify priorities.
(b) To specify accountability for delegated work.

17 Targets achieved or to be achieved in the future are identified.

To establish when to adjust, change or discontinue plans.

18 Agreed decisions are recorded.

To facilitate teamwork.

19 Resources are monitored and redirected as necessary.

(a) To prevent crises.
(b) To economize on effort and costs.

20 Areas of responsibility are documented.

In order to control the allocation of work.

21 Documenting the nursing process provides a basis for research by providing material for retrospective study.

In order to provide data from which description and evaluation of nursing activities can be constructed.

22 Documentation smooths transition between stages of work.

By ensuring that immediate action may be taken on identified needs or problems.

23 Nursing documentation identifies and maintains boundaries between work with different patients.

In order to individualize care.

24 Nursing documentation may be designed to make explicit a chosen model of care.

(a) To ensure continuity.
(b) To optimize the chosen model.

25 Patients' own views are recorded.

(a) To monitor the effects of nursing care.
(b) To summarize problems.
(c) To study outcomes.

26 Nursing documentation assigns patients to individual nurses.	(a) To develop nurses' skills and confidence in their use of selected interaction or assessment techniques. (b) To provide information for staff appraisal and clinical teaching. (c) To maximize the effective use of nurses based on their own records of their performance.
27 Nursing documentation monitors group processes in a ward or department.	To identify and prevent non-therapeutic occurrences such as scapegoating.
28 Nursing documentation keeps up-to-date information concerning patients.	To facilitate the transfer of responsibility for the care of patients. For example: when they are transferred or discharged.
29 The nursing documentation provides a professionally acceptable record.	To facilitate retrospective inquiry. For example: in the case of litigation.

REFERENCE MATERIAL
References
DHSS (1983) *Report of a Nursing Process Seminar*, DHSS, London.

Duncan, N. (1983) Doctors are under challenge from nurses' separate notes, *Pulse*, Vol. 43, no. 22, p. 12.

King Edward's Hospital Fund, *A Handbook for Nurse to Nurse Reporting*, KEHF, London.

Peplau, H. (1952) *Interpersonal Relations in Nursing*, Putnams, New York.

Wing, J.K., Cooper, J.E. and Sartorius, N. (1974) *Present State Examination*, Cambridge University Press.

Further reading
Baggaley, S. (1979) Deficiencies in traditional reporting and recording techniques, *Australian Nurses Journal*, Vol. 8, no. 9, pp. 30–1.

Baumann, B.A. (1977) The integrated process record, *Supervisor Nurse*, Vol. 8, no. 8, pp. 29–35.

Casper, E.S. (1987) A management system to maximise compliance with standards for medical records, *Hospital and Community Psychiatry*, Vol. 38, no. 11, pp. 1191–4.

Cowan, V. (1987) Documentation, *Nursing*, Vol. 3, no. 14, pp. 527–9.

Cushing, M. (1985) Incident reports: for your eyes only?, *American Journal of Nursing*, Vol. 85, pp. 873–4.

Farndale, W.A.J. (1978) The law relating to medical records, *Nursing Times*, Vol. 74, no. 28, pp. 1163–4.

Flood, N. and Saunders, M. (1984) The process of recording, *Nursing Mirror*, Vol. 158, no. 22, p. 37.

Garfinkel, H. (1967) 'Good' organizational reasons for 'bad' clinic records, in H. Garfinkel (ed.) (1984) *Studies in Ethnomethodology*, Polity Press, Cambridge.

Gilbert, K.J. (1983) The integrated approach: in-patient records and discharge summaries, *Australian Nurses Journal*, Vol. 13, no. 2, pp. 50–1.

Gwynne, A.L. (1978) The legal importance of nursing notes, *Nursing Times*, Vol. 74, no. 28, pp. 1162–3.

Holdich, R.J. (1978) The importance of patient care records, *Nursing Times*, Vol. 74, no. 28, pp. 1159–60.

Krause, K. (1983) Documentation of the physical, psychological and social needs of the patient/client, in E. Hamrin (ed.) *Research: A Challenge for Nursing Practice*, Swedish Nurses Association, Stockholm.

Nursing 78 Books (1978) *Documenting Patient Care Responsibly*, Intermed Communications, Horsham, Pa.

Oliver, J.E. and Buchanan, A.H. (1979) Generations of maltreated children and multiagency care in one kindred, *British Journal of Psychiatry*, Vol. 135, pp. 289–303.

Raffel, S. (1979) *Matters of Fact*, Routledge & Kegan Paul, London.

Rector, A.L. *et al.* (1981) *Innovations in Medical Records in the UK*, King Edward's Hospital Fund, London.

Report of a Working Group (1980) *Documentation of the Nursing Process*, WHO, Copenhagen.

Schmidt, A. (1981) Predicting nurses' charting behaviour based on Fishbein's model, *Nursing Research*, Vol. 30, no. 2, pp. 118–23.

Sklar, C. (1984) The patient's record, an invaluable communication tool, *Canadian Nurse*, Vol. 80, no. 5, pp. 50–2.

Smith, L. (1986) Talking it out, *Nursing Times*, Vol. 82, no. 13, pp. 38–9.

Standing Medical Advisory Committee (1965) *The Standardization of Hospital Medical Records*, HMSO, London.

Steckel, S.B. (1976) The use of reinforcement contracts to increase written evidence of the nursing assessment, *Nursing Research*, Vol. 25, no. 1, pp. 58–61.

Vaughn-Wroble, B.C. and Henderson, B.S. (1982) *The Problem-Oriented System in Nursing*, Mosby, St Louis, Mo.

Walker, V.H. and Selmanoff, E.D. (1964) A study of the nature and uses of nurses' notes, *Nursing Research*, Vol. 13, no. 2, pp. 113–21.

Weed, L.L. (1969) *Medical Records, Medical Education and Patient Care*, Case Western Reserve University, Chicago.

24

Visitors

DISCUSSION

Legislation relevant to the visiting of patients in hospital includes the Occupiers' Liability Act 1957. The charge nurse is the representative of the health authority, which occupies hospital premises in the terms of the Occupiers' Liability Act (Williams, 1977). As such, he or she has the necessary authority to decide who may visit and at what times. The charge nurse may ask any visitor to leave at any time. 'A visitor who refuses to leave becomes, in law, a trespasser [who] may be removed by reasonable force' (Finch, 1983a, p. 25). (The definition of reasonable force is discussed in Chapter 14.)

Visiting hours and regulating visiting

The establishing of visiting hours is constrained by a number of factors:

1 the wishes of individual patients;
2 treatment programmes of individual patients;
3 ward psychotherapy groups;
4 ward atmosphere;
5 ward space and accommodation.

While it is undesirable to operate inflexible restrictions on visiting, some regulation is necessary. Visiting which takes place solely at the discretion of the charge nurse is unsystematic and difficult to operate fairly or consistently. Negotiation with unexpected visitors can disrupt continuity of attendance at meetings by senior nurses. Rehabilitation programmes can be disrupted by unplanned visits. Patients can be disturbed by the unexpected entry of strangers into the ward. On the other hand, undue restrictions may result in the patient absconding, encouraged by the excluded visitor. Or the visitor may resent restrictions and refuse to leave when asked, thereby compounding the problem by becoming an unwanted and therefore unlawful visitor.

Hawker's (1984) historical study of hospital visiting illustrates the blurring of the distinction between what is good for patients and what is good for institutions. She

discusses the problems that arise because the charge nurse's duty to patients may be balanced against or with his or her duty of care to patients' visitors. She notes too the problems which occur when rules are enforced without the use of sanctions.

THE WISHES OF INDIVIDUAL PATIENTS

In general, visiting hours are designed to enable relatives and friends to visit patients in hospital as regularly and as often as suits the wishes and well-being of the patient. Patients are vulnerable to the conflict which can occur between their professional helpers, who are devising treatment programmes, and their visitors, who may be seen as disrupting them. Guidelines which are clear to both staff and visitors can enhance the co-operation which is necessary to facilitate the patient's eventual transition from hospital to home. The nurse who is primarily responsible for the nursing care of a group of patients is in an ideal position to liaise with them and their visitors in order to negotiate satisfactory arrangements.

TREATMENT PROGRAMMES

In most wards the patients' day is regulated partly by the hotel services and partly by treatment programmes. Establishing a routine is seen as desirable not only for the patient to attend meals or have the accommodation cleaned, but to support him or her in the task of restoring and maintaining his or her capacity for self-management.

WARD PSYCHOTHERAPY GROUPS

The principles of psychotherapy groups are dealt with in Chapter 31. Visiting during group times is strongly discouraged. It is made clear to patients and, if necessary, their visitors that if the groups are to work they must be ensured consistency of attendance, location, time, privacy, absence of interruptions and commitment by members to staying for the duration. Staff members who are seen to disregard these principles undermine the therapeutic effects of groups and risk precipitating unpredictable behaviour by patients.

WARD ATMOSPHERE

The ward atmosphere is influenced by events such as suicide, violence, self-destructive behaviour and accidents, by feelings of patients about one another and the staff. In such circumstances, it is reasonable to expect patients to plan for regular visiting hours, but unreasonable to expect them to tolerate random access to the ward by visitors.

WARD SPACE AND ACCOMMODATION

Where there are limited suitable areas in a ward for patients and their visitors to meet, visiting hours may be additionally restricted to times when the day areas are not being used for treatment activities. Disturbed behaviour by patients can be distressing for some visitors, especially children and the infirm. Disturbed patients cannot be excluded from the ward day areas because of their disturbance. However, if visiting hours are adhered to, it is possible and reasonable to negotiate with patients at such times, whereas it is unreasonable to do so if there is random access to the ward by visitors.

Pets

It is desirable for charge nurses to ensure that the patients' information booklet states clearly the hospital and ward policy on the presence of pets in the ward, given that many patients will keep animals or birds or both at home.

GUIDELINES: DEALING WITH VISITORS

Action	Rationale
1 Before admission, give the patient a leaflet which sets out the hospital policy on visiting and the visiting hours for the ward concerned.	Where there are not written guidelines it is unreasonable to expect people on admission to start negotiations about visiting.
2 Ensure that a copy of the leaflet is available in the ward for perusal by patients and their visitors.	It is important that people have time to absorb information – as they would in a hotel.
3 Explain and discuss visiting hours with the patient and with those accompanying him or her on admission.	In order to elicit any problems anticipated in conforming to the times, and to arrange alternatives.
4 Post in a prominent place in the ward a notice setting out the visiting hours.	To remind patients, their visitors and staff.
5 If visiting hours are planned in the evening (for example, 18:00–20:30), ensure that a suitable area is made available for patients and their visitors.	Restrictions to such times cannot otherwise be justified.
6 The charge nurse, primary and associate nurses introduce themselves to patients' visitors at the earliest opportunity.	(a) Common courtesy. (b) So that friends and relatives know whom to contact when they wish to talk to someone who knows the patient. (c) Observation of interaction between patients and visitors is less obtrusive if nurses make themselves known to visitors.

7 Primary and associate nurses supervise areas where visitors are present.

(a) In order to monitor any noise or disturbance and to intervene tactfully before it becomes unacceptable.

(b) To prevent access by visitors to private communal patient areas such as dormitories and bathrooms.

8 If a patient is not being visited try to find out why.
  (i) There may be an elderly relative or children who cannot be left. Ward staff may be able to help to make necessary arrangements.
  (ii) Visitors may have problems complying with visiting hours because of their jobs, say, and be reluctant to negotiate other times.

Rehabilitation will be easier if the patient maintains contact with his or her home.

9 It is made clear to visitors where their toilet facilities are.

It may be undesirable for visitors to use patients' lavatories because of the risk of access to dormitories, bedrooms and private storage facilities.

10 It is desirable for children and young people to visit accompanied by an adult.

They can otherwise sometimes find unsuitable diversions with which to pass the time.

11 Visits by children and young people may need to be arranged at times other than the visiting hours.

(a) It is essential to facilitate contact between parents and children.

(b) In order to reduce noise and disturbance at the usual times.

(c) To promote a more relaxed atmosphere for their visits.

12 Any decision to suggest restricted access by visitors is taken by the MDCT and discussed with the patient and relatives or friends by a senior member of the team.

(a) So that such decisions are taken only after careful consideration.

(b) It may be possible to negotiate alternatives, but this is possible only if done by a person with the necessary authority to make decisions.

13 Ward staff who wish to depart from the hospital policy negotiate first with their immediate manager.

So that hospital policies are administered consistently throughout the hospital.

14 Ensure that all visitors have left the ward before the day staff go off duty.

The reduced number of nurses at night makes supervision of visitors impossible.

15 Ensure that no visitor enters the patients' private accommodation unless they are accompanied by a nurse.

To prevent access to patients' private storage facilities.

REFERENCE MATERIAL
References
Finch, J. (1983a) Unwanted visitors, *Nursing Mirror*, Vol. 157, no. 4, p. 25.

Finch, J. (1983b) Children in hospital, *Nursing Mirror*, Vol. 157, no. 14, p. 32.

Hawker, R. (1984) Rules to control visitors 1746–1900, *Nursing Times*, Vol. 80, no. 9, pp. 49–51.

Williams, B. (1977) *Occupiers' Liability Act and the Liability of Hospitals*, Ravenswood, Beckenham.

Further reading
Barnes, S. (1982) Onwards from Platt, *Nursing Mirror*, Vol. 155, no. 18, pp. 49–51.

Bloomfield, K. (1986) Ask the family, *Nursing Times*, Vol. 82, no. 11, pp. 28–30.

Davies, J.M. (1987) Visiting acutely ill patients: a literature review, *Intensive Care Nursing*, Vol. 2, pp. 163–5.

DHSS (1971) HM(71)50, *Visiting of Patients by Children*, HMSO, London.

Doscher, P. (1986) When the relative is the nurse, *Nursing Times*, Vol. 82, no. 22, pp. 28–9.

Evans, D. (1986) Flying visits, *Nursing Times*, Vol. 82, no. 14, p. 64.

Fox, C. (1985) Dreaded visitation, *Nursing Mirror*, Vol. 161, no. 14, pp. 39–40.

Goodall, J. (1982) Children under 14 years are urged to visit these wards, *Nursing Times*, Vol. 78, no. 32, pp. 1366–7.

Hill, A. (1981) Care is relatives, *Nursing Times*, Vol. 77, no. 45, p. 1945.

Hughes, J. (1982) Helplessness and frustration: the relatives' dilemma, *Nursing Times*, Vol. 78, no. 23, pp. 960–1.

Rose, L.E. (1983) Understanding mental illness: the experience of families of psychiatric patients, *Journal of Advanced Nursing*, Vol. 8, pp. 507–11.

Sadler, C. (1981) Some thoughts on ward visiting, *Nursing Mirror*, Vol. 153, no. 11, p. 14.

25

Escorting Patients

DISCUSSION

These procedures distinguish between what is offered to the community by specialist nurses and units outside hospital and what is offered to the community by nurses from the inpatient units and wards. They deal with responsibilities of nurses in the second category. Health authorities are responsible for drawing up policies for referrals and consultations with community psychiatric nurses.

There is virtually no research in the field of escorting activities (Hermanstyne, 1984). Goering (1977) noted that the importance of ward-based nurses' activities in the community outside the hospital was increasing rapidly. Hoskins (1986) found a similar lack in a literature review for a study of escort duties in general hospitals. McKerrow (1976) discusses the difficulties of deciding when to escort inpatients, whether detained or informal, outside psychiatric hospitals. He notes the particular difficulties in balancing civil liberties of patients with the expectations of the general public. Escorting is linked with the issues of restraint and privileges for patients, but this commonly used procedure is based, not on research into these issues, but on accepted practice.

Categories of escort duty

The responsibilities for work in the community undertaken by nurses of the inpatient units and wards are inseparable from those of escort duties, and fall into seven categories.

1 Visits with inpatients to their homes in order to collect belongings and mail, to check on security, power and telephone supplies, to relocate or visit pets.
2 Visits with inpatients to enable the nurse to assess the patient's domestic conditions.
3 Accompanying patients who are carrying out treatment plans such as graded exposure to feared situations.

4 Visits to help the patient initiate any action needed before he or she is discharged and returns home.
5 Visits with inpatients to places other than their homes, such as law and housing centres, general hospitals or funerals.
6 Visits to patients who are not currently inpatients, but who are known to the ward team and about whose well-being there is concern.
7 Trips with patients either singly or in groups: for example, to the shops, the cinema or to seaside resorts.

Who should escort

An example of a policy might state that any member of the permanent ward nursing staff may be designated by the charge nurse to carry out duties in the seven categories, with the exception of student nurses as follows:

1 post-registered student nurses – not alone in the first six months of training;
2 basic three-year RMN course – not alone in the first year of training;

In general, it is inadvisable for a student nurse at any stage of training to be asked to carry out nursing duties outside the hospital alone. The principle of individualized patient care directed by a registered nurse precludes the delegation of work which cannot be readily supervised. Clinical experience suggests that visits to the local shops (that is, less than ten minutes' walk away) can be carried out by student nurses after personally supervised practice, but that student nurses who are allowed to escort patients further afield are being put at risk along with the patient.

Restrictions on patients leaving the hospital

When a patient is admitted to hospital, an implied agreement exists between him or her and the staff whereby he or she accepts certain restrictions to enable the hospital to run smoothly according to its policies and procedures. It is usually helpful to make aspects of this agreement explicit, especially in the case of those patients staff wish to remain accompanied outside the ward or unit.

To carry out a full assessment of patients safely, nurses may ask them to leave the hospital premises only in the company of a nurse. A wide range of caution and vigilance is expressed in this request, from a slight concern to major apprehension about an individual's capacity to keep him- or herself safe. It is not the student nurse's responsibility to conduct the assessment, which identifies how much restriction and observation the patient will be subject to, or to decide when that restriction or observation will be applied. The risk in allowing student nurses to accompany patients outside the hospital is that they are being asked to assume a responsibility which exceeds any authority that can be delegated to them, particularly if the reason for accompanying the patient is to do with doubts about his or her safety when alone.

GUIDELINES: ESCORTING A PATIENT

Action	Rationale
1 Determine whether the patient will be asked to refrain from leaving the ward alone.	In order that the team is clear about the responsibilities of supervising nurses.
2 Negotiate with the patient his or her agreement to any restrictions on his or her freedom of movement. Most patients accept the need to be accompanied during the early part of their admission.	Not all patients thought to be at risk are detained under sections of the Mental Health Act. The nurse can remind a patient who has agreed to refrain from leaving the ward unaccompanied. Such a reminder introduces further discussion with the patient about the management of the risk which he or she apparently presents. The discussion provides the opportunity to reassess the risk and the need for the patient to be accompanied or not when he or she leaves the ward.
3 Ensure that the nature of any restrictions are clearly recorded and are easily accessible in the nursing record.	In order that nurses taking over responsibility for the patient can confirm the nursing management.
4 Ensure that the record of any restrictions is reviewed and updated at least every seven days.	To respond to changes in the patient.
5 Ensure that the record is signed by a registered nurse and the patient's doctor.	To ensure proper delegation of authority.
6 When a patient requests to go out, check whether there is any restriction on his or her freedom of movement.	Patients often forget that they have agreed to be accompanied by a nurse on even short trips outside the ward.
7 Encourage the patient to make plans in advance for going out.	To avoid frustration and disappointment if there is no one available to accompany him or her.

8   Ensure that both patients and nurses know and understand the hospital policy restrictions on escorting of patients by learner nurses. The ward information booklet and the admission procedure may be used.

Nurses are more likely to be able later to negotiate successfully with patients arrangements for going out.

9   Adhere strictly to any hospital policy regarding the grades of nurses in training and of assistants who may be allowed to undertake escorting duties.

In order that only nurses who can be held accountable are made responsible for escorting patients.

10   If there is no nurse of the required category available, let the patient know immediately.

It is discourteous to keep a person waiting for a negative answer and it is likely to lead to management problems.

11   Nurses who are excluded by the hospital policy from escorting patients alone may go out with them provided that they are accompanied by a registered mental nurse on the permanent staff.

The preparation of learner nurses for Parts 1, 3, 5 or 8 of the register may be directed only by nurses qualified in that part of the register for which the student is preparing.

12   If the patient to be escorted is to travel by a privately hired car or taxi, the team will discuss how many nurses are required to carry out the escort.

More than one nurse may be needed because of the potential risk of a patient who might jump out of the car. This is less likely to be possible if a nurse sits either side of him or her.

13   The escorting nurse(s) will try to agree with the patient that he or she will refrain from absconding during the journey to be undertaken.

The patient's ability to agree to refrain from absconding provides the basis for deciding how safe it is to carry out the escort.

REFERENCE MATERIAL
References

Goering, P. (1977) A study of nursing staff off-ward community activities, *Journal of Psychiatric Nursing*, Vol. 15, no. 3, pp. 23–5.

Hermanstyne, L. (1984) Escorting mentally ill patients: ignored nursing function, *Dimensions*, Vol. 61, no. 12, pp. 30–1.

Hoskins, M.R. (1986) A study of escort duties undertaken by nursing staff accompanying patients outwith the hospital, *Nursing Research Abstracts*, Vol. 8, no. 3, p. 5.

McKerrow, L.W. (1976) The dilemma of psychiatric hospitals: patients' rights versus public safety, *Hospital Administration in Canada*, Vol. 18, no. 3, pp. 67–8.

Further reading

McIndoe, K.I. (1986) Why psychiatric patients go AWOL, *Journal of Psychosocial Nursing and Mental Health Services*, Vol. 26, no. 1, pp. 16–20.

26

Searching Patients' Property

DISCUSSION

In relation to being searched, patients have two rights which often conflict: the right not to be searched (common law sanctity of the person); and the right not to harm themselves when they appear not to be fully competent as a result of mental disorder (which is subject to the Mental Health Act 1983). An obligation which applies to both patients and staff is to ensure that no harm will be done to other people as a result of patients' actions. When suicide was decriminalized (Suicide Act 1961), the power of search by staff was significantly reduced, although it remains a criminal offence knowingly to assist a person to kill themselves.

The implied agreement between patients and staff

When patients are admitted to hospital, there is an implied agreement between them and the staff whereby they accept certain restrictions in order to enable the hospital to be run smoothly. Hospital staff may generally inspect patients' rooms to ensure that hotel services and hygiene can be maintained at required standards and to comply with statutes such as the Fire Prevention Act 1971. However, they may not routinely search patients or their belongings without consent.

Disruption of hospital routine by informal patients may be trying, but locking them up, restraining and searching them without consent are not permissible ways of preventing such disruption. Detention under the Mental Health Act 1983 does not in itself allow staff routinely to search detained patients.

Hospital policies can provide the means of preventing the build-up towards confrontation. The implicit agreement between staff and patients on admission could be made explicit, requiring selected patients to consent to regular searches of their belongings. Refusal to consent would result in withdrawal of the offer of admission or in discharge from hospital in the case of informal inpatients.

PATIENTS WHO DO NOT AGREE

The management of detained patients who do not consent to searches and will not comply with other hospital routines and policies is more problematic, since it is unlikely that they can be discharged so readily as informal patients. Nurses have a responsibility to make every effort to negotiate compliance as part of the planned nursing care of individual patients rather than by the imposition of rules and routine.

Fire and theft

In sleeping areas, the risk of fire carries with it the risk of loss of life if one breaks out. Hospital policy would require all patients to consent to refrain from smoking and from keeping matches and lighters in sleeping areas. Refusal to consent would result in withdrawal of the offer of admission or in discharge from hospital in the case of people who are already inpatients. Routine searches for matches, lighters and cigarettes cannot be conducted without the patient's consent. Again, nurses are responsible for negotiating with detained patients compromises between coercion and non-compliance.

There are circumstances when other patients may suffer thefts and call in police to investigate. Often patients will agree to nurses checking their property – searching it – in order to demonstrate their innocence. The police may be happy to leave this procedure in the hands of the ward nurses. The patient who makes the complaint of theft remains free to pursue the matter with the police regardless of the outcome of the nurses' check. The police require a warrant from a magistrate before they may search an inpatient's belongings.

The decision to search

To search patients and their belongings is a last resort when management policies and negotiation have failed to prevent a risk, and the risk is of serious harm to patients, the public or staff. It follows that the decision to search a patient may be taken only by the registered nurse in charge of the ward in consultation with a senior nurse manager and the patient's doctor or duty doctor. It is essential that the patient is asked for his or her consent to the procedure. Because withholding consent may result in the use of restraint by staff to carry out the search, nurses are responsible for ensuring that every effort is made to negotiate with the patient so that he or she consents to the search or agrees to hand over the dangerous articles which are the occasion of the search. Since the rights of patients not to be restrained or not to receive medical treatment without consent can be set aside only in clearly defined circumstances of danger, the use of force to carry out nursing interventions must be based on the same criteria as those which define these rights.

Use of restraint

The safety of the individual patient as defined by the nurse's duty of care must not be compromised by the requirement to search his or her property. The restraint must be the minimum required to allow the search to be carried out safely. It would not be reasonable to use force if no effort had been made to obtain the patient's consent to a search. It would not be reasonable to use force if the patient agreed not to interfere with the search. It would not be reasonable to define the search as urgent medical treatment and use this as justification for restraint. Secluding the patient in order to conduct the search would not be reasonable, nor would medicating the patient without his or her consent. Such procedures would greatly compound the degree of restraint and could not be argued as being necessary to achieve the objective of searching the patient's belongings. Forcible restraint and control of behaviour (Gostin, 1986) are most difficult to justify unless there is good evidence of the harm (as defined above) that would result to the patient or others if a search was not carried out.

Restraint of the kind used to manage a violent incident, lasting only so long as there was evidence of any danger, would be the maximum that was reasonable to allow nurses to carry out a search of a patient's property.

GUIDELINES: SEARCHING A PATIENT'S PROPERTY

Action

1   Any decision to search a patient is co-ordinated by the senior registered nurse on duty.

2   In order to decide whether to search a patient, the senior registered nurse on duty consults with the line manager, the patient's doctor, and any other member of the team as necessary.

3   Any search is carried out by the senior registered nurse on duty together with another registered nurse, whether a colleague from the ward or from elsewhere in the hospital.

4   The following criteria are used to decide whether to search a patient or his or her belongings:
   (i)   Has consent been given?
   (ii) Is serious harm feared for the patient, or any other person, including staff?

Rationale

Because of the legal problems which surround the procedure it is co-ordinated by the person who would be regarded as the person in charge of the ward and therefore accountable for decision-making.

A registered nurse is empowered under the Mental Health Act 1983 to detain a patient only until he or she is assessed by a doctor. Any other action requires a team decision.

(a)   A search is always conducted by two nurses.
(b)   Since the procedure can be seen as infringing a patient's rights, the nurses carrying it out have first-level qualifications and therefore access to professional indemnity insurance.

(a)   If consent has been given, the search can go ahead.
(b)   If consent has been withdrawn, the search can go ahead only if serious harm is feared and the MDCT agrees that search is necessary.

5 Before the patient is approached, the senior registered nurse on duty assembles the line manager, the patient's doctor, any other member of the MDCT as appropriate and extra nurses as needed.

(a) So that any necessary help is immediately available.
(b) So that there is no unnecessary delay between first approaching the patient and beginning the search.
(c) To safeguard both the patient and the other patients in the ward.

6 Before the patient is approached, the assembled staff work out an action plan, predicting possible outcomes and alternative strategies.

Indecisive behaviour by the staff will be perceived by the patient as threatening him or her.

7 If a search is to be conducted, the patient is asked again for his or her consent, or to surrender any dangerous items in his or her possession.

Clinical experience suggests that patients often agree to the procedure at this point.

8 The nurses conducting the search use the property retained book and the receipt and deposit book to record the possessions searched and any items removed for safe-keeping.

The search is a version of the property check carried out on admission, and requires the same safeguards.

9 If possible the search is conducted in the presence of the patient.

Clinical experience suggests that even resistant patients find this marginally more acceptable.

10 The nurse conducting the search explains as clearly as possible to the patient the reasons for carrying it out.

Patients who have immediate difficulties in accepting the explanation may later accept it after considering it further.

11 A search to find allegedly stolen property which is not believed to be dangerous may not be carried out without a patient's consent.

(a) Nurses do not have any authority to conduct such a search.
(b) Even if another patient has called the police in to investigate an alleged theft, the police have no authority to make a search without a warrant.

12 Any drugs removed from a patient's possession are taken to the pharmacy for disposal after consultation with the pharmacy manager.

No drugs other than ward stock may be stored in the ward drug cupboard.

13 Any weapons or similar are taken to the general office, deposited in the hospital safe and a receipt obtained.

When the patient is discharged from hospital the dangerous items will be returned to him or her in the presence of the police, who are then responsible for deciding what action to take if any.

REFERENCE MATERIAL
Reference
Gostin, L. (1986) *Institutions Observed*, King Edward's Hospital Fund, London.

Further reading
Alexis, A. (1986) Body searches and the right to privacy, *Journal of Psychosocial Nursing and Mental Health Services*, Vol. 24, no. 11, pp. 21–5.
George, J.E. (1980) Search and seizure, *Journal of Emergency Nursing*, Vol. 6, no. 3, p. 26.
Gostin, L. (1986) *Mental Health Services: Law and Practice*, Shaw and Sons, London.

27

Transferring Patients Within and Between Hospitals

DEFINITION

Transferring is defined as the planned movement of inpatients from the care of one ward or unit to another within the same hospital; or from the care of one hospital to another.

DISCUSSION

Not a great deal of nursing literature exists concerning the effects on psychiatric patients of transferring them between wards and between institutions. Investigations have been conducted into the effects of transfer to general medical or surgical wards from intensive care units. It is suggested that to move away from a place where nurses are visible and always available intensifies in patients any feelings of powerlessness. Transfer may be perceived by patients as an invasion of their privacy. Hare (1976) summarizes research which shows that groups assimilate newcomers more readily if the change has been expected, the group's life has been pleasant, and the newcomer is reasonably similar to other members. Other research summarized by Hare (1976) indicates the problems associated with role transition for individuals giving up one role for another. Such role transitions contribute to the accumulation of stressful experiences, and Wing and Brown (1970) note that relapse is common in long-stay patients who are transferred to rehabilitation wards, especially those patients who have received insufficient preparation. Muzekari (1970) distinguishes between 'transfer anxiety' which may be regarded as an understandable and normal response, and 'transfer trauma' which is a response to a procedure carried out abruptly and with minimal negotiation. Niskanen et al. (1974) in their study of suicides in Helsinki hospitals warned of the need to investigate the effects on proneness to suicide of transferring patients

between wards (p. 280). Park (1967) devised a patient transfer form intended, he said, to enable the nurse and physician to 'project themselves into the patient's new environment through information which affects his care' (p. 1665).

When patients are transferred between wards or between hospitals, nurses have often accumulated a good deal of information about them. When it is not possible to send sets of notes with the patient, the transfer form summarizes the information necessary for the nurses in the receiving ward safely to take over the responsibility for the nursing care of the patient. If necessary a special hazards form is completed, giving details of patients who may present particular nursing hazards. Examples of hazards include violence, suicide, infection such as HIV or hepatitis B, physical disability or frailty, mental retardation or impairment.

Shugar et al. (1986) identify four stages of the transfer process: planning, preparation, transfer, and adjustment. Using this framework they identified considerable dissatisfaction in patients and their families with existing transfer procedures.

The form to be used for transferring patients (see Figure 27.1 and guideline 7, p. 170) is largely self-explanatory. For the procedure to be carried out effectively, each section of the form must be completed.

One of the main reasons for fully and carefully completing the form is to ensure that a patient's rights under the Mental Health Act are not compromised (DHSS, 1987). If a person is detained and treated without consent it must be clearly and accessibly recorded when the detention started and when the treatment started within that period of detention, in order to comply with the restrictions on the duration of treatment without consent.

RECORD OF TRANSFER

PATIENT'S NAME

ADDRESS

TELEPHONE

HOSPITAL NO.

DATE OF ADMISSION

DETAINED/INFORMAL

DATE FROM WHICH DETAINED

SECTION NUMBER

NEXT OF KIN

ADDRESS

TELEPHONE

RELATIVE/FRIEND

ADDRESS

TELEPHONE

TRANSFERRED FROM   TO

REASON FOR TRANSFER

SPECIAL HAZARDS FORM COMPLETED?   YES/NO

CURRENT CARE PLAN

PROBLEM/NEED	OBJECTIVE	REVIEW DATE

CURRENT MEDICATION

DATE PRESCRIBED	MEDICATION	DOSE	FREQUENCY

DIETARY REQUIREMENTS

RELIGION

NEXT OF KIN INFORMED OF TRANSFER?   YES/NO

RELATIVE/FRIEND INFORMED OF TRANSFER?   YES/NO

PROPERTY TRANSFERRED

LIST ATTACHED?   YES/NO   NUMBER OF PIECES OF LUGGAGE

NAME OF TRANSFERRING NURSE   GRADE   DATE   SIGNATURE

Figure 27.1 Example of a transfer form

GUIDELINES: TRANSFERRING A PATIENT

Action	Rationale
1 The MDCT agrees who will initiate discussion of any proposed transfer with the patient.	(a) To give the patient warning. (b) So that he or she can plan any practical arrangements that are necessary.
2 If possible, the primary nurse from the transferring ward arranges for the patient to visit the receiving ward.	(a) It is likely that the patient's level of functioning will diminish temporarily following transfer. (b) If the patient has been able to meet his or her new primary nurse, it may be possible to reduce the extent and duration of this diminution.
3 If a visit by the patient is not possible, the primary nurse from the receiving ward visits the transferring ward.	In order to assess any special nursing problems that the patient may present (see Chapter 18).
4 If visits to or by nurses from the receiving ward are not possible, the primary nurse from the transferring ward describes it to the patient and answers any questions.	As for 1 and 2, above.
5 If the patient is detained, notify the Mental Health Act Administrator as soon as possible that the transfer has taken place.	(a) A great deal of administrative work is required for the section papers. (b) The Mental Health Act Administrator is required to keep accurate records of the number and whereabouts of all patients detained under the Mental Health Act 1983.
6 The nurses in charge of the transferring and receiving wards amend their bed-state reports: (i) stating the transfer; (ii) informing medical records.	So that the patient is not shown as occupying two NHS beds.
7 The primary nurse or the nurse in charge of the transferring ward completes a transfer form (see Figure 27.1) to accompany the patient and his or her nurse escort.	(a) The transfer form provides concise documentation of the planning process involved in transferring a patient. (b) It summarizes key information which may be needed if medical and nursing records do not accompany the patient.

REFERENCE MATERIAL
References

DHSS (1987) *Mental Health Act 1983: Memorandum on Parts I–VI, VIII and X*, HMSO, London.

Muzekari, L.H. (1970) The induction process: A method of choice in intrainstitutional transfers, *Journal of Nervous and Mental Disease*, Vol. 150, no. 6, pp. 419–22.

Niskanen, P., Lönnqvist, J., Achté, K. and Rinta-Mänty, R. (1974) Suicides in Helsinki hospitals 1964–1972, *Psychiatria Fennica*, pp. 275–80.

Park, W.E. (1967) Patient transfer form, *American Journal of Nursing*, Vol. 67, pp. 1665–8.

Shugar, G. (1986) Moving experiences: A model for inpatient transfer based on interviews with patients and their families, *Hospital and Community Psychiatry*, Vol. 37, no. 10, pp. 1035–40.

Wing, T.K. and Brown, G.W. (1970) *Institutionalism and Schizophrenia: A Comparative Study of Three Mental Hospitals 1960–1968*, Cambridge University Press.

Further reading

Fanslow, C. and Masset, E. (1979) Building staff rapport between institutions, *American Journal of Nursing*, Vol. 79, pp. 1441–5.

Lethbridge, B., Somboon, O. and Shea, H.L. (1976) The transfer process, *Canadian Nurse*, Vol. 72, no. 10, pp. 39–40.

Parnell, J. (1982) Continuity and communication 1, *Nursing Times*, Vol. 78, no. 9, pp. 33–6.

Parnell, J. (1982) Continuity and communication 2, *Nursing Times*, Vol. 78, no. 10, pp. 37–40.

Potterton, D. (1984) The yawning gap, *Nursing Times*, Vol. 80, no. 32, pp. 34–5.

Smith, B.A. (1986) When is 'confusion' translocation syndrome?, *American Journal of Nursing*, Vol. 86, pp. 1280–1.

Smith, D.S. (1985) Admitting, transfer and discharge: capturing savings from system design, *Nursing Management*, Vol. 16, no. 5, pp. 25–33.

Smith, M.C. (1976) Patient responses to being transferred during hospitalization, *Nursing Research*, Vol. 25, no. 3, pp. 192–6.

28

Patients who Die in Hospital

DISCUSSION

It is difficult to generalize about death and mental hospitals, because the necessary research into available data does not exist. Clinical experience suggests that there may be two broad categories: expected and sudden death. Examples of expected deaths include those of elderly mentally infirm patients, or of younger mentally disordered patients whose illness is characterized by an increased morbidity. Examples of sudden deaths are suicide, cardiac and respiratory arrests in younger patients in whom cardiovascular or other disease had been undiagnosed, and deaths by violence.

Expected deaths

When a patient's death is expected, nurses have available an extensive literature on which to base their preparation, and which stems, in the UK, from the work of Saunders (1959). Assessment of dying patients and their families is often based on one of the many models of stress which exist (Teesdale, 1985). Kübler-Ross's (1970) model of the stages of grief and dying is widely used by nurses to plan the care of dying patients and the interaction with their relatives. Hacking (1981) emphasizes the importance of communication skills in assessing patients' needs and implementing nursing care. Nurses may need help to identify and manage their own personal anxieties about death in order to be able to provide care for the dying person (Denton and Wisenbacker, 1977; Ross, 1978; Mood and Lakin, 1979; Stoller, 1980).

THANATOLOGICAL COUNSELLING

The nurse's work with families and friends of dying patients highlights the problem of who is a client and who is a patient. Work with relatives continues after the identified patient has died. The way in which nurses approach the practical tasks of helping relatives through the procedures of collecting the death certificate, sorting out property and monies and arranging the funeral is in itself a form of psychotherapy. These tasks can become the focus of much distress for relatives if handled by staff insensitively, inefficiently, or both (Wright, Cousins and Upward, 1988). Additionally, nurses may become involved in what has been termed thanatological counselling (Lego, 1984). Work with the dying person, exploration of anticipatory grief in the dying person and his or her friends and relatives, bereavement counselling, guided mourning and self-awareness work by nurses all form part of the spectrum of such counselling. The hospital chaplaincy or volunteer services are available to participate in team management of the care of dying patients. Unfortunately, there is evidence that the bereavement support available to friends and relatives in National Health Service hospitals is generally inadequate and unsatisfactory (Lamerton, 1980; Wright, Cousins and Upward, 1988).

Sudden death

The nature of the most common cause of sudden death in psychiatric hospitals is not known. Suicide presents nurses with tasks which arouse very strong feelings. Patients often go away from the hospital to kill themselves, but they may violently take their own lives near or in the hospital premises. Nurses may be faced with finding a patient's body that has been disfigured and damaged by the circumstances of death. They may have to identify a person who has been found nearby, say on a railway track, before the body is removed. The patient may have been missing for some time before his or her body is found. Additionally, the guilt experienced by staff as a result of a patient's suicide is intensified for relatives and friends. There is evidence that distressing emotional responses to suicide may persist for many years, and that counselling can be helpful (Soloman, 1981).

Other forms of violent death may be caused by

accidents or assault. If there is any doubt at all whether the cause of death is natural the police are informed, along with the hospital security service and hospital administration. Issues of negligence may be involved and nurses must be seen to co-operate fully with any investigation.

If the nurse works in a ward multidisciplinary setting where each professional takes responsibility for the cohesive functioning of the team and for the safety of the patients in its care, he or she will be supported by colleagues who share in the tasks of identifying bodies, dealing with their removal, participating in the debriefing process that such traumatic stress requires, and planning the support for relatives and friends of the patient.

The MDCT and the ward or department's nurse manager will meet immediately to decide who will be responsible for informing relatives, who will meet them and who will co-ordinate any continuing support. No nurse will be left on his or her own to decide priorities and perform tasks. Guilt among staff may be prominent. The team may need help from outside to facilitate discussion and working through of its responses to the patient's death. The hospital chaplaincy service and qualified psychotherapist staff are examples of skill resources which can be used to help the MDCT faced with death. After a patient's death it is helpful if the team meets to conduct a 'psychological inquest' into its management of the patient's care and treatment, and into the circumstances surrounding the death (Diller, 1979).

GUIDELINES: WHEN A PATIENT DIES IN HOSPITAL

Action

1 Even if the patient's spouse or nearest surviving relative is not the person the patient wanted to be informed in case of an emergency, details of their relationship, daytime and evening telephone numbers and address are, if possible, still recorded on the front sheet of the nursing record together with the details of those persons the patient wanted to be informed.

Rationale

(a) A wife or husband or nearest surviving relative is recognized by law as the next of kin.
(b) After death there may be matters for which the hospital administration requires the next of kin, such as dealing with property, valuables and a will.

2 If a patient's death is expected, his or her primary nurse will have established whom the patient would like present at the time of death, by discussion with the patient and the friends or relatives or both who are most closely involved.

(a) In order that the patient's wishes are respected.
(b) In order that relatives are helped to begin the bereavement process which will continue after the patient dies.

3 The primary nurse will have negotiated a care plan specifying the interventions required to meet the patient's identified needs and to deal with any problems:
  (i) demonstrating 'respect for the patient's religious and philosophical convictions';
  (ii) ensuring that the patient 'has a dignified death';
  (iii) recording the patient's wishes as well as those of relatives or friends or all.

In order that the guidelines of the Professional Code of Conduct may be met in an individualized and planned way.

4 The primary nurse will have regularly met with the patient and his or her relatives and friends.

(a) In order to build a relationship whereby they can help the patient meet the objectives in 3(i) and 3(ii).
(b) So that practical arrangements can be made in advance and in as an unhurried a way as possible.

5 The primary and associate nurses work closely within the MDCT responsible for the patient, including, when suitable, the chaplaincy service.

(a) The social worker will be experienced in working with families.
(b) The medical staff will be closely involved with the patient.
(c) The patient's doctor is usually responsible for providing necessary information to the patient's next of kin if the patient is thought to be terminally ill.
(d) To ensure that there is harmonious co-ordination between members of the team.

6 If the people are not present whom the patient nominated as those he or she wished to be contacted in an emergency, the primary nurse or the nurse in charge notifies them immediately that the patient has died.

(a) So that they may see the patient if they wish.
(b) So that they can take action such as informing other people, finding a will or contacting an undertaker.

7 The nurse in charge ensures that there are enough nurses available for two to prepare the body to go to the mortuary, one to make the necessary arrangements, and those required to provide nursing care for the other patients in the ward.

(a) Two nurses will identify the body and its container.
(b) Two nurses are required to check the patient's property.
(c) In order to provide the resources necessary for the nurses to work as closely as necessary with the patient's friends and relatives and with any other members of the ward team and the chaplaincy service.

8 Nurses refrain from moving or disturbing the patient's body if it appears that death was the result of suicide or the circumstances are suspicious, and the police are informed immediately.

So that the coroner's office may be immediately informed.

9 The primary nurse or the nurse in charge notifies the patient's doctor or the duty doctor immediately that the patient has died.

(a) To confirm that the patient is dead before the body is removed from the ward.
(b) To sign the death certificate.
(c) To report the death to the coroner if:
  (i) the cause of death is uncertain;
  (ii) a general anaesthetic was administered within the last forty-eight hours;
  (iii) death is sudden, unexplained or in suspicious circumstances;
  (iv) death is thought to be by suicide;
  (v) death is the result of alcohol or drug abuse;
  (vi) death may have been the result of industrial disease, accident, violence, neglect, abortion or poisoning;
  (vii) the patient was a foster child.

10 The nurse in charge notifies the duty clinical nurse manager.

The duty nurse manager will control how information concerning the death is spread.

11 The primary nurse or the nurse in charge informs the patient's minister of religion immediately if he or she is not present when the patient dies.

(a) Special care of the body is required if the patient was:
  (i) Jewish;
  (ii) Muslim;
  (iii) Hindu.
(b) Respect for their religious convictions is a right of patients.

12 If last offices are to be performed by the patient's family or minister of religion or other member of the same religion, they are provided with the necessary privacy to carry out the procedure.

So that ritual observances can be made.

13 The primary nurse or the nurse in charge informs the hospital chaplain of the patient's death.

Even if the patient had no religious convictions the chaplain may be able to help and support both relatives and staff.

14 During office hours the nurse in charge notifies the hospital manager immediately that the patient has died.

(a) So that the necessary preparations can be started to transfer the patient's property to his or her next of kin.
(b) To administer the statutory requirements in relation to the death certificate, police investigations or coroner's inquiry.
(c) To deal with any press inquiries.

15 The nurse in charge informs the portering staff that the patient has died.

To arrange for the transfer of the body to the mortuary.

16 The primary nurse or the nurse in charge checks whether any of the patient's organs are to be donated.

(a) If it is recorded that the patient has said in the presence of two witnesses that he or she wishes to donate any organ, the necessary steps may be started.
(b) The regional transplant co-ordinator will advise as necessary.

17 The nurse in charge confirms with the patient's next of kin that he or she will consent to the removal of any organs for transplant.

The next of kin may not wish to agree to the removal of organs.

18 If the patient was HIV antibody positive, the nurse in charge obtains the necessary plastic bag.

The patient's body is placed in such a bag in order that cross-infection will not occur during transport, storage and handling.

19 The nurse in charge completes the hospital's notices of death.

(a) So that a record of death will stay in the ward.
(b) So that a copy can be sent to the hospital administrator.
(c) So that one can be securely attached to the outside of the shroud or the plastic body bag.

20 The nurses preparing the patient's body for transfer to the mortuary screen off the area.

To ensure privacy.

21 If the patient was HIV antibody positive, they wear gloves and a plastic apron.

To prevent cross-infection.

22 They use identified clinical waste bags to dispose of rubbish such as dressings, swabs or cloths.

So that the bags will be incinerated using the necessary precautions.

23 If the patient was Jewish, Muslim or Hindu and there is no person of the same religion who can carry out last offices, the nurses wear gloves.

In order to avoid direct contact with the patient's body.

24 They remove pillows and bedding in order to lay the patient's body flat on its back with the legs straight and arms extended by the sides if possible.

So that when the body stiffens during rigor mortis the limbs and head will not become contorted.

25 If the patient was Muslim and there is no Muslim relative present, the nurses turn his or her head towards the right shoulder before rigor mortis occurs.

The patient will be buried facing Mecca, and this movement is meant to prepare for such positioning.

26 They close the patient's eyes before rigor mortis occurs.

Because the patient's relatives and friends may wish to see his or her body, closing the eyes is a convention which is meant to make the experience less disturbing.

27 If the patient was Muslim, Jewish or Hindu and there is no member of the same religion who can carry out last offices the nurses wrap the patient's body in a plain sheet.
  (i) They then continue with 33, below.

Many hospital shrouds bear a crucifix, which is not appropriate for members of non-Christian religions.

So that a member of the patient's religion can carry out last offices in the mortuary.

28 If possible the nurses remove all jewellery from the patient's body.

To be placed in safe custody.

29 They drain the patient's bladder.

To prevent leaking of possibly infected urine during transport of the body.

30 They remove any dressings, taking care not to abrade the skin, and resecuring them with low-adhesive tape or bandage.

(a) In order to re-dress wounds.
(b) The skin rapidly loses its elasticity and becomes extremely vulnerable to abrasion.

31 They wash the patient's body, following the procedures for bathing in bed and mouth care.

(a) In order to prepare the body to be seen by relatives and friends.
(b) To ensure that the body is hygienically prepared for transfer to the mortuary.

32 After cleaning any false teeth they replace them in the patient's mouth.

In preparation for when the relatives and friends come to see the patient's body.

33 If necessary they secure the patient's limbs so that the legs remain straight and together and the arms by the side.

If the patient's limbs are not secure they may be damaged when the body is moved.

34 They complete and place identity bands on the patient's wrist and ankle.

The patient's body will not be removed from the ward unless the information on the labels on the wrist and ankle agrees with that on the death notice, a copy of which is attached to the shroud, plain sheet wrapping or plastic bag.

35 They check the notices of death against the details on the identity bands.

So there will be no misidentification of the body.

36 They place the patient's body in the shroud, plain sheet or plastic bag.

For transfer to the mortuary.

37 They tape securely the notice of death to the outside of the shroud or plastic bag.

Tape will not damage either the body, its container, or anyone handling them.

38 They label the plastic bag prominently: HIGH RISK – DANGER OF INFECTION.

To ensure that appropriate care will be taken by those subsequently handling the body.

39 As soon as they have wrapped and labelled the patient's body, they call the porters.

To transfer the body to appropriate storage conditions in the mortuary.

40 Two nurses remove and check the patient's property against the property retained record.

So that the property retained record can be amended if necessary.

41 They lock the property in safe custody.

In preparation for transfer to the hospital manager and collection by the patient's next of kin.

42 The nurse in charge sends the second notice of death to the hospital administrator.

(a) So that preparations for the issue of the death certificate and property to the patient's next of kin can be made.
(b) So that preparations for any post-mortem and inquest can be made.

43 The staff meet to talk with the patient's relatives.

To begin to deal with the bereavement.

44 The primary nurse or the nurse in charge or both explain to the patient's next of kin how to go about obtaining the death certificate, the patient's property and preparing for the funeral; arranging, if necessary, an appointment with the hospital manager, and if necessary accompanying them to the administrator's office to provide help.

(a) The hospital manager will deal with issuing the death and burial or cremation certificates, and any property.
(b) The hospital manager will give help and advice regarding undertakers, the funeral arrangements and registration of the death.

45 The primary nurse or the nurse in charge arranges, if necessary, for the patient's relatives to see his or her body:
(i) arranging an appointment for them to go to the chapel of rest;
(ii) accompanying them if necessary;
(iii) liaising with the staff in charge of the mortuary.

To ensure that they are able to see the body privately and without being disturbed.

46 The primary nurse notifies the welfare officer of the death.

(a) So that the welfare officer can deal with any pensions or other allowances that the patient was receiving while in hospital.
(b) The welfare officer may be able to help with an application for the death grant.
(c) If the patient's affairs were administered by the Court of Protection the welfare officer will assist the receiver if necessary. (See Chapter 21.)

47 The primary nurse or the nurse in charge arranges with the hospital chaplain the preparation for the chapel of rest (the viewing room) for the patient's relatives and friends to be with his or her body.

(a) The relatives and friends may wish to have a religious service.
(b) So that appropriate religious symbols and decorations are displayed, or not displayed at all if necessary.

48 If the death is to be reported to the coroner (see 9 above) the primary nurse or the nurse in charge tells the patient's relatives how to contact the coroner's office.

(a) The coroner collects the body in order to conduct a post-mortem.
(b) The coroner issues a death certificate when the cause of death is known.
(c) An inquest is held if the post-mortem shows that the death was not naturally caused.
(d) A death certificate is not issued until after the inquest verdict.

49 If necessary, the primary nurse informs the patient's community nurse that he or she is dead.

In order for the community nurse to take any action necessary.

50 If there are no next of kin, the primary nurse informs the hospital administrator and the patient's social worker.

(a) The hospital administrator will arrange the patient's funeral.
(b) The social worker will arrange for the administration of the patient's estate.

51 The staff meet for a personal debriefing and to plan how to manage further contact with the dead patient's relatives.

(a) If work with the relatives before the patient's death failed to help their anticipatory grief, the nurses may encounter difficulties with their expressions of grief after the death.
(b) If the death was unexpected, the relatives may blame the staff.
(c) Meetings with the relatives may be joint ones with other disciplines, or with nurses alone, or both.

52 The nurses who carry out the procedures write an account of them in the patient's nursing record.

So that it is clear when the necessary tasks have been completed.

53 The primary nurse completes an account of the events leading to the patient's death.

To facilitate any psychological or coroner's inquest into the patient's death.

54 The nurse in charge completes the bed-state return for the medical records department, showing the patient's death, and if he or she was detained under the Mental Health Act 1983, the relevant section number.

(a) Medical records staff notify the welfare officer who will deal with any property held on the patient's behalf and with any organizations from which money was being claimed on the patient's behalf.
(b) They will inform the Mental Health Act Administrator that the patient has died.

55 The multidisciplinary team holds a special meeting to discuss the death of the patient and any relevant matters.

Team functioning is enhanced by 'psychological inquests' into critical incidents.

REFERENCE MATERIAL
References

Denton, J.A. and Wisenbacker, V.B. (1977) Death experience and death anxiety among nurses and nursing students, *Nursing Research,* Vol. 26, no. 1, pp. 61–4.

Diller, J. (1979) The psychological autopsy in equivocal deaths, *Perspectives in Psychiatric Care,* Vol. 16, no. 5–6, pp. 156–61.

Hacking, M. (1981) Dying and bereavement, *Nursing,* Vol. 1, no. 27, pp. 1168–70.

Kübler-Ross, E. (1970) *On Death and Dying,* Tavistock, London.

Lamerton, R. (1980) *Care of the Dying,* Penguin, Harmondsworth.

Lego, S. (ed.) (1984) *The American Handbook of Psychiatric Nursing,* Lippincott, Philadelphia.

Mood, D.W. and Lakin, B.A. (1979) Attitudes of nursing personnel towards death and dying: 2, linguistic indicators of denial, *Research in Nursing and Health,* Vol. 2, pp. 95–9.

Ross, C.W. (1978) Nurses' personal death concerns and responses to dying-patient statements, *Nursing Research,* Vol. 27, no. 1, pp. 64–8.

Saunders, C. (1959) *Care of the Dying,* Nursing Times, London.

Soloman, M.I. (1981) Bereavement from suicide, *Canadian Journal of Psychiatric Nursing,* Vol. 22, no. 3, pp. 18–19.

Stoller, E.P. (1980) Effect of experience on nurses' responses to death and dying in the hospital setting, *Nursing Research,* Vol. 29, no. 1, pp. 35–8.

Teesdale, J. (1985) Stress and coping mechanisms in families of children with cancer, *Nursing,* Vol. 2, no. 43, pp. 1280–2.

Wright, A., Cousins, J. and Upward, J. (1988) *Matters of Death and Life,* King Edward's Hospital Fund, London.

Further reading

Advisory Committee on Dangerous Pathogens (1986) *LAV/HTLV III – The Causative Agent of AIDS and Related Conditions – Revised Guidelines,* HSE and DHSS, London.

Bell, I. (1984) Bereavement in continuing care wards, *Nursing Times,* Vol. 80, no. 37, pp. 51–2.

Benoliel, J.Q. (1983) Nursing research on death, dying and terminal illness: development, present state and prospects, *Annual Review of Nursing Research,* Vol. 1, pp. 101–30.

Chodil, J.J. and Dulaney, P.E. (1984) Continuing education on dying and death, *Journal of Continuing Education in Nursing,* Vol. 15, no. 1, pp. 5–8.

Demi, A.S. and Miles, M.S. (1986) Bereavement, Annual Review of Nusing Research, Vol. 4, pp. 105–23.

Dracup, K.A. and Breu, C.S. (1978) Using nursing research findings to meet the needs of grieving spouses, *Nursing Research,* Vol. 27, no. 4, pp. 212–16.

Field, D. (1984) We didn't want him to die on his own: nurses' accounts of nursing dying patients, *Journal of Advanced Nursing,* Vol. 9, pp. 59–70.

Field, D. and Kitson, C. (1986) The practical reality, *Nursing Times,* Vol. 82, no. 12, pp. 33–4.

Formby, Fr J. (1978) Christian teaching concerning death, *Nursing Times,* Vol. 74, no. 21, pp. 58–60.

Freihofer, P. and Relton, G. (1976) Nursing behaviours in bereavement: an exploratory study, *Nursing Research,* Vol. 25, no. 5, pp. 332–7.

Fulton, R. and Gottlesman, D.J. (1980) Anticipatory grief: a psychosocial concept reconsidered, *British Journal of Psychiatry,* Vol. 137, pp. 45–54.

Green, R.M. (undated) *A Guide to Mourners,* Reform Synagogues of Great Britain, London.

Hare, A.P. (1976) *Handbook of Small Group Research,* Free Press, New York.

Henley, A. (1986) *Good Practice in Hospital Care for Dying Patients,* King Edward's Hospital Fund, London.

Hopping, B.L. (1977) Nursing students' attitudes toward death, *Nursing Research,* Vol. 26, no. 6, pp. 443–7.

Keck, V.E. and Walther, L.S. (1977) Nurse encounters with dying and non-dying patients, *Nursing Research,* Vol. 26, no. 6, pp. 465–9.

Lally, M.M. (1978) Last rites and funeral customs of minority groups, *Midwife Health Visitor and Community Nurse,* Vol. 14, no. 7, pp. 224–5.

Lunt, B. and Jenkins, J. (1983) Goal-setting in terminal care: a method of recording treatment aims and priorities, *Journal of Advanced Nursing,* Vol. 8, pp. 495–505.

Mufti Abdul Baqui (1979) Muslim teaching concerning death, *Nursing Times,* Vol. 75, no. 14, pp. 43–4.

National Association of Health Authorities (1987) *Care of the Dying: a Guide for Health Authorities,* NAHA, Birmingham.

Pedder, J.R. (1982) Failure to mourn and melancholia, *British Journal of Psychiatry,* Vol. 141, pp. 329–37.

Pennington, E.A. (1978) Postmortem care, *American Journal of Nursing,* Vol. 78, pp. 846–7.

Pett, D. (1979) Grief in hospital, *Nursing Times,* Vol. 75, no. 17, pp. 709–12.

Pritchard, M.A. (1980) A concept of continuing care, *Nursing Times,* Vol. 76, no. 4, pp. 169–72.

Rabinowicz, H. (1979) The Jewish view of death, *Nursing Times,* Vol. 75, no. 18, p. 757.

Shady, G., Brodsky, M. and Staley, D. (1979) Validation of the multidimensionality of death anxiety as supported by differences between volunteers and non-volunteers, *Psychological Reports,* Vol. 45, p. 255–8.

Telban, S.G. (1981) Death anxiety and knowledge about death, *Psychological Reports*, Vol. 49, p. 648.

Ward, B. and Houghton, J. (eds.) (1988) *Good Grief: Talking and Learning about Loss and Death*, Cruse/Bereavement Care, London.

Webster, M.E. (1981) Communicating with dying patients, *Nursing Times*, Vol. 77, no. 23, pp. 999–1002.

Williams, A. (1986) *Procedures Following Deaths in Hospitals*, Institute of Health Service Management, London.

29

Discharging Patients

DISCUSSION

The experience of patients and their families at the time of leaving a psychiatric hospital has been called the 'discharge crisis' (Leavitt, 1975). Her research demonstrated that the communication between a sample of families and nursing staff was insufficient to prepare the families for their relatives' discharge from hospital – which may be experienced by patients as rejection, confirmation that they cannot be helped or abandonment. Ecock-Connelly's review (1978) of research found that continuing compliance by patients was associated with continuity of care and with the quality of their relationships with nurses.

Patients may see their families as being accustomed to being without them, and their families may indeed have evolved different patterns of activity without them. They may be apprehensive about returning to work. Money may be short. After discharge they may be transferred to the care of another team in the hospital, to a community psychiatric nurse, to a general practitioner, to a hostel or to another hospital. They may be moving to a home which is different from the one they left on admission. The rate of suicide is increased in patients who are about to leave or who have just left hospital. Preventive discharge programmes by psychiatric nurses are little documented, but LaDuke et al. (1980) implemented an educational rehabilitation programme designed to cover four aspects of patients' transition to the community: independent living, leisure education, general education, and work-related activities. Their preliminary evaluation of the programme indicates that it effectively achieves its aims.

Kitto and Dale (1985) found that in a surgical ward it was not possible to standardize discharge assessment and planning using existing methods. The variety and number of needs of different patients led to poor timing and preparation for discharge. Silver and Wilcox (1986) found that inefficient admission practices in an acute care hospital were related to part and late completion of discharge procedures. As a result of research in a surgical unit, Smeltzer (Smeltzer and Flores, 1986) recommends that pre-admission assessments are used to identify patients who, when discharged, are likely to be at risk of problems additional to those caused by their illness.

In 1987 the government published a White Paper on the organization of primary health care (CM249). While the detailed proposals are not relevant to this chapter, the philosophy, which emphasizes consumerism and choice, is pertinent. Patients will not merely be transferred like a parcel to another agency in the community, but will be involved in negotiating the referral process. The Report of the Community Nursing Review (1986) concluded that the community nurse excels at considering holistically the well-being of individuals. The illness-oriented emphasis of hospital will need to be adjusted when ward-based nurses refer patients to community psychiatric nurses and set up any liaison necessary to support patients at home.

The practical aspects

Completion of the practical details, such as withdrawing valuables and money, arranging benefits, setting up social service support, settling on any revised medication, being accepted at a day centre or hostel, negotiating when to start work, may take several weeks. They require detailed planning and extensive liaison between the agencies involved in such a way that the patient is able to retain autonomy and responsibility for what is happening.

THE INVOLVEMENT OF OTHERS

Family meetings, meetings with other professionals and meetings with colleagues from work may need to be set up in order to facilitate the transition period. Where the nursing work is organized in a system such as primary

---

To: Medical Records Officer

Name of Patient........................ Hospital No. .... Ward.................. Section................

LEAVE OF ABSENCE – I have granted the above-named patient leave of absence between the following dates (inclusive):

From .... To .... /indefinite period (Maximum 6 months)

Signed .... Date ....
(responsible medical officer)

ABSENCE WITHOUT LEAVE – The above-named patient has today been recorded as being absent without leave. I have instructed the Ward to notify you of the date of patient's return

Signed .... Date.................... (MRO USE ONLY: Returned................)

RELEASE FROM SECTION – I have today removed the above-named patient from Section restrictions. The patient will remain in hospital as an informal patient. I confirm that the nearest relative has been

informed by_____*

Signed .... Date ....
(responsible medical officer)

DISCHARGE FROM HOSPITAL – I have today discharged the above-named patient from hospital and from Section (NOT applicable to patients detained on a hospital order with restrictions). The patient is not liable to recall under this section. I confirm that the nearest relative has been informed by_____*

Signed .... Date ....
(responsible medical officer)
* indicate if not applicable

Figure 29.1   An example of a form for notification of discharge or leave of absence of a patient held under a Section of the Mental Health Act 1983

---

nursing, which ensures fully individualized patient care, the primary nurse can undertake the co-ordination and liaison of the different agencies and members of the team. The primary nurse reports back to the meetings of the multidisciplinary care team.

The social worker is likely to facilitate negotiation with families, social services and after-care services. The occupational therapist will schedule therapy appropriate to the patient's occupation on discharge. The medical staff regulate and stabilize medication and other treatments well before discharge. The psychologist will plan any cognitive or behavioural treatments thought to be necessary to achieve discharge. If a patient is detained under the Mental Health Act 1983 the hospital managers are required to inform the nearest relative within seven days of discharge. In practice the nearest relative is likely to be involved well before discharge of the patient. Although the responsible medical officer completes the Notification of Discharge Form (Figure 29.1), nurses will be responsible for liaison with relatives. Patients detained under sections 3, 37, 47 and 48

are provided for in section 117 of the Mental Health Act 1983, which refers to the requirements for aftercare. Figure 29.2 is an example of a check-list for these requirements.

THERAPEUTIC GROUP
If nurse–patient meetings (therapeutic groups) are held in the ward or unit, they demand skill and leadership from the nurses in order to facilitate examination of the mixed feelings both of the patients remaining and of the patient who is about to leave. Staff and patients may pin their hopes on the person who is to leave, so that he or she is unable to voice personal misgivings about the prospects outside hospital. Some people express their envy of the patient perceived as 'better' by decrying his or her achievements, predicting disaster, with the same effect of preventing the person from expressing any worries. Effective intervention in the so-called discharge crisis requires skilled assessment, since the way in which it manifests itself will vary with each patient.

(Consultant/Responsible medical officer to arrange for completion of the checklist for patients detained under Sections 3, 37, 47 & 48 who cease detention and leave hospital – and, if thought useful, for informal patients).

NAME: .... HOSPITAL NO: .... SECTION: ....

Is there any aspect of this aftercare plan with which the patient disagrees?
Do others interested (below) agree?

	CONTACTABLE – HOW?	CONTACTED?
ADDRESS:	....	Yes/No
GP	....	Yes/No
RELATIVE/FRIEND?......................	....	Yes/No
WARD KEY WORKER?	....	Yes/No
COMMUNITY PSYCHIATRIC NURSE?.....	....	Yes/No
SOCIAL WORKER?........................	....	Yes/No
ANY APPOINTMENT?.....................	....	Yes/No
CLINICAL PSYCHOLOGIST?..............	....	Yes/No
PROBATION OFFICER?	....	Yes/No
ANY DAY CARE? WHERE.................	....	Yes/No

ANY HOME VISIT? BY WHOM?................ WHEN? ....

OUTPATIENT APPOINTMENT? .... WHEN? ....

WITH WHOM? ....

SOCIAL SECURITY BENEFITS ARRANGED?   Yes/No

MEDICATION?..

.... FROM WHOM IN FUTURE? ....

....

IF CONTACT IS BEING LOST, WHAT ACTION?...

.... BY WHOM?..

IF READMISSION BECOMES NECESSARY, HOW BEST EFFECTED?..

....

....

.... BY WHOM?..

SIGNED: CAPITALS   DESIGNATION: DATE:

CHECK LIST FOR AFTER-CARE PLANS

Section 117 of the Mental Health Act (1983) reads:

(1) This section applies to persons who are detained under Section 3 above, or admitted to a hospital in pursuance of a Hospital Order made under Section 37 above, or transferred to a hospital in pursuance of a Transfer Direction made under Section 47 or 48 above, and then cease to be detained and leave the hospital.

(2) It should be the duty of the District Health Authority and of the local Social Services Authority to provide, in co-operation with relevant voluntary agencies, after-care services for any person to whom this section applies until such time as the District Health Authority and the local Social Services Authority are satisfied that the person concerned is no longer in need of such services.

(3) In this section 'the District Health Authority' means the District Health Authority for the District, and 'the local Social Services Authority' means the local Social Services Authority for the area in which the patient concerned is resident or to which he is sent on discharge by the hospital in which he was detained.

Figure 29.2   An example of a discharge check list (Section 117 – Aftercare) (With permission Bethlem Royal and Maudsley Hospital)

Discharge against medical advice

Krakowski (1985) surveyed discharges against medical advice ('AMAs'). He notes that AMAs are considered to be at higher risk than patients who leave hospital in agreement with the staff, but there is little evidence to support or refute this opinion.

Nevertheless, the possibility that it may, in the long run, be thought to be beneficial for a patient to take control of his or her treatment by discharge against medical advice does not absolve the nurse of responsibility for conducting an accurate assessment at the time of self-discharge (Withersty, 1977).

A patient who wishes to leave hospital without going through the usual procedures requires immediate and accurate mental state assessment followed by multidisciplinary consideration of the alternative courses of action available to the team. If the patient's family or friends can be involved, it is possible that their support will help the patient navigate the return home safely. Alternatively, their advice could help the hospital staff persuade a vacillating patient to stay. If the staff make an equivocal decision that is supported by the family, it is less likely to be open to adverse criticism when examined later.

GUIDELINES: DISCHARGING A PATIENT

Action	Rationale
1 The discharge date is negotiated between the patient and all members of the MDCT and the patient's relatives if necessary.	(a) The patient needs to be the active subject of any discharge plan if it is to succeed. (b) Because of the seven-day requirement for nearest relatives to be informed of a person's discharge, it is preferable to set up plans well in advance. (c) So that any programme of family meetings thought to be necessary can be arranged.
2 During the period leading up to discharge the patient goes on increasing periods of leave from the ward or unit.	To identify any difficulties which may occur.
3 As agreed with the patient and employer the patient returns to work from the ward.	(a) To establish a working routine within the security of the ward. (b) Because of his or her behaviour before admission the patient's colleagues may take time to accept him or her again. (c) To assess the effects of any medication.
4 The primary nurse liaises with the patients' services officer (welfare officer).	(a) To ensure that the patient will have money on discharge. (b) To ensure that the patient will continue to receive benefits to which he or she is entitled.
5 The primary nurse checks that the patient's doctor has booked an outpatient appointment and has given the patient an appointment card.	Lapse of follow-up may put the patient's life as well as health at risk.

6 If, after discussion by the multidisciplinary team, it is decided to refer the patient to the community psychiatric nurse (CPN) the primary nurse completes the referral.

(a) So that the CPN can meet the patient before discharge.
(b) So that the primary nurse can fit detailed discharge plans with the CPN's recommendations.
(c) So that the CPN will be fully informed about any potential hazards presented by the patient. Examples of hazards include violence, self injury, infection such as HIV or hepatitis B, physical disability or frailty, mental retardation or impairment.

7 The patient and his or her nurses arrange a timetable for withdrawing valuables and money from safe custody.

(a) Notice to the hospital treasury may be required for withdrawal of monies.
(b) So that the patient takes as much responsibility as possible for an orderly departure.

8 The primary nurse liaises with the patient's doctor to have medication dispensed and stored in the ward drug cupboard on the day before the patient's departure.

(a) In order that the primary nurse and doctor can confirm with the patient that he or she understands the drug regimen.
(b) So that the patient is not kept hanging around on the day of discharge.
(c) So that any dispensing errors can be rectified before the day of discharge.

9 The primary nurse checks that the patient's doctor has completed a discharge medical certificate.

(a) The discharge certificate is needed by the patient in order that he or she can claim the increased benefits payable to outpatients.
(b) The working patient will need the certificate for his or her employers.

10 The patient completes a final self-evaluation with the help of his or her nurses if necessary.

(a) In order to evaluate the nursing care given.
(b) To measure his or her satisfaction.
(c) To compare with other evaluations of the nursing care.

11 The primary nurse completes a discharge nursing summary.

In order to summarize outcomes of the nursing care and to document plans for the future.

12 The patient gives the primary nurse a forwarding address and telephone number.

(a) For the discharge particulars required by the medical records department.
(b) So that any mail can be forwarded.

13 On the day of discharge the patient gives the nurse his or her locker and wardrobe keys and strips the bed.

To enable preparation for the next person admitted to that bed.

14 The primary nurse or nurse in charge of the ward gives the patient medicines to take away just before he or she leaves.

(a) Medicines are administered by a registered nurse.
(b) To prevent the possibility of mislaying the drugs in the ward.

15 The primary or associate nurse checks that the patient's storage facilities are empty before departure.

(a) So that the patient takes his or her property safely away.
(b) Property left and not reclaimed may be disposed of by hospital administrators.

16 The patient's nurses and the nurse in charge of the ward take leave of the patient before he or she departs.

(a) Ordinary courtesy.
(b) To make a last assessment of the person's well-being.

17 After the patient has left, the primary nurse or the nurse in charge of the ward arranges with the domestic staff for the bed area and storage facilities to be cleaned and for the bed to be made with clean linen.

(a) To enable preparation for the next person admitted to that bed.
(b) The nurses are responsible for monitoring the hotel services to the ward or unit.

18 The patient's nurse updates the relevant ward lists and documentation as soon as the person has left.

So that all patients actually in the ward or unit can be accurately accounted for in case of emergency.

19 The prescription card, nursing record and all other relevant nursing information are filed by the patient's nurse in the correct order in the medical notes and locked in the ward's medical notes cupboard.

It is the responsibility of all staff to ensure that records are properly filed.

Discharge against medical advice

20 If a patient wishes to leave hospital where this has not been planned, and a doctor is not present, the nurse assesses whether to implement section 5(4) of the Mental Health Act 1983.

The conditions for implementing section 5(4) provide the yardstick by which to measure any attempts to persuade a person to stay in hospital.

21 If the nurse decides not to implement section 5(4) he or she suggests to the patient that if discharge from hospital is to be beneficial, it is better to have made suitable plans, for example with friends and relatives, and with the team responsible for his or her care.

A patient may agree not to discharge her- or himself immediately if the nurse refrains from coercion and confrontation.

22 If the nurse has decided not to detain the patient in hospital, he or she refrains from getting into an argument with the patient.

(a) An argument where the participants are angry is not a suitable means of rational decision-making.
(b) There is no evidence that patients who leave hospital against medical advice do any worse than patients who are discharged routinely.

23 The nurse will suggest that it is in the patient's best interests to make plans for discharge, and that if he or she wants to leave in the near future, then it should be planned accordingly.

It is preferable that the patient takes responsibility for planning his or her discharge.

24 The nurse will discuss with the patient whom he or she would like to talk to in order to expedite any arrangements for discharge; such as the ward doctor, welfare officer, next of kin, friend or partner.

In order to convey that the patient's wishes are respected.

25 The nurse obtains advice from a senior nurse manager and the ward doctor as soon as is practicable during the discussion with the patient.

(a) In order to have support.
(b) In order to confirm the nurse's judgement about the decision not to detain the patient.

26 The nurse helps the patient make arrangements to meet with people to discuss his or her plans for leaving hospital as soon as possible.

It may be that the patient has concerns which he or she is unwilling to disclose to the nurse, which are worrying to the extent of obliging them to leave hospital, but which might be sorted out if they could take someone into their confidence.

27 If the patient insists on leaving, the nurse explains that a sudden decision to leave without taking advice or making plans is unlikely to benefit the patient, and that the nurse advises him or her to stay in hospital for the time being.

In order to make the nurse's position absolutely clear. That is, the nurse will not force the patient to stay, but advises him or her to do so.

28 If the patient still leaves, the nurse immediately informs the nurse manager and doctor and the patient's next of kin, if they were not present.

So that any further action can be jointly planned in the light of the evaluation of the nurse's actions.

29 The nurse writes a full account of the incident in the patient's record, narrating what he or she said to the patient and the patient's responses and, in addition, explains the reasons for:
   (i) deciding to implement or not to implement section 5(4);
   (ii) informing or not informing the nurse manager, doctor or next of kin.

(a) So that it is clear on what grounds the patient discarded the advice.
(b) To facilitate any future inquiries and evaluation of the episode.

REFERENCE MATERIAL
References

Ecock-Connelly, C. (1978) Patient compliance: a review of the literature with implications for psychiatric-mental health nursing, *Journal of Psychiatric Nursing*, Vol. 16, no. 10, pp. 15–18.

Kitto, J. and Dale, B. (1985) Designing a brief discharge planning screen, *Nursing Management*, Vol. 16, no. 9, pp. 28–30.

Krakowski, A.J. (1985) Patients who sign against medical advice, *Psychiatric Journal of the University of Ottowa*, Vol. 10, no. 4, pp. 254–9.

LaDuke, D.L. *et al.* (1980) Operation homeward bound – a military psychiatric transition programme, *Journal of Psychiatric Nursing*, Vol. 18, no. 7, pp. 22–8.

Leavitt, M. (1975) The discharge crisis: the experience of families of psychiatric patients, *Nursing Research*, Vol. 24, no. 1, pp. 33–40.

Report of the Community Nursing Review (1986) *Neighbourhood Nursing – A Focus for Care*, HMSO, London.

Silver, K. and Wilcox, P.A. (1986) Admission: the consumer's first impression, *Journal of Nursing Administration*, Vol. 16, no. 9, pp. 14–17.

Smeltzer, C.H. and Flores, S.M. (1986) Preadmission discharge planning: organization of a concept, *Journal of Nursing Administration*, Vol. 16, no. 5, pp. 18–24.

Withersty, D.J. (1977) Patient responsibility and the AMA discharge: one-year follow-up study, *American Journal of Psychiatry*, Vol. 134, no. 12, pp. 1442–3.

CM249 (1987) *Promoting Better Health*, HMSO, London.

Further reading

Altschul, A.T. (1984) Safe journey home, *Nursing Times*, Vol. 80, no. 10, pp. 18–19.

Barnett, D. (1985) The information exchange, *Nursing Times*, Vol. 81, no. 9, pp. 27–9.

Barnett, D. (1986) Smooth passage home, *Journal of District Nursing*, Vol. 5, no. 3, pp. 4–6.

Battle, E.H., Halliburton, A. and Wallston, K.A. (1982) Self medication among psychiatric patients and adherence after discharge, *Journal of Psychosocial Nursing and Mental Health Services*, Vol. 20, no. 5, pp. 21–8.

Bowling, A. and Betts, G. (1984) Communication on discharge, *Nursing Times*, Vol. 80, no. 32, pp. 31–3.

Bowling, A. and Betts, G. (1984) Communication on discharge, *Nursing Times*, Vol. 80, no. 33, pp. 44–6.

Brookes, D.J. (1981) A behavioural approach to psychiatric rehabilitation, *Nursing Times*, Vol. 77, no. 9, pp. 367–70.

Buckwalter, K.C. and Kerfoot, K.M. (1982) Teaching patients self care: a critical aspect of psychiatric discharge planning, *Journal of Psychosocial Nursing and Mental Health Services*, Vol. 20, no. 5, pp. 15–20.

Demlo, L.K. and Campbell, P. (1981) Improving hospital discharge data: lessons from the national hospital discharge survey, *Medical Care*, Vol. 19, no. 1, pp. 1030–41.

Derdiarian, A. and Clough, D. (1976) Patients' dependence and independence levels on the prehospitalization–postdischarge continuum, *Nursing Research*, Vol. 25, no. 1, pp. 27–33.

Freeman, H.L., Fryers, T. and Henderson, J.H. (1985) *Mental Health Services in Europe: 10 Years On*, WHO, Copenhagen.

Gay, P. and Pitkeathley, J. (1979) *When I Went Home: A Study of Patients' Discharge from Hospital*, King Edward's Hospital Fund, London.

Giberson, D. (1981) Factors that affect patient compliance with psychiatric follow-up therapy after hospital discharge, *Nursing Research*, Vol. 30, no. 6, pp. 373–5.

Gilbert, K.J. (1983) The integrated approach: in-patient records and discharge summaries, *Australian Nurses Journal*, Vol. 13, no. 2, pp. 50–1.

Glover, J.C. (1981) Reducing discharge planning paperwork with a pocket-sized discharge planning record, *Nursing*, Vol. 11, no. 12, pp. 50–1.

Hartigan, E.G. and Brown, D.J. (eds.) (1985) *Discharge Planning for Continuity of Care*, National League for Nursing, New York.

Krausova, L. and Hemsley, D. (1976) Discharge from a therapeutic community, *British Journal of Medical Psychology*, Vol. 49, pp. 199–204.

Mezzanotte, E.J. (1980) A checklist for better discharge planning, *Nursing*, Vol. 10, no. 11, p. 64.

Mitchell, S.F. and Birley, J.L.T. (1983) The use of ward support by psychiatric patients in the community, *British Journal of Psychiatry*, Vol. 142, pp. 9–15.

Northrop, C.E. (1986) Don't overlook discharge teaching about drugs: lessons from the law, *Nursing*, Vol. 16, no. 11, p. 43.

Parnell, J. (1982) Continuity and communication 1, *Nursing Times*, Vol. 78, no. 9, pp. 33–6.

Parnell, J. (1982) Continuity and communication 2, *Nursing Times*, Vol. 78, no. 10, pp. 37–40.

Price, B. (1986) Giving the patient control, *Nursing Times*, Vol. 82, no. 20, pp. 28–30.

Romankiewicz, J.A. *et al.* (1978) To improve patient adherence to drug regimens: an interdisciplinary approach, *American Journal of Nursing*, Vol. 78, pp. 1216–19.

Schurr, M. (1984) The extent of caring, *Nursing Focus*, Vol. 5, no. 4, p. 8.

Sechrist, K.R. (1979) The effect of repetitive teaching on patients' knowledge about drugs to be taken at home, *International Journal of Nursing Studies*, Vol. 16, no. 1, pp. 51–8.

Smith, D.S. (1985) Admitting, transfer and discharge: capturing savings from system design, *Nursing Management*, Vol. 16, no. 5, pp. 25–33.

Smith, J.A., Buckalew, J. and Rosales, S.M. (1979) Coordinating a workable system, *American Journal of Nursing*, Vol. 79, pp. 1439–40.

Stone, M. (1979) Discharge planning guide, *American Journal of Nursing*, Vol. 79, pp. 1448–54.

Tilden, V.P. and Gustafson, L. (1979) Termination in the student–patient relationship: use of a teaching tool, *Journal of Nursing Education*, Vol. 18, no. 8, pp. 9–13.

Turns, D. and Quinlan, M. (1975) Emergency discharges: their outcome, *Journal of Psychosocial Nursing and Mental Health Services*, Vol. 13, no. 5, pp. 7–10.

Waters, K.R. (1987) Discharge planning: an exploratory study of the process of discharge planning on geriatric wards, *Journal of Advanced Nursing*, Vol. 12, pp. 71–83.

Webster, S. (1984) Perfect discharges, *Journal of District Nursing*, Vol. 3, no. 5, pp. 12–13.

Wells, R. and Snee, N. (1981) Life beyond the hospital, *Nursing Mirror*, Vol. 152, no. 8, pp. 22–4.

Youssef, F.A. (1983) Compliance with therapeutic regimens: a follow-up study for patients with affective disorders, *Journal of Advanced Nursing*, Vol. 8, pp. 513–17.

Part Four

Psychological Interventions

30

Psychotherapy

DEFINITIONS

This chapter is based on the classification of the levels of psychotherapy developed by Cawley (1976) and subsequently in his unit (Ritter, 1988). It is a classification of psychotherapeutic techniques in order to identify those applicable to each category. The classification is being used as the basis for research into training of community psychiatric nurses and is linked with the conversational model of psychotherapy (Goldberg *et al.*,1984; Faugier and Reilly, 1986).

P1 Psychotherapy

Psychotherapy in its widest sense is coextensive with the doctor – or nurse–patient relationship. It is required in all clinical situations.

P2 General psychotherapy

General psychotherapy is required by all psychiatric patients. This includes aspects of treatment elsewhere described as supportive, directive, non-directive, focal, client-centred and distributive. The common factor is the development and use with therapeutic intent of a professional relationship whose form and content are tailored to the needs and reality situation of the patient as perceived by the patient and the nurse, doctor or other therapist, and to the time and facilities available. The objectives are as diverse as the patient's problems and there is no unitary theoretical basis. All members of the multidisciplinary care team (MDCT) need to be competent in the practice of general psychotherapy.

P3 Formal psychotherapy

Formal psychotherapy depends on establishing a transference relationship within which the therapist offers to the patient a series of interpretations relating the transactions within this relationship to present and past experiences. It identifies and interprets unconscious conflicts and in so doing dismantles defences and evokes anxiety in the short term, with the aim of resolving it more permanently.

P4 Behavioural and cognitive psychotherapy

Behavioural and cognitive psychotherapy are based on aspects of experimental psychology, mainly learning theory, and of social and cognitive psychology. In behaviour therapy, observable behaviours are taken as the main unit of focus, and behavioural principles are used in an attempt to change maladaptive behaviour directly. Cognitive therapy focuses on distortions and bias in the patient's thinking about him- or herself and others around him or her. It is hypothesized that once these cognitions are elicited and identified, they can be restructured in a systematic programme of interviews, practice tasks and homework. Both behavioural and cognitive therapy require specific training.

The four definitions P1–P4 are based on Cawley (1976), Cawley *et al.* (1980) and Ritter (1988).

DISCUSSION

Distinguishing between the levels of psychotherapy

A problem is that much of the terminology of three of the techniques defined above (formal, behavioural and cognitive) is used as nursing jargon – for example, defences, reinforcement, feedback. Although many interpersonal techniques of levels P3 and P4 can be taught and used in levels P1 and P2, it is essential that psychiatric nurses are clear about the distinction between being a psychotherapist and behaving in a psychotherapeutic way.

For the purposes of this chapter it is assumed that psychiatric nurses are not qualified in any of the categories of formal, behavioural or cognitive psychotherapy.

An overview of recent developments

At the time of writing, practitioners of nursing are searching for scientific status, partly through the development of models and theories, partly through research. This search is paralleled in much of the history of psychotherapy, the developments of which remain a strong influence on the practice of psychiatric nursing. However, prescriptive writing by nurses tends to discuss, recommend or condemn psychotherapy as if it were a unitary phenomenon.

Discussions of the efficacy of psychotherapy seldom distinguish between the kinds of psychotherapy being evaluated or between types of patients who are the subjects of the research, and who range from volunteer college students to inpatients with diagnoses of schizophrenia. A 'placebo treatment' is often included in research trials and ranges from reading books to interviews designed to be non-specific and non-interventionist (Prioleau, Murdock and Brody, 1983). Attempts to identify a placebo effect similar to that noted in drug trials have further complicated the issue. The case for or against 'psychotherapy' remains unproven.

In a brief view of psychotherapy outcome studies, Wilkinson (1984, p. 23) notes 'our substantial ignorance of the epidemiological and social context of psychotherapy'. As to the effects of psychotherapy, Erwin (1983, p. 290) argues cautiously, 'we are still not entitled to infer that there is no evidence that psychotherapy with real patients is better than no treatment'.

The growth of behaviour therapy in the 1960s and 1970s led to the development of a 'new clinical role for psychiatric nurses' (Bird, Marks and Lindley, 1979, p. 321). But the practice of behaviour therapy has not tended to be integrated into the repertoire of ward-based nurses. The problem noted by Barker (1982) of an apparent incompatibility between behaviour therapy and psychoanalytic psychotherapy still exists.

Lego's historical review (1980) of the development of ideologies and frameworks for structuring the nurse–patient relationship demonstrates comprehensively how little psychiatric nurses have built on one another's work. Nurse therapists, if they practise autonomously, tend to practise independently of other nurses. Pockets of development, whether in psychiatry generally or in psychiatric nursing particularly, have tended to grow in isolation from conventional practice, despite conclusive proof of desirable outcomes for patients (Mason, 1986). An example of the former is the work being done in a number of centres in the UK on short-term psychotherapy by psychiatrists or other mental health care professionals trained in a selection of psychotherapeutic techniques (Goldberg et al., 1984; Maguire et al., 1984). An example of the latter is the work on short-term courses in behaviour therapy for psychiatric nurses, and

training in aspects of psychotherapy for community nurses (Milne, 1984, 1985a, 1985b, 1986; Barker, 1986; Faugier and Reilly, 1986).

An attempt to generalize the principles and practice of behavioural and cognitive therapeutic techniques was presented to a conference on 'advanced nursing practice' (Barker, 1985). The title of advanced practice obscures its value as an example of meticulously applied psychiatric nursing skills as defined in the current mental nursing syllabus.

The therapeutic environment

In 1960 Bettelheim (1970, p. 26) describes milieu therapy as 'the creation of a purposefully designed total environment, apt to help in achieving radical personality changes in persons who could not be reached by psychoanalysis'. The therapeutic milieu has tended to be described in terms of psychoanalytic theory, but some of the most persuasive evidence for learning theories comes in the form of studies which describe the unintended social engineering by nurses that creates distinctly non-therapeutic milieux (Shipley, 1977). Milne (1986) has approached changes in nursing practice by measurement of the ward atmosphere in order to gauge the effects of introducing new methods.

Del Campo (1978, p. 35) defines psychiatric nurses as 'people engaged in giving nursing care to the psychiatric patient and functioning simultaneously in the creation of a therapeutic environment'. She notes, as does Lego (1980), the central influence of Peplau (1952), but she considers also the psychoanalytic developments of the post-Freudians and the humanistic therapies of followers of Rogers (1965). Recent developments in psychiatric nurse education emphasize holistic approach philosophies. Much of the literature on the therapeutic milieu shares and has built on these foundations (Wolf, 1978).

If the notion of the therapeutic milieu is accepted it is possible to define the psychiatric nurse's role in terms of adjuvant therapy. That is, the work of the psychiatric nurse is a form of psychological therapy in its own right, which complements the therapies provided by other mental health care professionals, so that the sum of the whole care offered to a patient is greater than its parts. Adjunct therapy (Barker, 1985) implies an assistant role for the nurse rather than an autonomous one. However, observational studies have shown that nurses often avoid patients and spend time talking instead to each other (Shipley, 1977). In the chapter on suicide, evidence is cited that patients often give warnings that are not heeded before they kill themselves. Such evidence contributes to the argument for a framework within which nurse–patient interaction fulfils the aims of spending time with patients, listening to their concerns and helping to devise care plans to deal with these concerns, thus being valued as a form of treatment in itself.

To arrive at a conception of this role for the psychiatric nurse it is necessary to consider in detail the definitions of psychotherapy and the different skills required for the various techniques and in different settings, which are described at the beginning of this chapter.

GUIDELINES: CONDUCTING PSYCHOTHERAPY SESSIONS

Action	Rationale
1 The primary nurse attends all meetings which discuss his or her assigned patient.	To define the primary nurse's role in relation to any psychotherapy that is being planned.
2 At these meetings the primary nurse presents carefully documented nursing assessments and evaluations of plans.	In order to contribute to decision-making about the nature of any psychotherapy to be offered.
3 The primary nurse notes whether the patient is prepared to make and keep appointments, to perform agreed activities independently, to take initiative in problem-definition and problem-solving.	(a) In order to help the patient and team decide what kind of psychotherapy is likely to be beneficial. (b) A patient's behaviour in these areas indicates his or her potential for engaging with a psychotherapist.
4 Primary nurses discuss with their supervisors their role in any therapy of their patients.	(a) In order to benefit from clinical teaching and supervision. (b) In order to formulate the differences between the nursing work and the other levels of psychotherapy. (c) In order to define the nature of the adjuvant therapy to be offered by the nurses.
5 The primary nurse books the room or area to be used by the patient's therapist.	(a) So that the patient has space and privacy for his or her treatment. (b) The nurse is the ward-based colleague of a therapist who may be based outside the institution.
6 When the therapist arrives, the primary nurse or the nurse in charge of the ward shows him or her to the booked area and escorts the patient there.	(a) To ensure that the room or area is ready. (b) So that the therapist can make any preparations necessary for the session.
7 The primary nurse or the nurse in charge of the ward makes him- or herself available at the end of the session.	(a) Safety may need attention if the patient is distressed. (b) To exchange information with the therapist.
8 If the primary nurse wishes to discuss the patient in detail with the therapist, he or she makes the arrangements to do so independently of the patient's session times.	(a) The therapist may be unwilling to breach confidentiality. (b) To maintain psychological as well as physical privacy round the nurses' and therapists' sessions.

9 The primary nurse discusses any difficulties in managing the patient first with his or her supervisor, then with the MDCT.

10 The nurse undertakes any form of psychotherapy only after discussion with the MDCT, his or her supervisor and, if necessary, tutor, and with the guarantee of supervision of the work by a qualified therapist.

Sometimes distressed patients are able to provoke and are provoked by conflict and interference with or between members of staff.

(a) Levels P3 and P4 psychotherapy require extensive training and supervision for therapists to become qualified or accredited.

(b) Attention to the transference is required in general psychotherapy as well as in level P3 psychotherapy. Supervision is intended to monitor the effects of the transference.

(c) Supervision is intended to ensure that the skills of nurses and therapists are used effectively.

REFERENCE MATERIAL
References

Barker, P. (1982) *Behaviour Therapy Nursing*, Croom Helm, Beckenham.

Barker, P. (1985) *Patient Assessment in Psychiatric Nursing*, Croom Helm, Beckenham.

Barker, P. (1986) Mechanical faults, *Nursing Times*, Vol. 82, no. 39, pp. 55–6.

Bettelheim, B. (1970) *The Informed Heart*, Paladin, London.

Bird, J., Marks, I.M. and Lindley, P. (1979) Nurse therapists in psychiatry: developments, controversies and implications, *British Journal of Psychiatry*, Vol. 135, pp. 321–9.

Cawley, R.H. (1976) Assumptions and preconceptions about psychotherapy, *Association of University Teachers of Psychiatry Newsletter*, pp. 4, 15–23.

Cawley, R.H. *et al.* (1980) *Ward Six Procedures* (unpublished).

Del Campo, E.J. (1978) Psychiatric nursing therapy: philosophy and methods, *Journal of Psychiatric Nursing*, Vol. 16, no. 8, pp. 34–7.

Erwin, E. (1983) Psychotherapy, placebos, and wait-list controls, *The Behavioural and Brain Sciences*, Vol. 6, pp. 289–90.

Faugier, J. and Reilly, S. (1986) Taking time to talk, *Nursing Times*, Vol. 82, no. 18, pp. 52–4.

Goldberg, D.P. *et al.* (1984) The clarification and assessment of a method of psychotherapy, *British Journal of Psychiatry*, Vol. 144, pp. 567–75.

Lego, S. (1980) The one-to-one nurse–patient relationship, *Perspectives in Psychiatric Care*, Vol. 18, no. 2, pp. 67–89.

Maguire, G.P. *et al.* (1984) Evaluating the teaching of a method of psychotherapy, *British Journal of Psychiatry*, Vol. 144, pp. 575–80.

Mason, P. (1986) Behaviour therapy: mainstream or slipstream?, *Nursing Times*, Vol. 82, no. 21, pp. 55–6.

Milne, D. (1984) The development and evaluation of a structured learning format introduction to behaviour therapy for psychiatric nurses, *British Journal of Clinical Psychology*, Vol. 23, pp. 175–85.

Milne, D. (1985a) Review and replications of a 'core-course' in behaviour therapy for psychiatric nurses, *Journal of Advanced Nursing*, Vol. 10, pp. 137–48.

Milne, D. (1985b) An observational evaluation of the effects of nurse training in behaviour therapy on unstructured ward activities and interactions, *British Journal of Clinical Psychology*, Vol. 24, pp. 149–58.

Milne, D. (1986) Planning and evaluating innovations in nursing practice by measuring the ward atmosphere, *Journal of Advanced Nursing*, Vol. 11, pp. 203–10.

Peplau, H. (1952) *Interpersonal Relations in Nursing*, Putnams, New York.

Prioleau, L., Murdock, M. and Brody, N. (1983) An analysis of psychotherapy versus placebo studies, *The Behavioural and Brain Sciences*, Vol. 6, pp. 275–310.

Ritter, S.A.H. (1988) Care plan for an anxious person, based on Cawley's Levels of Psychotherapy, in B. Collister (ed.) *Person-to-Person*, Edward Arnold, London.

Rogers, C. (1965) *Client-Centred Therapy*, Houghton Mifflin, Boston, Mass.

Shipley, R.H. (1977) Applying learning theory to nursing practice, *Nursing Forum*, Vol. 16, no. 1, p. 83–94.

Wilkinson, G. (1984) Psychotherapy in the market place, *Psychological Medicine*, Vol. 14, pp. 23–6.

Wolf, M.S. (1978) The effect of education on nurses'

views of a therapeutic milieu, *Journal of Psychiatric Nursing*, Vol. 16, no. 8, pp. 29–33.

Further reading

Bandura, A. (1977) Self-efficacy: toward a unifying theory of behavioural change, *Psychological Review*, Vol. 84, pp. 191–215.

Barker, P. (1980) Behaviour therapy in psychiatric and mental handicap nursing, *Journal of Advanced Nursing*, Vol. 5, pp. 54–69.

Brown, D. and Pedder, J. (1979) *Introduction to Psychotherapy*, Tavistock, London.

Chevron, E.S. and Rounsaville, B.J. (1983) Evaluating the clinical skills of psychotherapists, *Archives of General Psychiatry*, Vol. 40, pp. 1129–32.

Cormack, D. (1982) Custodian or counsellor?, *Nursing Mirror*, Vol. 154, no. 4, pp. ii–v.

Crown, S. (1983) Contraindications and dangers of psychotherapy, *British Journal of Psychiatry*, Vol. 143, pp. 436–41.

Davis, H. (1985) Training professionals in behaviour modification, *British Journal of Medical Psychology*, Vol. 58, pp. 241–8.

Denford, J. *et al.* (1983) Selection and outcome in inpatient psychotherapy, *British Journal of Medical Psychology*, Vol. 56, pp. 225–43.

Drake, R.E. and Sederer, L.I. (1986) Inpatient psychosocial treatment of chronic schizophrenia: negative effects and current guidelines, *Hospital and Community Psychiatry*, Vol. 37, no. 9, pp. 897–900.

Farhood, L. (1975) Choosing a partner for co-therapy, *Perspectives in Psychiatric Care*, Vol. 13, no. 4, pp. 177–9.

Faugier, J. (1985) Throwing down the gauntlet, *Nursing Times*, Vol. 82, no. 20, p. 63.

Fraser, D. and Cormack, D. (1975) The nurse's role in psychiatric institutions 1, *Nursing Times*, Vol. 71, no. 51, pp. 125–7.

Fraser, D. and Cormack, D. (1975) The nurse's role in psychiatric institutions 2, *Nursing Times*, Vol. 71, no. 52, pp. 129–32.

Gardner, K.G. (1977) Levels of psychiatric nursing practice in an ambulatory setting, *Journal of Psychiatric Nursing*, Vol. 15, no. 9, pp. 26–9.

Getz, W.L. *et al.* (1983) *Brief Counselling with Suicidal Persons*, Heath, Lexington, Mass.

Hardin, S.B. and Durham, J. (1985) First rate, *Journal of Psychosocial Nursing and Mental Health Services*, Vol. 23, no. 5, pp. 9–15.

Heron, J. (1986) *Six Category Intervention Analysis*, Human Potential Research Project, University of Surrey, Guildford.

Hobson, R.F. (1984) *Forms of Feeling*, Tavistock, London.

Kennedy, R., Heymans, A. and Tischler, L. (1987) *The Family as In-Patient*, Free Association Books, London.

Leibenluft, E. and Goldberg, R.L. (1987) Guidelines for short-term inpatient psychotherapy, *Hospital and Community Psychiatry*, Vol. 38, no. 1, pp. 38–43.

Macaskill, N. (1986) Working out the problem, *Nursing Times*, Vol. 82, no. 42, pp. 42–3.

Marks, I. *et al.* (1977) *Nursing in Behavioural Psychotherapy: An Advanced Clinical Role for Nurses*, RCN, London.

McCann, J. (1979) Termination of the psychotherapeutic relationship, *Journal of Psychiatric Nursing*, Vol. 17, no. 10, pp. 37–46.

Morrison, E.F. (1987) Determining social and therapeutic rules for psychiatric inpatients, *Hospital and Community Psychiatry*, Vol. 38, no. 9, p. 994–5.

Ployé, P.M. (1977) On some difficulties of inpatient individual psychoanalytically oriented therapy, *Psychiatry*, Vol. 40, pp. 133–45.

Quinn, P. (1985) Open minds, *Nursing Times*, Vol. 81, no. 26, pp. 36–7.

Rachman, S.J. and Wilson, G.T. (1980) *The Effects of Psychological Therapy*, Pergamon, Oxford.

Reavley, W. and Herdman, L.F. (1985) Training nurses in behavioural psychotherapy, *British Journal of Medical Psychology*, Vol. 58, pp. 249–56.

Royal College of Psychiatrists, Royal College of Nursing and British Psychological Society (1980) *Behaviour Modification*, HMSO, London.

Ruch, M.D. (1984) The multidisciplinary approach: when too many is too much, *Journal of Psychosocial Nursing and Mental Health Services*, Vol. 22, no. 9, pp. 18–23.

Russell, G.F.M. and Hersov, L. (1983) *Handbook of Psychiatry*, Vol. 4, Cambridge University Press.

Woods, D. (1985) The age of the specialist, *Nursing Mirror*, Vol. 160, no. 24, pp. 23–4.

31

Therapeutic Groups

DEFINITIONS

It is useful to employ a framework of categories of therapeutic groups similar to that used in Chapter 30, in order to define the kinds of staff–patient groups that may be offered as methods of treatment in a psychiatric ward.

Category 1

The ward 'community' corresponds to the basic nurse–patient relationship identified as level P1 of individual psychotherapy. Each nurse is responsible for monitoring the ward atmosphere, participating in group decision-making, carrying out interventions within the community and evaluating them with other nurses and patients. The setting is the ward as a whole, and groups which meet may comprise part or all of the ward community, meeting more or less spontaneously in the course of a day's activities or programme.

Category 2

This category refers to nurses' use with therapeutic intent of group meetings comprising patients and nurses. It is likely that most 'morning meetings' or 'community meetings' fall into this category. There is no unitary theoretical base and interventions by nurses may be characterized by a variety of techniques derived from several theoretical stances. The number of nurses in such groups will fluctuate according to the duty rota. The size of the group as a whole will depend on the patient population in the ward. The content of the group discussion will be as varied as individual patients' concerns, often shaped by the here-and-now issues within the ward community.

Category 3

Formal group psychotherapy is carried out by one or two, but not usually more, conductors. The size of the group will not usually exceed twelve members. It is informed by a specific theory which assigns particular significance to the concept of a group dynamic process, which may be described in terms of a group matrix (Foulkes, 1964), or a group mentality (Bion, 1961), and in psychoanalytic terms (Malan *et al.*, 1976.)

It is assumed that interactions within the group shed light on or correspond to significant relationships in the patient's past or present, and that change within the group can be carried over into ways of relating with other people outside the group. Therapists may interpret such phenomena as transference in terms of the individual or the group depending on their theoretical base.

Two essential factors distinguish formal psychotherapeutic groups. First, therapists are trained or have personal experience in training groups. Second, if unqualified, they attend regular supervisions by qualified group psychotherapists. Groups may be closed or open. Closed groups have fixed membership and meet over a specified duration of time agreed in advance by the members. Open groups have fluid membership whereby patients join for varying lengths of time.

Category 4

This category comprises behaviourally, cognitively, and behavioural-cognitively oriented groups. The therapist(s) agree with group members specific targets or objectives, the number of meetings and group size. Unlike analytic groups, which meet for twelve months or more, cognitive or behavioural groups are limited to not more than six months, and more usually three months. Examples are social skills groups, coping skills groups and anxiety management groups. Training for therapists is necessary because of the skills required to identify target problems, to negotiate objectives to deal with them and to translate this planning into actions utilizing specific techniques.

DISCUSSION

This chapter will focus on therapeutic groups from category 2. Aspects of the theory of groups in categories 2, 3 and 4 will be briefly described before principles of practice for category 2 are listed.

Category 2

Attention to the therapeutic milieu of psychiatric hospitals resulted from influential descriptions of practice in therapeutic communities, and of psychoanalysts' and psychologists' involvement in treatment of patients in ward settings (Searles, 1965; Jones, 1968). These studies identified the strong effects of the nurse as an agent of change for good and bad. Nurses who wished to improve their practice were influenced by the interpersonal theories of Sullivan (1953) as mediated by nurse teachers such as Peplau (1952). These theories depended to a great extent on the work of Freud, and his systematic account of unconscious mental processes. Recent developments are owed to the humanistic or personal growth perspective, characterized by the work of Rogers (1965) and Heron (1977, 1986).

A major assumption of therapeutic communities is that day-to-day social encounters can be used to help patients understand themselves in psychodynamic terms, and that this understanding will lead to improved mental health. Community meetings or groups are used to explore relationships between patients and between staff and patients, in order to promote understanding and personal development. As therapeutic communities developed, sociological accounts of the harmful effects of institutions for the mentally ill provided extra impetus for apparently more humane treatment methods which would aim to foster independence rather than dependence (Goffman, 1961; Spitzer and Denzin, 1968).

Many inpatient units, unable because of their organizational settings to adopt therapeutic community practices such as self-governance, borrowed aspects such as the focus on interpersonal relationships in groups. However, there is a danger that patient members of such groups will be subjected to conflicting demands: of being expected to participate freely and even lead in meetings; and of being expected to comply without too much question with treatment regimens devised by a hierarchically managed team. It is also likely that if a community meeting includes all the patients and nurses of a unit, a fairly large number of people will be involved: larger than the eight or so thought to be the optimum for a psychotherapy group (Yalom, 1983). These factors mean that to be effective, careful planning is required both of the role of the staff and of the purpose of the community meeting.

There is evidence that if staff are inadequately prepared, the meetings can become unpleasant if not harmful, in terms of staff morale and of patients' mental states (Bernard, 1983). According to Yalom (1983) the main danger of the variety of community meetings which exists in inpatient units is that it fosters an 'everyperson-for-her-or-himself' attitude among staff: that is, a supposition that any approach will do. The resulting lack of coherence has prevented development either of theory or practice for these kinds of groups.

Category 3

In the UK three main strands of formal group psychotherapy exist. Bion (1961) has not founded a particular school of group psychotherapy, but several of his theories about group functioning, such as the 'work group', the 'group mentality' and 'basic assumptions', have been very influential. The so-called Tavistock approach was developed at the Tavistock Clinic in London, and adapted psychoanalysis to the group setting, interpreting anxiety or the transference as group phenomena rather than as individual responses. The group analytic approach was formulated by Foulkes, who summed it up as 'psychotherapy by the group of the group, including its conductor' (de Maré, 1983, p. 229). The group is conceived as a matrix, network or web within which individuals form nodal points. The conductor facilitates the group's attention to the nature of communications within this network.

Category 4

As behavioural therapies were shown to be effective from the 1960s, they were adapted to the group setting. The areas that have been found to be useful include social skills and anxiety management. Unlike the groups in the other three categories, participation in groups in category 4 is based on previous negotiation of specific, measurable behavioural targets. Sessions are task-oriented and group members are commonly required to complete tasks between sessions. Progress is evaluated by using measures carried out before, during and after treatment. The theoretical basis derives from social learning theory and cognitive approaches, the latter particularly as applied to disorders of affect such as depression, which have traditionally been medicalized (Bandura, 1977; Beck et al., 1979).

Aim of the chapter

The aim of this chapter is to guide nurses in the practice of groups in category 2. It is assumed that if groups from categories 3 and 4 are used in the inpatient setting they are conducted by people who have had the necessary training, and receive the necessary supervision from qualified therapists.

Principles

Staff members or conductors of a group are responsible for:

1 ensuring that the group has a location in which to take place and that this is the same for each meeting;
2 ensuring privacy;
3 ensuring confidentiality within the multidisciplinary clinical team;
4 making known to patients that material may be communicated to colleagues within the MDCT;
5 writing a record of each group meeting;
6 ensuring that groups start and finish on time;
7 ensuring that groups are not encroached on by and do not encroach on other ward or department activities;
8 ensuring that the number of chairs available corresponds to the number of group members;
9 ensuring that group members can make eye-contact with each other, which, in practice, generally means being seated in a circle;
10 ensuring that patients are given at least three sessions' warning of absences of staff members or of breaks.

Unless there is an emergency, staff members do not leave the group before it is due to finish, nor do they arrive after it is due to start.

Patients are not excluded from groups unless this has been agreed between the nurse in charge of the ward and the rest of the multiprofessional team.

No patient at risk is left alone during group meetings, whether as a result of refusing to come in the first place or of leaving the group while it is in progress.

Groups do not meet unless there is the same registered mental nurse experienced in conducting groups available for each session. It is preferable to have no meetings at all rather than ones characterized by fluctuating attendance by different nurses or by nurses who are not experienced in groups, or who are not registered mental nurses.

Staff members of groups attend supervision based on their written records of sessions.

Yalom (1983) gives detailed guidance on ways of structuring inpatient groups, along with clinical examples of strategies and interventions that can be used to deal with various eventualities such as absenteeism, 'bolting' from the group, sleeping, anger, patients who act rather than talk and psychotic patients.

GUIDELINES: CONDUCTING THERAPEUTIC GROUPS

Action

1 The senior registered nurse in the ward attends all category 2 meetings unless there is another registered nurse acknowledged to have the required skills and experience and who is available to attend every group.

2 The objectives of all groups of whatever level are agreed with the MDCT, documented and reviewed at regular intervals by the team as a whole.

3 All nurses who attend therapeutic groups also attend regularly supervision of those groups.

Rationale

(a) Consistency of attendance by experienced nurses is essential for patients to be able to continue work from meeting to meeting.
(b) Patients may respond to what they see as lack of cohesion among nurses by behaving in disturbed and disruptive ways.
(c) To ensure clinical teaching and modelling to less experienced staff.

(a) To ensure a consistent and harmonious approach by team members.
(b) To prevent conflict between staff about treatment regimens or individual patients.

(a) To maintain consistent standards of practice by nurses.
(b) To monitor the practice of individual nurses.
(c) To ensure that nurses receive necessary clinical teaching.

4   Group supervision follows the same principles as other groups.

Absenteeism from the supervision group is potentially detrimental to the safety of the therapeutic group because it makes the interventions of nurses unpredictable and difficult to support.

5   Nurses take turns to write notes on each group, starting with a detailed seating plan, date and time of the group.

(a) To share what otherwise can become a tedious chore.
(b) To provide specific material for group supervision.
(c) To provide the basis for individual clinical teaching.
(d) To provide a continuing record for nurses who are off duty, so that they can maintain safe practice after periods away from the group.
(e) To provide material for retrospective evaluation of process and outcomes of ward groups.

6   Patients who are to attend such groups are selected beforehand for suitability.

To ensure that the objectives of the group are matched to the needs of its members.

7   The purpose of ward group meetings is explained to each patient on admission and again as necessary.

(a) So that patients are aware from the beginning of an admission that groups are a treatment method in their ward.
(b) So that the nursing staff demonstrate a coherent rationale for the groups.
(c) So that group interactions are integrated into individual nursing care programmes.
(d) The patient's consent is required.

8   Individual patients' nurses ensure that other meetings are not scheduled at the same time as category 2, 3, or 4 groups.

(a) To demonstrate commitment by nurses to a treatment method in which they participate.
(b) To prevent conflict between staff.
(c) Common courtesy.

9   The chosen model of group psychotherapy is made explicit in the ward objectives and agreed with the multiprofessional team.

(a) In order that teaching to nurses of skills specific to the model may take place.
(b) In order that evaluation and comparison of the model in use can be carried out.

10 Nurses ensure that patients who decline to attend a group are observed during the time it takes place.

(a) To ensure safety.
(b) To communicate that the patient remains part of the group even when not actually physically present.
(c) To communicate that the whole team is committed to the group.

11 Patients who consistently do not attend ward groups are discussed in detail as soon as possible with the MDCT.

(a) So that the team can discuss and examine its own attitudes to the ward groups.
(b) To decide whether the patient is being helped by the ward milieu as it is being managed.
(c) To provide a forum for the patient to discuss his or her priorities for treatment with members of the team who do not attend the groups.

12 Before a group meeting the nurses discuss the ward atmosphere and decide on any precautions to be taken in relation to safety.

(a) So that problems may be anticipated.
(b) So that a nurse may be allocated and prepared to intervene.
(c) So that another nurse may be prepared to support the first.

13 A nurse member of the group prepares the room in which the meeting is to take place.

So that it is clear that nurses are taking responsibility for the therapy they are offering.

14 If the group is a category 2 group, the nurses decide beforehand who will call time at the end of the meeting.

So that responsibility for finishing on time is not diffused among the nurse members.

15 Nurses arrive in good time and sit spaced at regular intervals round the room.

(a) To avoid sitting in a line-up
(b) To be prepared for eventualities such as absconding or violence.
(c) To distribute experienced and inexperienced staff.

16 Nurses maintain a posture of relaxed and open attention during the group.

To demonstrate receptiveness to what other members of the group have to say.

17 Nurses warn the meeting if they are likely to have to leave the group, say, because they are detailed to carry an emergency bleep.

(a) So that if they suddenly leave their behaviour is explicable even if it is disruptive.
(b) Common courtesy.

18 Nurses refrain from leaving the room unless there is an emergency.

(a) To model adaptive ways of dealing with tension.
(b) To demonstrate regard for and attention to patients' concerns.
(c) To maintain privacy and structure within the group.

19 Nurses refrain from smoking or taking drinks into category 2, 3 or 4 group meetings.

(a) To comply with hospital policy.
(b) To demonstrate that such groups are different from ordinary social interaction.
(c) To model adaptive methods of dealing with tension.

20 Nurses deal firmly with interruptions outside the room where the meeting is being held.

(a) To maintain privacy for the group.
(b) To provide a sense for group members that their concerns are foremost within the group.

21 There is a discussion of not less than ten and not more than fifteen minutes immediately following the meeting, between the nurse members in private, leaving a nurse with the patients if necessary.

(a) To allow ventilation by nurses of any difficulties experienced during the meeting.
(b) To check out between nurses that perceptions and judgements are shared with colleagues.
(c) To decide on any immediate nursing actions which may be required in the light of patients' disclosures during the meeting.
(d) To provide a basis for the nurse writing the group record that day.

22 When a patient does not have an assigned nurse on duty on a particular day, the senior first-level nurse in the meeting writes a brief account of the patient's behaviour during the group in the patient's record as well as in the group record.

(a) To fulfil the requirement of a daily entry in the nursing record.
(b) To base this entry on personal interaction.

REFERENCE MATERIAL
References
Bandura, A. (1977) *Social Learning Theory*, Prentice-Hall, Englewood Cliffs, NJ.

Beck, A.T. *et al.* (1979) *Cognitive Therapy for Depression*, Guilford Press, New York,

Bernard, H.S. (1983) Anti-therapeutic dimensions of a community meeting in a therapeutic milieu, *Psychiatric Quarterly*, Vol. 55, no. 4, pp. 227–35.

Bion, W. (1961) *Experiences in Groups*, Tavistock, London.

De Maré, P. (1983) Michael Foulkes and the Northfield experiment, in M. Pines (ed.) *The Evolution of Group Analysis*, Routledge & Kegan Paul, London.

Foulkes, S.H. (1964) *Therapeutic Group Analysis* (1984 reprint) Maresfield Reprint, London.

Goffman, E. (1961) *Asylums: Essays on the Social Situation of Mental Patients and Other Inmates*, Doubleday-Anchor, New York.

Heron, J. (1977) *Dimensions of Facilitator Style*, HPRP and BPMF, Guildford.

Heron, J. (1986) *Six Category Intervention Analysis*, Human Potential Research Project, University of Surrey, Guildford.

Jones, M. (1968) *Beyond the Therapeutic Community*, Yale University Press, New Haven.

Malan, D.H. *et al.* (1976) Group psychotherapy: a long-term follow-up study, *Archives of General Psychiatry*, Vol. 33, pp. 1303–15.

Peplau, H. (1952) *Interpersonal Relations in Nursing*, Putnams, New York.

Rogers, C. (1965) *Client-Centred Therapy*, Houghton Mifflin, Boston, Mass.

Searles, H.F. (1965) *Collected Papers on Schizophrenia and Related Subjects*, Hogarth, London.

Spitzer, S.P. and Denzin, N.K. (1968) *The Mental Patient: Studies in the Sociology of Deviance*, McGraw-Hill, New York.

Sullivan, H.S.S. (1953) *The Interpersonal Theory of Psychiatry*, W.W. Norton, New York.

Yalom, I.D. (1983) *Inpatient Group Psychotherapy*, Basic Books, New York.

Further reading
Adrian, S. (1980) A systematic approach to selecting group participants, *Journal of Psychosocial Nursing and Mental Health Services*, Vol. 18, no. 2, pp. 37–41.

Affonso, D.D. (1985) Therapeutic support during inpatient group therapy, *Journal of Psychosocial Nursing and Mental Health Services*, Vol. 23, no. 11, pp. 21–5.

Alfaro, R.R. (1970) A group therapy approach to suicide prevention, *Bulletin of Suicidology*, Vol. 6, pp. 56–9.

Authier, J. and Gustafson, K. (1976) Group intervention techniques: a pratical guide for psychiatric team members, *Journal of Psychiatric Nursing*, Vol. 14, no. 7, pp. 19–22.

Benton, D.W. (1980) The significance of the absent member in milieu therapy, *Perspectives in Psychiatric Care*, Vol. 18, no. 1, pp. 21–5.

Berczeller, E. (1984) A new format for the community meeting, *Psychiatric Quarterly*, Vol. 56, no. 1, pp. 35–44.

Bloch, S., Crouch, E. and Reibstein, J. (1981) Therapeutic factors in group psychotherapy: a review, *Archives of General Psychiatry*, Vol. 38, pp. 519–26.

Duffey, M. (1979) Factors contributing to the development of a cohesive adolescent psychotherapy group, *Journal of Psychiatric Nursing*, Vol. 17, no. 1, pp. 21–4.

Ernst, C., Vandezyl, S. and Salinger, R. (1981) Preparation of psychiatric inpatients for group therapy, *Journal of Psychosocial Nursing and Mental Health Services*, Vol. 19, no. 7, pp. 28–33.

Licker, L. *et al.* (1976) It's the staff that keeps the patients talking, *Journal of Psychiatric Nursing*, Vol. 14, no. 5, pp. 11–14.

MacKenzie, K.R. and Livesley, W.J. (1984) Development stages: an integrating theory of group psychotherapy, *Canadian Journal of Psychiatry*, Vol. 29, pp. 247–51.

Maratos, J. and Kennedy, M.J. (1974) Evaluation of ward group meetings in a psychiatric unit of a general hospital, *British Journal of Psychiatry*, Vol. 125, pp. 479–82.

McMahon, N. and Links, P.S. (1984) Cotherapy: the need for positive pairing, *Canadian Journal of Psychiatry*, Vol. 29, pp. 385–9.

Palmer, J. (1976) Group psychotherapy in a state hospital: who needs it?, *Journal of Psychiatric Nursing*, Vol. 14, no. 3, pp. 19–22.

Pelletier, L.R. (1983) Interpersonal communications task group, *Journal of Psychosocial Nursing and Mental Health Services*, Vol. 21, no. 9, pp. 33–6.

Ross, D.M. *et al.* (1980) The impact of group and individual therapy on socialization of residents in an institutional setting, *Issues in Mental Health Nursing*, Vol. 2, no. 4, p. 33–42.

Ryle, A. and Lipschitz, S. (1976) An intensive case study of a therapeutic group, *British Journal of Psychiatry*, Vol. 128, pp. 581–7.

Sattin, S.M. (1975) The psychodynamics of the 'holiday syndrome', *Perspectives in Psychiatric Care*, Vol. 13, no. 4, pp. 156–62.

Smith, P.B. (ed.) (1980) *Small Groups and Personal Change*, Methuen, London.

Spitz, H.I. (1984) Contemporary trends in group psychotherapy: a literature survey, *Hospital and Community Psychiatry*, Vol. 35, no. 2, pp. 132–42.

Trauer, T. (1979) The relationship between large group meetings and patients' estimates of ward tension, *British Journal of Medical Psychology*, Vol. 52, pp. 205–13.

Trauer, T. (1980) Correlates of patient participation in the large group meeting of a therapeutic community, *British Journal of Medical Psychology*, Vol. 53, pp. 109–16.

Van Servellen, G.M. and Dull, L.V. (1981) Group psychotherapy for depressed women: a model, *Journal of Psychosocial Nursing and Mental Health Services*, Vol. 19, no. 8, pp. 25–31.

Williams, R.A. (1976) A contract for co-therapists in group psychotherapy, *Journal of Psychiatric Nursing*, Vol. 14, no. 6, pp. 11–14.

Wolf, M.S. (1977) A review of literature on milieu therapy, *Journal of Psychiatric Nursing*, Vol. 15, no. 5, pp. 26–33.

32

Time-Out

DEFINITIONS

Time-out

In this chapter the term 'time-out' refers to the withdrawal of a patient with his or her consent from positive reinforcement, or the withdrawal of positive reinforcement from the patient, applied consistently, clearly and contingent on the undesired behaviour.

Withdrawal of positive reinforcement is designed to reduce undesirable behaviour.

Positive reinforcement

A positive reinforcer is an event which strengthens the behaviour upon which it is contingent.

DISCUSSION

A good deal of behaviour therapy is based on organizing positive reinforcers so that desired behaviours will produce them. The target behaviour is identified, in steps if necessary, and positive reinforcement supplied when the desired behaviour or a specified component of it occurs. At first this will be each time it occurs. As the behaviour is strengthened the reinforcement may be given intermittently.

It is necessary to quantify the target behaviour, the amount of reinforcement and the length of time allowed to elapse between the behaviour and the reinforcer. In treatment programmes the reinforcer will usually follow the desired behaviour immediately. If it does not follow immediately it may act as reinforcement to a different and undesired behaviour.

Classifying reinforcers

Part of the detailed assessment required is the identification of events which act as positive reinforcement for the behaviours of a given patient. Classifications exist of typical reinforcers.

PRIMARY REINFORCER

Primary reinforcers require no learning in order to be effective. They include food and sleep.

SECONDARY REINFORCER

Secondary reinforcers are those which have been effectively associated with primary reinforcers and gradually have become reinforcing in themselves. Attention and money are examples of secondary reinforcers.

GENERALIZED REINFORCER

Generalized reinforcers are secondary reinforcers which have become effective in many different settings, originally through being associated with existing reinforcers. Expressions of praise and acknowledgement are examples of generalized reinforcers which strengthen a wide variety of social behaviours. One of the most powerful general reinforcers is social attention from another person. The nurse, then, as several studies have shown, is usually a powerful reinforcer in the ward setting.

Reinforcers may be immediately usable, or they may be accumulated in order to acquire other reinforcers which cannot be immediately used, such as going out. Examples of reinforcers which can be immediately used are food and cigarettes. Points or tokens are examples of generalized reinforcers used in behaviour therapy which can be collected and exchanged for primary and other secondary reinforcers.

A person's own behaviour may be used as a reinforcer by making it contingent on the occurrence of another behaviour. For example, going swimming being made contingent on completing homework.

RESPONSE COST

Response cost is the procedure whereby positive reinforcers are removed as a result of a behaviour. It may involve, for example, fining of tokens or cigarettes.

Positive reinforcement and nursing

It has been noted that nurses' application of positive reinforcement is rarely planned or systematic outside a specific behaviour programme. The structure of management of most multidisciplinary clinical teams ensures that such programmes are carried out by the clinical psychologist or a behaviour therapist. Nurses need to be aware that during apparently informal interactions their responses to patients may reinforce patients' behaviour for the better or the worse. An example will be found in Chapter 13, where it is noted that the attention paid to fear-inducing behaviours may have the effect of positively reinforcing them. Other undesired behaviours may also be maintained by reinforcement, often intermittent, such as talking to a patient who is in bed at times when he or she has an occupational therapy programme. Staff are not necessarily aware of the ways in which their attention acts as reinforcement for undesirable behaviours, or in which attention or praise for desirable behaviours can be aversive for a patient. Careful observation and self-awareness are required to assess reinforcement patterns.

The principle behind the use of time-out is that the positive reinforcers are withdrawn in a systematic way in order to reduce unwanted behaviour. Time-out has been shown to be effective with children, mentally retarded adults and adolescents (White, Nielson and Johnson, 1972; Pendergrass, 1972; Sachs, 1973). Little research evidence is available about its efficacy with adults in psychiatric institutions.

Time-out procedure

A time-out procedure can be effectively carried out if the necessary detailed behaviour assessment has been made, target behaviours and reinforcers identified, and a plan agreed with the patient. The procedure does not require the patient to be put in a special room for positive reinforcement to be withdrawn. Broome, Weaver and Kat (1978) note that many patients from their study who were put into a side room after undesirable behaviour began to enjoy staying in bed and would behave disruptively in order to go in the room. Paul and Lentz (1977) also found that in certain circumstances time-out could become a positive reinforcer that was stronger than the effect of losing other reinforcers, and so had to use additional aversive measures to control undesired behaviour.

The effectiveness of time-out can be quickly assessed provided that the necessary records are kept. A health authority's ethical committee may review the practice of wards and departments which use time-out, so that it is implemented only in the context of a planned treatment programme for which consent has been obtained. Time-out is thus distinguished from seclusion, which is a procedure that is unlikely to be carried out with a patient's consent and that usually involves physical restraint.

A treatment programme which includes time-out from positive reinforcement requires, therefore, a ward environment where staff–patient relationships are clearly defined, where all patients have individually negotiated care plans containing patient-centred objectives and which specify the desired behaviours and the patient and nursing actions designed to achieve them. Otherwise the uncertainty about causes and effects will invalidate a time-out programme.

It is often especially difficult for nurses to develop the skills of apparently disattending behaviour while maintaining the necessary observation and intervening in as low-key way as possible if safety becomes compromised.

GUIDELINES: IMPLEMENTING TIME-OUT

Action	Rationale
1 The hospital ethical committee decides which wards and departments may practise time-out from positive reinforcement.	The committee will include members from the health authority, representatives of the community as well as senior professionals in the hospital, thereby providing independent monitoring of the procedure.
2 The patient consents to time-out as part of a treatment programme designed to help him or her change undesired behaviour.	Consent is required from all patients for treatment (see Chapter 10).

3 The treatment plan specifies the behaviours as a consequence of which time-out will be implemented.

(a) So that the patient knows what he or she is consenting to.
(b) In order to be effectively withdrawn, positive reinforcement must be identified together with the exact behaviour on which it is contingent.

4 The patient's primary nurse, together with any other member of the MDCT thought appropriate, explains to the patient that no warning will be given of the implementation of time-out.

In order to be effective, withdrawal of positive reinforcement must immediately follow the undesired behaviour.

5 They explain that if a specified behaviour occurs, positive reinforcement as specified in the care plan will be withdrawn.

So that the patient will be able to predict when time-out will occur.

6 They explain that time-out will last for a time specified in the care plan but not more than three minutes.

So that both parties are clear that time-out is an intervention which is effective over short periods of time.

7 As the programme is implemented, it will be necessary to identify the amount of time that is effective, usually one or two minutes.

It is not easy to predict the exact duration of time-out for individual patients until it has been implemented a few times.

8 A member of the patient's treatment team will be on duty at all times.

So that someone familiar with the plan will be able to respond immediately to behaviours specified in the plan.

9 All staff agree to co-operate with the withdrawal of positive reinforcement even though they may experience some anxiety when carrying out the intervention.

(a) To be effective, withdrawal of reinforcement must be complete.
(b) It is often used to reduce bizarre and disruptive behaviours which staff generally tackle by increased rather than decreased attention. Withdrawal of this attention can cause staff to feel that they are doing nothing, rather than that they are carrying out a particularly skilled intervention.

10 If the patient behaves in a way specified in the plan the member of the treatment team reminds him or her that the consequence of such behaviour is time-out:
   (i) without making eye contact;
   (ii) without touching the patient;
   (iii) making the link between the undesired behaviour and its consequence;
   (iv) without rebuking or otherwise criticizing the patient.

The aim is to remove any kind of positive reinforcement for the patient's behaviour.

11 While the nurses withdraw positive reinforcement they maintain unobtrusive observation of the patient's behaviour.

(a) To ensure the patient's safety.
(b) To determine whether time-out is effective.
(c) To determine the best duration of time-out for that patient.

12 At the end of the time stated in the treatment plan the patient's nurse or other treatment team member invites the patient to return to the activity interrupted by the undesired behaviour.

Sticking to the agreed time makes the sequence of events predictable and therefore more likely to achieve desired change.

| **13** | The patient's nurse completes any documentation required by the hospital ethical committee. | So that regular review of standards can take place. |
| **14** | The patient's nurse writes a detailed account of the procedure in the nursing record, describing the events leading to its implementation, how it was implemented, and what the consequences were. | So that the effectiveness of the procedure can be assessed. |

REFERENCE MATERIAL

References

Broome, A.K., Weaver, S.M. and Kat, B.J.B (1978) Some patterns of disturbed behaviour in a closed ward environment, *Journal of Advanced Nursing*, Vol. 3, pp. 51–63.

Paul, G.L. and Lentz, R.J. (1977) *Psychosocial Treatment of Chronic Mental Patients: Milieu Versus Social-Learning Programmes*, Harvard University Press, Cambridge, Mass.

Pendergrass, V.E. (1972) Timeout from positive reinforcement following persistent, high-rate behaviour in retardates, *Journal of Applied Behaviour Analysis*, Vol. 5, pp. 85–91.

Sachs, D. (1973) The efficacy of time-out procedures in a variety of problems, *Journal of Behaviour Therapy and Experimental Psychiatry*, Vol. 4, pp. 237–42.

White, G.D., Nielson, G. and Johnson, S.M. (1972) Timeout duration and the suppression of deviant behaviour in children, *Journal of Applied Behaviour Analysis*, Vol. 5, pp. 111–20.

Further reading

Berry, P., Leonhardt, W.B. and Stuhm, G. (1982) Differential reinforcement: practical applications to reduce aggressive and disruptive behaviour, *Canadian Journal of Psychiatric Nursing*, Vol. 23, no. 3, pp. 16–18.

Finch, B.E., Wallace, C.J. and Davis, J.R. (1976) Behavioural observations before, during, and after brief isolation (time out), *Journal of Nervous and Mental Disease*, Vol. 163, no. 6, pp. 408–13.

Gelfand, D.M. (1984) *Child Behaviour Analysis and Therapy*, Pergamon, New York.

Roberts, M.W., Hatzenbuehler, L.C. and Bean, A.W. (1981) The effects of differential attention and time out on child noncompliance, *Behavioural Therapy*, Vol. 12, pp. 93–9.

Yule, W. and Carr, J. (eds.) (1987) *Behaviour Modification for People with Mental Handicaps*, Croom Helm, Beckenham.

33

Treatment Agreements

DEFINITION

Treatment agreements are a more formal method of involving patients in plans for their care than the routinely negotiated care plans described in Chapter 2.

DISCUSSION

Aims and advantages of treatment agreements

By planning patient care on a continuum which ranges from less to more formal agreements, nurses provide a climate in which opportunities exist for patients to take responsibility for the smooth running of their care plans. Formal agreements tend to be advocated when there is conflict between nurses and patients and can appear punitive rather than educative.

Treatment agreements have been found to be useful in managing the nursing care of certain groups of patients including some with non-psychotic mental disorders, some in general hospital and community settings. Caution is necessary when defining treatment agreements. In this chapter it is proposed to avoid the term 'contract' because it has a misleadingly legal sound. No treatment agreement could be legally binding because neither the nurse nor the patient has the legal capacity to make a contract for treatment. Moreover, the nurse cannot exact a price for his or her nursing care.

Some views of treatment agreements

In Langford's (1978) account of 'establishing a nursing contract' she suggests that the development of nursing contracts makes explicit the rights and responsibilities of patients within the nurse–patient relationship. The European Parliament's statement of the rights of patients (Resolution, 1984) includes:

1 the right to available treatment and care appropriate to the illness;
2 the right to prompt treatment.

Another right implied by the present structure of the

British National Health Service is the right to health care without charge at the point of use. No treatment agreement can override these rights.

A different way of looking at treatment agreements is that they identify and make explicit the values and preferences of the people agreeing them, at the same time as stating the objectives towards which the negotiators agree to work (Pettit, 1980, p. 148; Artinian, 1983). The agreement describes things as they are at present; it sets out the conditions which constrain things as they are; and it specifies the means (nursing and patient actions) by which a different state of affairs can be achieved. That is, by indicating the conditions which limit nurses within a relationship, it identifies what the patient must do in order to be able to effect a change or to reach a given objective. It also makes clear the specific obligations of the nurse.

This view of a treatment agreement is closer to Campbell's (1984) view of a covenant. Campbell suggests that covenants often define a set of interlocking obligations, and that reciprocity in a caring relationship is necessary in order to avoid paternalism and coercion. A treatment agreement spells out the reciprocal actions to be taken by the patient and nurse.

Negotiating the agreement

The negotiation of treatment agreements hinges on the patient's consent. The agreement itself is a form of treatment to be explained in the same way as any other treatment. The patient is free to accept or decline it at any time. A treatment agreement cannot be used to enforce compliance with any other form of treatment. Provisions for treatment without consent are strictly controlled by the Mental Health Act 1983, which does not mention agreements between staff and patients. However, if the negotiation of a treatment agreement is thought to be the correct treatment by a multidisciplinary care team and a patient declines such treatment, the team may suggest that the patient seeks a second opinion from another treatment facility.

The procedures for carrying out the different stages of the nursing process are intended to enhance reciprocity by involving patients as much as possible in the planning and evaluation of their nursing care. Patients who have difficulty in negotiating care plans may sometimes be helped by the specificity of a treatment agreement, which may be used as an intermediate step towards their participating fully in negotiating care plans.

GUIDELINES: SETTING UP A TREATMENT AGREEMENT

Action	Rationale
1 If a patient presents nursing problems for which a treatment agreement is thought to be potentially helpful, the primary nurse discusses the issues involved with his or her supervisor, the rest of the nursing team, and the multidisciplinary team.	Sometimes problems between nurses and patients can be resolved by improving communication between the staff, so that a treatment agreement may not be necessary.
2 If the multidisciplinary team agrees that a treatment agreement may be helpful, the primary nurse discusses the issues with the clinical psychologist.	The clinical psychologist will have experience of setting behavioural objectives and can help to clarify priorities.
3 The nurse agrees with the MDCT who will work with the patient on the agreement.	A multidisciplinary approach sets out to supply more various and more imaginative solutions to the problems than would one person alone.
4 When his or her priorities have been clarified, the primary nurse meets with the patient to discuss his or her values and preferences about treatment and nursing care.	In order to identify the areas where the nurses' and patient's priorities agree and where they conflict.
5 The primary nurse explains that a treatment agreement is being considered in order to resolve conflict between the nurses' and the patient's objectives.	In order to introduce the idea of reciprocity within the nurse–patient relationship.
6 After the preliminary meetings alone with the patient, the primary nurse and the nominated member of the multidisciplinary team meet with the patient to negotiate a draft agreement, bearing in mind that the process is likely to take some time, especially if the problems to be tackled are long-standing ones.	Prolonged and careful consideration of the patient's problems is not only desirable in itself, but also helps to ensure that the provisions of any agreement are coherent and logical.
7 When a draft agreement has been made it is discussed with the nursing and multidisciplinary teams.	To confirm that it can be implemented.
8 The nurse and the other members of the MDCT prepare the version of the agreement that is proposed, bearing in mind that the agreement may have to be renegotiated quite soon, depending on how effective it turns out to be.	To design an agreement which will facilitate co-operation between the patient and staff, rather than attempt to coerce him or her.

[*Named staff members*] on behalf of [*named multidisciplinary care team*] agree with [*named patient*] to provide the necessary assistance for [*named patient*] to achieve the following objective:

_____

_____

_____

[*Named patient*] will achieve the objective by carrying out the following actions:

_____

_____

_____

[*Named staff*] will assist [*named patient*] to achieve the objective by carrying out the following actions:

_____

_____

_____

If [*named patient*] or [*named staff*] fail to keep any part of this agreement, it will be renegotiated as soon as is practicable. The agreement will, in any case, be reviewed in [*state meeting*] at [*state time*] on [*state date*] in [*state location*] by [*state who will review*].

Signed on behalf of [*named multidisciplinary care team*] by:
[*signature*] [*name in blocks*] and [*signature*] [*name in blocks*]

Signed by:
[*signature*] [*patient's name in blocks*]
Date:

Figure 33.1 An example of a treatment agreement

---

9 An outline agreement is shown in Figure 33.1.

10 The date on which the review will be carried out is clearly stated.

So that the patient knows for how long he or she must expend effort on the agreement's objective.

11 It is made clear to the patient that he or she can request to renegotiate the agreement with the staff members who implemented it.

So that the patient will take the initiative in renegotiating any aspects of the agreement which dissatisfy him or her.

12 The treatment agreement states only the specific objective designed to resolve a specific problem of conflict between the patient's and the team's objectives.

If more global aims are included in the agreement the patient is likely to become discouraged by the difficulties in achieving them.

13 The treatment agreement states not more than one objective.

To give the patient a chance of achieving something.

14 The objective is patient-centred, states the conditions under which it will be achieved, the standard expected, and the time available within which to achieve it.

So that it is clear what, how, and by when the patient will expect to achieve the objective.

15 The nursing interventions and patient actions are spelt out in detail.

(a) So that it is clear what help the patient can expect.
(b) So that the patient knows how much responsibility he or she expects to assume.

16 The agreement states that it is between the patient and the MDCT as represented by the staff members negotiating it.

To discourage the patient from approaching other staff in order to circumvent the provisions of the agreement.

REFERENCE MATERIAL
References

Artinian, B. (1983) Implementation of the inter-system patient-care model in clinical practice, *Journal of Advanced Nursing*, Vol. 8, pp. 117–24.

Campbell, A. (1984) *Moderated Love: A Theology of Professional Care*, SPCK, London.

Langford, T. (1978) Establishing a nursing contract, *Nursing Outlook*, Vol. 26, no. 6, pp. 386–8.

Pettit, P. (1980) *Judging Justice*, Routledge & Kegan Paul, London.

Resolution on a European charter on the rights of patients (1984) *Official Journal of the European Communities*, c46/104.

Further reading

Cooklin, A.L. (1973) Consideration of the 'contract' between staff and patient and its relationship to current hospital practice, *British Journal of Medical Psychology*, Vol. 46, pp. 279–85.

Helgeson, D.M. and Berg, C.L. (1985) Contracting: a method of health promotion, *Journal of Community Health Nursing*, Vol. 2, no. 4, pp. 199–207.

Loomis, M.E. (1985) Levels of contracting, *Journal of Psychosocial Nursing and Mental Health Services*, Vol. 23, no. 3, pp. 9–14.

McEnany, G.W. and Tescher, B.E. (1985) Contracting for care: one nursing approach to the hospitalized borderline patient, *Journal of Psychosocial Nursing and Mental Health Services*, Vol. 23, no. 4, pp. 11–18.

O'Brien, P., Caldwell, C. and Transeau, G. (1985) Written treatment contracts can help cure self-destructive behaviours of the borderline patient, *Journal of Psychosocial Nursing and Mental Health Services*, Vol. 23, no. 4, pp. 19–23.

Parsons, V. (1972) Contact vs contract: the process of taming, *Journal of Psychiatric Nursing*, Vol. 10, no. 3, pp. 18–20.

Rosen, B. (1978) Contract therapy, *Nursing Times*, Vol. 74, no. 3, pp. 119–21.

Steckel, S.B. (1980) Contracting with patient-selected reinforcers, *American Journal of Nursing*, Vol. 80, pp. 1596–9.

Zangari, M.-E. and Duffy, P. (1980) Contracting with patients in day-to-day practice, *Amercian Journal of Nursing*, Vol. 80, pp. 451–5.

34

Seclusion

DEFINITION

Seclusion is the forced isolation of a person for an arbitary period of time (Thorpe, 1980).

DISCUSSION

A critical examination finds that seclusion tends to be used to remove a patient from social contact of any kind in order to prevent or control undesirable behaviour. It is often carried out without necessarily measuring the unwanted behaviour or measuring in detail the results of the seclusion or of its duration. Seclusion is a method of restraint which often dispenses with nurse–patient interaction (Whaley and Ramirez, 1980; Grigson, 1984; Way, 1986; Hammill, 1987).

If a patient consents to seclusion as a means of controlling his or her behaviour the question whether the procedure is a form of medical treatment or not is less of a problem than when the patient withholds consent. To be lawfully carried out without the patient's consent seclusion must be unequivocally a treatment for which there is no medical alternative.

Restraint

The issues of restraint are discussed in detail in Chapter 10. It is emphasized that the decision to implement seclusion is extremely grave.

Restraint of patients is permissible in the limited circumstances described in Chapter 10. The provisions of the Mental Health Act are repeated here. Restraint is permissible:

1 when consent has been given (for instance, to a treatment programme involving restraint or seclusion as a response to specific behaviours); this consent must be written, and may be withdrawn at any time;
2 to *prevent*, using 'reasonable' force, a crime;
3 to *prevent*, using 'reasonable' force, a breach of the peace – the definition of a breach of the peace involves

the threat of violence which is likely to harm another person or his or her property;
4 in self-defence, defence of the employer's property, or (more problematically) defence of another person;
5 to *prevent*, by the use of 'reasonable' force, harm to a person who appears to be so mentally disordered as not to be competent to keep him or herself safe and who appears likely to cause harm to others.

Detained as well as informal patients need not consent to 'urgent treatment':

(a) which is immediately necessary to save the patient's life; or
(b) which [not being irreversible] is immediately necessary to prevent a serious deterioration of his condition; or
(c) which [not being irreversible or hazardous] is immediately necessary to alleviate serious suffering by the patient; or
(d) which [not being irreversible or hazardous] is immediately necessary and represents the minimum interference necessary to prevent the patient from behaving violently or being a danger to himself or others.

(Mental Health Act 1983, section 62)

Because seclusion is used to restrain and control behaviour it is difficult to justify under Part II of the Act which includes sections 57, 59, 60 and 62, referring to the urgent medical treatment of informal and detained patients. It is less a method of treatment than a means of restraining disruptive patients.

The nature and purpose of seclusion

There is very little research into the nature or efficacy of the procedure as practised by different hospitals. It is likely that there is wide divergence in practice. It is a problematic procedure to carry out with any ethical or legal justification. Its effects require comparison with the use of mechanical restraints and of time-out and there is little in the way of controlled studies (Wadeson and Carpenter, 1976; Grassian and Friedman, 1986). It is described by those who practise it as an intervention of last resort, to be used when other measures have failed to control unwanted behaviour that is thought to be dangerous to other people. By this definition it is the culmination of increasing efforts to take control of a person's behaviour and so is difficult to distinguish from retaliation and punishment.

The purpose of seclusion, in summary, is to prevent a mentally disordered patient from harming him- or herself or others. It is not clear at what point the prevention most effectively starts; whether at a stage where the patient's behaviour is becoming disorganized or potentially threatening or both; or at a stage where uncontrollable violence is unequivocally threatened.

Such problems beset all aspects of seclusion. Researchers agree that there is disagreement about the duration and the effectiveness of different periods of seclusion. It is not clear whether seclusion is more effective when used alone, or when combined with other treatment methods. It is not clear which treatment methods are most effective when used in combination with seclusion. There is evidence that hospital staff tend to respond to violence with a single choice of treatment (Whitman, Armao and Dent, 1976; Way, 1986). Wide variations exist in the rates of use of seclusion even in the same hospitals. There is little evidence which explains why this is so; whether patients vary from area to area; whether staff–patient ratios have an influence; whether different treatment-philosophies have an influence.

Seclusion is, therefore, a treatment to be used with the utmost caution and with scrupulous attention to the civil liberties of patients and to the mental health law governing the administration of treatment without consent.

GUIDELINES: IMPLEMENTING SECLUSION

Action	Rationale
1 The nurse in charge of a ward or unit, who will be a registered mental nurse, ensures that the room to be used for seclusion is prepared according to the following criteria.	In order to achieve a balance between the requirements for the safety and well-being of the patient who is secluded and the conditions necessary for the procedure to be effective.
2 The whole interior of the room may be observed from outside.	If a patient is left alone in the room it is essential that he or she can be observed by nursing and medical staff in case of self-injury or an untoward response to any medication that has been administered.
3 The room affords privacy to anyone inside it whenever they are not being observed by staff.	A person's disturbed behaviour is likely to be reinforced by conditions which differ from the norms which usually govern social interaction.
4 The door of the room opens outwards.	So that the person being secluded is unable to barricade the door.
5 The door of the room is lockable by a standard hospital key.	(a) That is, the door is not self-locking. (b) It is possible for a special key to be mislaid, so that the door could not be opened in an emergency.
6 The furnishings and fittings of the room are checked for possible risks. For example: (i) electrical fittings; (ii) breakable items such as lampshades; (iii) feather pillows.	So that they cannot be used by a person to injure him- or herself or others.

7 The room is heated or ventilated or both as dictated by the weather and the clothing worn by the patient. This implies that the regulating mechanism is outside the room.

So that the patient's body temperature remains within normal limits, especially if intramuscular neuroleptic drugs have been administered.

8 The person being secluded has ready access to toilet facilities.

To maintain normal personal hygiene.

9 The person being secluded has ready access to reading or writing material or other means of recreation.

To offer an alternative to destructive or disorganized behaviour.

10 If available, an emergency team is summoned, assembling a nurse manager, a doctor, another trained nurse, and another nurse, whether qualified or not.

If the patient's behaviour is so dangerous as to need treatment by seclusion, staff are required in sufficient numbers to carry out the procedure effectively.

11 The nurse in charge checks whether the patient has consented to the use of seclusion as a treatment. Such consent will be in the patient's medical records.

(a) Consent is required for both informal and detained patients.
(b) General consent by the patient is insufficient. Consent to this particular administration of treatment must be requested.

12 If the patient has not consented and will not consent to seclusion, the nurse in charge ensures that the duty clinical nurse manager and the duty doctor agree to carry out the treatment without consent.

(a) Although in an emergency a decision can be made by the doctor alone, agreement by the different disciplines present helps to ensure that individual members of the team fulfil their responsibilities both to the team and to the hierarchies of their own discipline.
(b) It is possible that the patient's disturbed and dangerous behaviour can be treated by methods other than seclusion.

13 If seclusion is to be carried out, the nurse in charge of the ward directs the procedure.

So that instructions are clearly given by one person and are immediately followed.

14 If there are fewer than eight members of staff present, the duty clinical nurse manager will summon help from elsewhere (see Chapter 14, 'Managing violence').

(a) Up to six people will be needed to carry out the procedure.
(b) At least two nurses, one of whom is a RMN must be available to look after the patients in the ward.

15 Away from the clinical area the nurse in charge briefly outlines the situation that has led to the emergency.

Preparation is done away from the clinical area so that the nursing team appears united and decisive when it is time to act.

16 The nurse in charge outlines generally what is to be done.

(a) So that the team knows who the patient is;
(b) who the ward staff are;
(c) who has been brought in to help.
(d) In order to understand the risks.

17 Members of staff remove personal jewellery, badges and pens.

To prevent injury to the patient and to themselves.

18 The nurse in charge assigns to four nurses the task of immobilizing the patient by taking control of his or her limbs.

(a) The nurses are trained and practised in the techniques of restraining and immobilizing patients.
(b) This is a fall-back in case the patient refuses to consent to seclusion.

19 Each nurse is responsible individually or jointly for immobilizing a specific part of the patient's body.

(a) So that a method will be selected which meets the requirements of the present emergency.
(b) So that each nurse knows from which side to approach the patient.

20 The nurse in charge nominates a nurse to fetch any equipment needed, such as mattress, blankets, pillows, sheets.

(a) A mattress or pillow may be used as protection against a knife.
(b) Blankets or sheets may be used to immobilize the patient.
(c) Pillows may be needed to protect the patient if he or she is on the floor.

21 The nurse in charge maintains contact with the nurses supervising the patient.

In order to know where the patient is.

22 If necessary the nurse in charge describes the location of the seclusion room.

So that the team knows where the patient is to go.

23 The nurse in charge nominates a nurse to check the seclusion room.

To ensure that it meets the necessary standards (see 2–9 above).

24 The nurse in charge instructs the team members, stating:
  (i) timings;
  (ii) how the patient will be approached;
  (iii) where the team members will position themselves;
  (iv) what the patient is likely to do;
  (v) any other risks which may be present. For example, an infected patient.

So that when the time comes they will act in collaboration, having anticipated what needs to be done.

25 The nurse in charge confirms with the doctor and the clinical nurse manager what their roles will be.

So that support and help will be available if needed.

26 The nurse in charge confirms with the remaining nurses in the ward what their role will be.

So that the other patients in the ward will be safely looked after.

27 The nurse in charge says what his or her words of command will be.

So that team members know when to act.

28 The nurse in charge confirms that the members of the team understand their role.

The resulting co-ordination will increase confidence in each other.

29 The nurse in charge asks for any questions from team members.

To confirm finally that the action to be taken is understood by all.

30 The team approaches the patient, led by the nurse in charge.

To make it clear that the patient now does not have a choice about the need to control his or her behaviour.

31 The nurse in charge asks the patient to desist from the dangerous or violent behaviour.

To offer the patient a last chance to take control of his or her behaviour.

32 If the patient refuses, the nurse in charge asks if he or she will consent to seclusion, explaining that consent to seclusion is a means of regaining control of his or her behaviour.

The aim of treatment by seclusion is to prompt the patient to control his or her behaviour without coercion if at all possible.

33 If the patient refuses to consent to seclusion, the nurse in charge gives the prearranged command and the team moves quickly to either side and immobilizes the patient as planned. Depending where the patient is, this might be on the floor, in a chair or on a bed.

In order to prevent further violence or injury to the patient which would result from a prolonged struggle.

34 The nurse in charge remains by the patient's head, restraining it if necessary, and talking continuously to him or her.

The effect of one person talking quietly can help to reduce fear and anger, especially in perplexed patients.

35 The team quickly and gently lifts the patient, using a recognized technique, and transfers him or her to the seclusion room.

In order to prevent a struggle during which the patient could be injured.

36 When the patient is in the seclusion room the team remains in position, the nurse in charge talking to the patient until it is confirmed that he or she is calm enough to be released. This may take some time.

Psychotic patients are especially vulnerable to being suddenly released after being immobilized and may become violent again.

37 One or two nurses who know the patient undertake maximum supervision. Two nurses may remain in the room with the patient. One nurse may supervise the patient from outside the room.

(a) To observe the effects of any medication that has been given.
(b) To judge when seclusion may cease.

38 The team returns to the ward office to meet together with the duty clinical nurse manager and the doctor.
(i) Each member of staff will evaluate his or her own role.
(ii) Each member of staff will evaluate the work of the team as a whole.
(iii) Any points for improvement are noted by the nurse in charge.

In order to debrief from the incident, and plan for the future.

39 The nurse in charge completes the documentation required by the hospital managers.

(a) The Mental Health Act Commissioners review all episodes of seclusion.
(b) Accurate figures are required of the use of seclusion in order to facilitate comparison and research.

40 The nurse in charge writes an account of the procedure in the patient's nursing record.

To ensure that if necessary the incident can be evaluated after the lapse of some time.

41 The doctor writes in the medical record an account of the patient's mental state before and after seclusion.

In order for seclusion to be a treatment there must be evidence of the patient's psychopathology and that the mental state changed for the better as a result of seclusion.

42 If the procedure was carried out without consent the nurse in charge ensures that the steps required by the Mental Health Act 1983 are begun: such as the obtaining of a second medical opinion or consulting with the Mental Health Act Commissioners or both.

In order to protect so far as possible the civil liberties of the patient, and to ensure the propriety of actions taken by staff to control the behaviour of the patient.

REFERENCE MATERIAL
References

Grassian, S. and Friedman, N. (1986) Effects of sensory deprivation in psychiatric seclusion and solitary confinement, *International Journal of Law and Psychiatry*, Vol. 8, pp. 49–65.

Grigson, J.W. (1984) Beyond patient management: the therapeutic use of seclusion and restraints, *Perspectives in Psychiatric Nursing Care*, Vol. 22, no. 4, pp. 137–42.

Hammill, K. (1987) Seclusion: inside looking out, *Nursing Times*, Vol. 83, no. 5, pp. 38–9.

Mental Health Act 1983, HMSO, London.

Thorpe, J.G. (1980) Time out or seclusion?, *Nursing Times*, Vol. 76, no. 14, p. 604.

Wadeson, H. and Carpenter, W.T. (1976) Impact of the seclusion room experience, *Journal of Nervous and Mental Disease*, Vol. 163, no. 5, pp. 318–28.

Way, B.B. (1986) The use of seclusion and restraint in New York State Psychiatric Centres, *International Journal of Law and Psychiatry*, Vol. 8, pp. 383–93.

Whaley, M.S. and Ramirez, L.F. (1980) The use of seclusion rooms and physical restraints in the treatment of psychiatric patients, *Journal of Psychosocial Nursing and Mental Health Services*, Vol. 18, no. 1, pp. 13–16.

Whitman, R.M. Armao, B.B. and Dent, O.B. (1976) Assault on the therapist, *American Journal of Psychiatry*, Vol. 133, no. 4, pp. 426–9.

Further reading

Apostoles, F.E., Little, M.E. and Murphy, H.D. (1977) Developing a psychiatric nursing audit, *Journal of Psychiatric Nursing*, Vol. 15, no. 5, pp. 9–15.

Baradell, J.G. (1985) Humanistic care of the patient in seclusion, *Journal of Psychosocial Nursing and Mental Health Services*, Vol. 23, no. 2, pp. 9–14.

Block, B. (1976) Preparing students for physical restraint, *Journal of Psychosocial Nursing and Mental Health Services*, Vol. 14, no. 10, pp. 9–10.

Davidson, N.A., Hemmingway, M.J. and Wysocki, T. (1984) Reducing the use of restrictive procedures in a residential facility, *Hospital and Community Psychiatry*, Vol. 35, no. 2, pp. 164–7.

Ecock-Connelly, C. (1978) Patient compliance: a review of the research and implications for psychiatric mental health nursing, *Journal of Psychiatric Nursing*, Vol. 16, no. 10, pp. 15–18.

Gerlock, A. and Solomons, H.C. (1983) Factors associated with the seclusion of psychiatric patients, *Perspectives in Psychiatric Care*, Vol. 21, no. 2, pp. 46–53.

Grassian, S. (1983) Psychopathological effects of solitary confinement, *American Journal of Psychiatry*, Vol. 140, no. 11, pp. 1450–4.

Guirguis, E.F. and Durost, H.B. (1978) The role of mechanical restraint in the management of disturbed behaviour, *Canadian Psychiatric Association Journal*, Vol. 23, pp. 209–13.

Gutheil, T.G. (1978) Observations on the theoretical bases for seclusion of the psychiatric inpatient, *American Journal of Psychiatry*, Vol. 135, no. 3, pp. 325–8.

Kendrick, D.W. and Wilber, G. (1986) When in seclusion, *American Journal of Nursing*, Vol. 86, p. 1117.

Kendrick, D.W. and Wilber, G. (1986) Seclusion: organizing safe and effective care, *Journal of Psychosocial Nursing and Mental Health Services*, Vol. 24, no. 11, pp. 26–8.

Kilgallen, R.K. (1977) The effective use of seclusion, *Journal of Psychiatric Nursing*, Vol. 15, no. 1, pp. 22–6.

Mattson, M.R. and Sacks, M.H. (1978) Seclusion: uses and complications, *American Journal of Psychiatry*, Vol. 135, pp. 1210–13.

McCoy, S.M. and Garritson, S. (1983) Seclusion: the process of intervening, *Journal of Psychosocial Nursing and Mental Health Services*, Vol. 21, no. 8, pp. 9–15.

Mental Health Act Commission (1987) *Second Biennial Report*, HMSO, London.

Morrison, J. *et al.* (1987) Formulating a restraint use policy, *Journal of Nursing Administration*, Vol. 17, no. 3, pp. 39–42.

Oldham, J.M., Russakoff, M. and Prusnofsky, L. (1983) Seclusion patterns and milieu, *Journal of Nervous and Mental Disease*, Vol. 171, no. 11, pp. 645–50.

Pilette, P.C. (1978) The tyranny of seclusion: a brief essay, *Journal of Psychosocial Nursing and Mental Health Services*, Vol. 16, no. 10, pp. 19–21.

Plutchik, R. *et al.* (1978) Toward a rationale for the

seclusion process, *Journal of Nervous and Mental Disease*, Vol. 166, pp. 571–9.

RCN Society of Psychiatric Nursing (1979) *Seclusion and Restraint in Hospitals and Units for the Mentally Disordered*, RCN, London.

Redmond, F.C. (1980) Study on the use of the seclusion room, *Quality Review Bulletin*, Vol. 6, no. 8, pp. 20–3.

Richardson, B.K. (1987) Psychiatric inpatients' perceptions of the seclusion room experience, *Nursing Research*, Vol. 36, no. 4, pp. 234–8.

Roper, J.M. *et al.* (1985) Restraint and seclusion: a standard and standard care plan, *Journal of Psychosocial Nursing and Mental Health Services*, Vol. 23, no. 6, pp. 18–23.

Schwab, P.J. and Lohmeyer, C.E. (1979) The use of seclusion in a general hospital psychiatric unit, *Journal of Clinical Psychiatry*, Vol. 40, pp. 228–31.

Soloff, P.H. (1979) Physical restraint and the non-psychotic patient: clinical and legal perspectives, *Journal of Clinical Psychiatry*, Vol. 40, pp. 302–5.

Soloff, P.H., Gutheil, T.G. and Wexler, D.B. (1985) Seclusion and restraint in 1985: a review and update, *Hospital and Community Psychiatry*, Vol. 36, pp. 652–7.

Soloff, P.H. and Turner, S.M. (1981) Patterns of seclusion, *Journal of Nervous and Mental Disease*, Vol. 169, pp. 37–44.

Strutt, R. *et al.* (1980) Seclusion: can it be justified?, *Nursing Times*, Vol. 76, no. 37, pp. 1629–33.

Weekly Hansard (1982) Debates 6 December, no. 1261, col. 398.

Winston, F. (1977) Restraints in delirium tremens, *American Journal of Psychiatry*, Vol. 134, p. 98.

Part Five

Somatic Interventions

35

Administering Medicines

DISCUSSION

This chapter is intended to identify the principles behind the administering of medicines and to indicate where the nurse will find detailed guidance and information.

UKCC guidelines

In April 1986 the United Kingdom Central Council for Nursing, Midwifery and Health Visiting issued an advisory paper on the administration of medicines (UKCC, 1986). The advisory paper's subtitle was: 'a framework to assist individual professional judgement and the development of local policies and guidelines'. The framework comprises the legislative aspect, the prescribing role of the doctor, the dispensing role of the pharmacist, the administering role of the nurse and the receiving role of the patient. See Appendix E for details of these guidelines.

Official standards
THE BRITISH PHARMACOPOEIA AND BRITISH NATIONAL FORMULARY

The *British Phamacopoeia* (DHSS, 1980), derived from the *European Phamacopoeia*, is the reference for the standards and composition of all medicines, listed according to their non-proprietary (generic) names. The *British Pharmaceutical Codex* (Pharmaceutical Society, 1979) is the standard reference for the composition of dressings, along with drugs. The *British National Formulary* (Joint Formulary Committee, 1988) is described as a pocket-book for rapid reference. It describes in detail nearly all the preparations likely to be prescribed in wards and departments, and summarizes the relevant legislation regarding prescriptions and controlled drugs. It summarizes, among other topics, drug interactions, prescribing in pregnancy, intravenous additives and the emergency treatment of poisoning. It is regularly up-

dated and reissued by the British Medical Association and the Pharmaceutical Society of Great Britain. Each nurse is responsible for familiarizing him- or herself with it.

DATA SHEET COMPENDIUM

The *Data Sheet Compendium* (Association of the British Pharmaceutical Industry, 1986) is published annually by the pharmaceutical companies, and consists of manufacturers' data sheets for their products, which are subject to regulation under the Medicines Act. It may be used to supplement the material to be found in the *BNF*, bearing in mind that the *Compendium* is a form of promotion and advertising by the pharmaceutical companies as well as an information service.

The nurse's responsibility

Nurses who administer medicines require a good working knowledge of basic pharmacology, anatomy and physiology, and of disease processes in order to be able to evaluate accurately the effects of any drugs they give to patients. *The nurse is expected to use his or her own knowledge and judgement when reading a prescription, so that deviations from usual practice, dosages or frequency may be checked with a doctor before administering the medicine. If necessary, the medicine is withheld until the nurse is satisfied that it is safe to administer.* Knowledge of the patient, of disease processes and the actions of drugs is essential in order to evaluate whether an apparently routine prescription is having, or will have, acceptable effects (DeGennaro *et al.*, 1981). The standard of multidisciplinary team practice must be such that there is adequate written and verbal communication, while at the same time the patient is kept informed about and involved in decisions about medication (Brands and Brands, 1983).

Medicines Act 1968

The hospital prescription card is the means by which a

doctor directs a nurse to administer medicines. The policies and rules of hospitals ensure that prescribing practice conforms to the requirements of the Act.

The *BNF* contains guidance about cautionary and advisory labels (Joint Formulary Committee, 1988, p. 463). Particular attention is paid to the quantity, strength, batch or lot reference and expiry date of a given container of medicines. Medicines for external use are supplied in fluted bottles, which are recognizable by touch, except that bottles with a capacity greater than 1.14 litres need not be fluted, and ear and eye drops may be supplied in a plastic container.

The Poisons Act 1972

This Act classifies and regulates the sale, supply and storage of 'non-medicinal poisons'. The relevance of the Poisons Act to this procedure is the need for nurses to know about storage, labelling and transport of poisons and where to find information about poisonous substances. Any nurse can obtain information on any poison by telephone twenty-four hours a day from a regional poisons information centre:

    Belfast: Royal Victoria Hospital – 0232 40503
    Cardiff: Royal Infirmary – 0222 492233
    Dublin: Jervis Street Hospital – 0001 745588
    Edinburgh: Royal Infirmary – 031–229 2477
    Leeds: General Infirmary – 0533 32799
    London: Guys Hospital – 01–955 5000.

The Misuse of Drugs Act 1971

This Act was passed as a result of the greatly increased social problems in the 1950s and 1960s caused by the abuse of drugs hitherto regarded as harmless enough to be widely prescribed in single or combined preparations, as well as of drugs classified as 'dangerous' under existing legislation. The Misuse of Drugs Act created four schedules of 'controlled drugs'. In practice, the controlled drugs most likely to be administered by nurses are those in Schedule 2, which regulates the opiates, cocaine, amphetamines and codeine. They are subject to strict rules about storage and record-keeping (The Misuse of Drugs [Safe Custody] Regulations, 1973).

The Classifications Packaging and Labelling of Dangerous Substances Regulations (1986)

A selected list of prescribed dangerous substances will be found in the most recent edition of *Medicines and Poisons Guide* (Pearce, 1984). Its relevance to this chapter is the need for nurses to know the names of, the general and particular risks associated with and the precautions required for certain commonly used substances.

STORAGE OF POISONS

Containers of poisons must be stored in locations reserved solely for the storage of poisons and separated from the remainder of the premises on which they are kept. In a ward or department of a hospital this means a locked cupboard to which patients and unauthorized persons do not have access.

Dealing with medicines

PRESCRIBING

Detailed general recommendations on prescribing can be found in the *BNF* (Joint Formulary Committee, 1988, pp. 2–3). The UKCC suggests that certain medicines from the general sales list or the pharmacy medicines, such as mild laxatives or analgesics, may be the subject of local written hospital policies agreed between doctors, nurses and pharmacists to allow nurses to administer selected named medicines at their discretion and without a prescription.

DISPENSING

The pharmacist can help nurses greatly in the following ways:

1 by visiting the ward or department regularly at a time agreed with the charge nurse to check stocks and plan the ordering schedule so that unplanned trips to the pharmacy may be avoided;
2 by negotiating with the charge nurse stock levels for each drug so that minimum stocks are kept in the ward, thus keeping down costs as well as reducing waste;
3 by dispensing all medicines to be taken out by patients going on leave no matter how short the duration of leave;
4 by providing advice and information about storage, doses and formulations of medicines and other preparations;
5 by providing advice and information about methods of administering medicines and other preparations;
6 by meeting regularly with the nurses of the ward or department in order to evaluate the service being provided to patients;
7 by monitoring safety aspects of prescribing by the medical staff;
8 by using a system of labelling which not only fulfils statutory requirements but is also easily and safely read by the nurse(s) administering the medicines.

ADMINISTERING

The purpose of the UKCC's advisory paper (1986) was to draw to the attention of nurses how professional judgement and professional responsibility are exercised according to the competencies laid down in rule 18 of the

Nurses' Rules (1983). The possibility that medication may have to be withheld implies that only a nurse who is competent to assess the patient and make the necessary judgement will administer the medicine.

The UKCC is quite clear that a first-level nurse may administer medicines on his or her own. A second-level nurse may administer medicines *only under the direction of a first-level nurse*, who remains responsible for the procedure. Although local circumstances, training requirements or clinical needs may result in a second person being involved in administering medicines, the first-level nurse is responsible both for directing and carrying out the procedure. Under no circumstances are nursing assistants, auxiliaries or aides involved in administering medicines.

The procedure takes account of the possibility that a learner may already be a registered first-level nurse.

RECEIVING
The UKCC advisory paper (1986) emphasizes the need for the patient to be an informed participant in the use of medicines, whether administered by a nurse or self-administered. The paper stresses that the patient's consent is required for the administration of all medicines. For the purposes of this procedure it is assumed that the nurse has, as part of an educative and collaborative process, sought the patient's informed consent to the medication prescribed. (See Chapters 10 and 37.)

HIV-positive and hepatitis B antigen-carrying patients
Because the human immunodeficiency virus (HIV) and the hepatitis B virus are present in blood and other body fluids, precautions are necessary when medication is administerd parenterally: that is, by intramuscular or intravenous injection. Provided that nurses know and follow the most recent guidelines for managing contact with HIV-positive individuals or people thought to be HIV-positive, the risks of transmitting infection by the human immunodeficiency virus will be reduced (DHSS, 1986; USDHSS, 1988). The same is true of hepatitis B (USDHSS, 1988). It is generally recommended that nurses whose own immune responsiveness is lowered for any reason do not come into contact with HIV-positive or hepatitis B antigen-carrying individuals. Because it appears that the human immunodeficiency virus has to travel through the blood-stream in order to reach the tissues which it infects, as does the hepatitis B virus, nurses who have skin lesions of any kind should either cover them with a waterproof dressing before carrying out an invasive procedure with an HIV-positive or hepatitis B antigen-carrying individual, or refrain from carrying it out at all. Conversely, it must be borne in mind that lesions on the skin of infected individuals are a potential source of infection.

GUIDELINES: ADMINISTERING MEDICINES

Action

1 The following actions are subject to the proviso that in each case, the nurse deemed to be responsible for administering medicines can identify the patients for whom they are intended.

2 If medicines are to be administered by two nurses, at least one must be a first-level nurse.

Rationale

Since the first-level nurse is in law competent to administer medicines alone and is therefore responsible for doing so, or for withholding them if the patient's condition warrants it, it is essential that he or she knows the patient in order to make the necessary assessments before and after giving the drugs.

Although a first-level nurse is in law competent to administer medicines on his or her own, the nature of the patients and of the medicines used in psychiatric hospitals may require a more cautious approach to the question of safety.

3 Where possible, medicines are administered from a central point such as a treatment room housing the medicine cupboard.

(a) In order to have a consistent policy throughout the hospital.
(b) Because most patients are mobile and relatively free to move round wards or units.
(c) In order to keep the prescription cards and references such as the *BNF* readily available near the medicine cupboard and the place where medicines are administered.
(d) To be near a telephone in case of emergency.

4 The times when medicines are administered conform to a routine common to all wards.

In order to fit in with other centrally planned services and activities such as meal times and changeovers of staff, as well as timing requirements of specific medicines.

5 If medicines are to be administered from a central area, it is prepared so that there is a physical barrier, such as a half-door or shelf, between the open drug cupboard and the patients.

(a) Although a determined patient could get through or over a barrier, the precaution of having two nurses carry out the procedure means that it is more likely that the cupboard could be locked in an emergency.
(b) Staffing levels may preclude the administration of drugs individually by patients' primary or key nurses.

6 If a drug trolley is used, it is moved to and from points at which it can be secured at all times.

It may be all a nurse could do to lock the trolley itself, without also attempting to secure it, if an emergency occurred which obliged him or her to leave the trolley unattended.

7 Under no circumstances are medicines borrowed from other wards or departments.

(a) Because, out of office hours, the duty doctor can, if necessary, dispense medicines from the pharmacy.
(b) Borrowing cannot be formally recorded and accounted for.
(c) If an error was made, the nurses concerned would have doubly breached their duty of care to the patient.

8 If, while two nurses are administering medicines to several patients in turn, one of the nurses has to leave the room, the drug cupboard or trolley is immediately locked.

To prevent forcible access to the drugs while only one nurse is present.

9 Each prescription on the prescription card for prescription-only medicines, pharmacy or general sales list medicines fulfils the following criteria:
(i) written legibly;
(ii) in ink or typed;
(iii) dated not more than a week previously;
(iv) signed by the prescriber;
(v) bearing the patient's full name, hospital number, age, ward, and date of admission;
(vi) full non-proprietary name of the medicine to be administered;
(vii) quantity of the drug;
(viii) frequency of administration, written in English and unabbreviated;
(ix) times of administration;
(x) length in days of treatment required;
(xi) route of administration.

(a) So that the requirements of the Medicines Act 1968 for health prescriptions are fulfilled.

(b) In lieu of the patient's home address.

10   Any discontinued prescriptions are clearly cancelled with the signature of the doctor cancelling, and the date cancelled.

So that such medicines will not be administered.

The following instructions (11–25) apply to the administration of oral medicines

11   Before any patients are summoned, the following equipment is assembled:
   (i)   clean jug of fresh drinking water;
   (ii) a bottle of fruit squash;
   (iii) clean, dry medicine measures;
   (iv) 5-ml spoons;
   (v)   a bowl in which patients put used measures and spoons;
   (vi) clean, dry tumblers;
   (vii) paper tissues;
   (viii) indelible ink writing instrument.

It is discourteous to keep people hanging around while the medicine room is prepared.

12   Where two nurses are carrying out the procedure, they agree who will give the medicines to the patients and who will record the procedure.

In order that the tasks are clearly allocated, bearing in mind that the senior of the two nurses remains responsible for the entire administration.

Although actions 13–24 refer to two nurses, the principles hold good if one nurse carries out the procedure

13   The procedure begins at the time expected by the patients, and as detailed in their drug regimens.

In order to promote compliance by patients with their drug regimens.

14   Both nurses wash their hands before beginning to administer medicines.

Scrupulous personal hygiene is necessary when handling food and drugs.

15   Both nurses assume comfortable positions from which they can observe that patients indeed swallow their medicines and they can check and record administration.

(a) In order that patients do not feel pressurized; and
(b) the nurses can give the impression of unhurried attention.

16   Both nurses greet each patient by name.

In order to confirm identity.

17   The recording nurse reads aloud each item on the prescription, noting the presence of each component required, as stated in 9 above.

To ensure that the Medicines Act 1968 has been complied with.

18   The administering nurse takes the container required and reads the label aloud, noting if it is the patient's 'own' or a 'stock' medicine.

(a) In order to check that the drug, and its strength and form (e.g. tablets or syrup) are those stated in the prescription.
(b) To check any expiry date.
(c) To re-order, if necessary.

19   The administering nurse decants the required tablet(s) into the cap of the container and shows the label and the tablet(s) to the recording nurse.

(a) The tablets are not touched by hand for hygienic reasons and because some medicines can cause an allergic reaction.
(b) To confirm that the medicine and the dose conform to the prescription.

20 When the two nurses agree, the tablet(s) is placed in a medicine measure and the container closed and replaced in the cupboard.

It could be confusing to accumulate medicine containers in use outside the drug cupboard, even if the same ones are used for several patients.

21 In the case of liquids the administering nurse complies with any instructions on the label after reading it aloud, such as 'shake if necessary'.

Failure to do so may result in, for instance, different dilutions of the medicine being given if the bottle is not shaken properly.

22 The administering nurse decants the correct amount of medicine into a clean dry measure which has been placed on a flat surface at eye level within easy reading distance of both nurses.

(a) It is easier to pour the correct amount first time if the measure is already in position.
(b) So that the thumb nail may be used as a guide to read the lower line of the meniscus when the measuring glass is at eye level.

23 When both nurses have agreed that the measure contains the correct medication, the administering nurse gives it to the patient as both nurses watch.

So that both nurses have confirmed that it is the correct medicine before it is given to the patient.

24 The administering nurse encourages the patient to drink at least a tumbler of fluid with the medicine.

(a) To prevent oesophagitis from the irritant effect that some neuroleptic drugs can have.
(b) The patient is more likely to have swallowed the medicine with plenty of fluid.

25 The recording nurse enters the details of the medicine(s) administered in the space provided on the prescription card.

(a) So that the effects can be reliably monitored.
(b) So that there is no chance of duplication if the procedure is interrupted and different nurses take over.

The following instructions (26–52) apply to the administration of injectable medicines

26 Injections are administered at the end of the medicine procedure or at other times negotiated between the patient and his or her primary or key nurse.

(a) So that nurses can give the patient as much time and individual attention as necessary.
(b) In order that any precautions may be taken in an unflurried and effective manner for high-risk patients, such as those who are infectious or potentially violent or both.

27 For each patient in turn, the following equipment is assembled:
   (i) a clean receiver containing;
   (ii) a sterile disposable syringe;
   (iii) two sterile disposable needles;
   (iv) two sterile injection swabs;
   (v) indelible ink writing instrument;
   (vi) the size of needle will depend on the nature of the injection and the nutritional state, age and build of the patient.

(a) It may cause patients anxiety to assemble their injections in front of them.
(b) Each injection is prepared individually, not in batches.

28 Where two nurses are carrying out the procedure, they agree who will give the injection to the patient and who will record the administration.

In order that the tasks are clearly allocated, bearing in mind that the senior of the two nurses remains responsible for the procedure.

Although actions 29–52 refer to two nurses, the principles hold good if one nurse carries out the procedure

29 The administering nurse explains to the patient that he or she will give the patient's injection in five minutes' time.

To give the patient time to prepare. For example, to go to the lavatory or have a cigarette.

30 Both nurses go to the treatment room.

So that both nurses are present when the drug cupboard is unlocked.

31 The recording nurse reads aloud the prescription, noting that each required component is present, as stated in 9 above.

To ensure that the Medicines Act 1968 has been complied with.

32 The administering nurse takes the container required and reads the label aloud, noting if it is the patient's 'own' or a 'stock' medicine.

(a) In order to check that the drug, and its strength and form are those stated in the prescription.
(b) To check any expiry date.
(c) To re-order, if necessary.

33 Both nurses independently calculate and then agree the amount required to be drawn up.

To confirm that the medicine and the dose conform to the prescription.

34 The nurses agree with the patient which site to use for the injection, having explained its nature and bearing in mind the patient's physique.

So that the patient can choose, say, in which buttock a regularly administered injection will be sited.

35 The administering nurse washes his or her hands and draws up the drug, wearing unused protective gloves and plastic apron if necessary. Each apron and pair of gloves is discarded between each patient's injection.

(a) This is a clean procedure.
(b) The gloves are worn in case of an allergic reaction, as well as in case of infection.

36 When the syringe is airfree and the needle has been changed if necessary, both nurses check the syringe and medicine container while the recording nurse again reads aloud the prescription.

In order to double check that the correct medication and dose have been drawn up.

37 When both nurses are satisfied that they have drawn up the correct amount of medicine, the recording nurse locks the drug cupboard.

The drug cupboard is locked while a patient is in the treatment room to prevent his or her access to other medicines.

38 The recording nurse collects the patient.

In order to provide the patient with privacy for the treatment.

39 The administering nurse washes his or her hands again if necessary.

This is a clean procedure.

40 The administering nurse explains where he or she will give the injection, and asks the patient to choose which side, right or left.

In order to confirm that the patient consents to the injection.

41 The patient assumes as comfortable a position as possible and exposes the injection site.

It is desirable that the patient feels able to control aspects of this invasive procedure.

42 If health authority policy permits, the administering nurse cleans the site with a circular rubbing movement, using an isopropyl alcohol BP injection swab or similar antiseptic agent as approved by health authority policy, and allows it to dry.

(a) The friction may be experienced by the patient as reducing painful effects even though its value in reducing infection is questionable.
(b) So that the antiseptic is not driven into the skin by the needle.

43 The nurse warns the patient before inserting the needle to its full extent less 5 mm.

(a) So that the patient is not startled and so moves suddenly.
(b) To allow removal should it break.

44 The nurse withdraws the plunger slightly.

To observe whether the needle is in a blood vessel.

45 If the needle is in a blood vessel it is withdrawn and direct pressure applied.

To stop any bleeding.

46 If the needle is not in a blood vessel, the injection is given steadily and without force.

Excessive force causes pain, and is likely to cause tissue damage, possibly muscle necrosis.

47 If more than 4 ml is to be given intramuscularly, the nurse slightly withdraws and resites the needle, again ensuring that it is not in a blood vessel.

Large volumes injected into muscle are not absorbed and can cause abscess.

48 The nurse withdraws the needle in a swift movement, supporting the surrounding skin with a finger on an injection swab.

Thereby causing no pain.

49 If there is any bleeding, the nurse applies direct pressure with a sterile swab until it ceases, explaining to the patient what is happening.

(a) It could be distressing for a patient later to find that his or her underwear is bloodstained.
(b) Blood may transmit infection.

50 The patient replaces his or her clothing.

In order to leave the treatment room in a composed way.

51 The administering nurse confirms with the patient whether he or she is satisfied.

To evaluate the procedure.

52 The recording nurse enters the details of the medicine(s) administered in the space provided on the prescription card.

(a) So that the effects can be reliably monitored.
(b) To prevent duplication.
(c) To ensure that the next injection is given at the correct time.

53 All debris is disposed into a sharps bin for incineration, using a separate bin labelled High Risk for waste from HIV-positive or hepatitis B antigen-positive patients, and ensuring that the bins are sealed for disposal when partly full.

(a) To prevent injury during disposal of the waste.
(b) To prevent any cross-infection.
(c) If the bins are used until they are full, there is a risk of injury and infection from contact with contaminated needles and other waste.

54 If the injection was the 'patient's own', the empty box, if available, is returned to pharmacy with an order for resupply.

So that when the injection is next due, the necessary medication will be available.

REFERENCE MATERIAL
References

Association of the British Pharmaceutical Industry (1986) *ABPI Data Sheet Compendium 1986–1987*, Datapharm, London.

Brands, A.J. and Brands, A.B. (1983) Drug therapy and monitoring: a team responsibility, *Family and Community Health*, Vol. 6, no. 3, pp. 63–71.

Classification, Packing and Labelling of Dangerous Substances Regulations (1984) S.I. No. 1244, HMSO, London.

DeGennaro, M.D. *et al.* (1981) Psychotropic drug therapy, *American Journal of Nursing*, Vol. 81, pp. 1303–34.

DHSS (1980) *British Pharmacopoeia*, HMSO, London.

DHSS (1986) *Information and Guidance on AIDS (Acquired Immune Deficiency Syndrome) for Local Authority Staff*, DHSS, London.

Joint Formulary Committee 1987–1988 of the British Medical Association and the Pharmaceutical Society of Great Britain (1988) *British National Formulary Number 16*, BMA and Pharmaceutical Press, London.

Medicines Act 1968, HMSO, London.

Misuse of Drugs Act 1971, HMSO, London.

Misuse of Drugs (Safe Custody) Regulations (1973) S. I. No. 798, HMSO, London.

Nurses, Midwives and Health Visitors Rules Approval Order (1983) (S.I. 873), HMSO, London,

Pearce, M E. (1984) *Medicines and Poisons Guide*, Pharmaceutical Press, London.

Pharmaceutical Society of Great Britain (1979) *British Pharmaceutical Codex*, Pharmaceutical Press, London.

Poisons Act 1972, HMSO, London.

UKCC (1986) *Administration of Medicines*, UKCC, London.

US Department of Health and Human Services (1988) Update: Universal precautions for prevention of transmission of human immunodeficiency virus, hepatitis B virus, and other blood borne pathogens in health-care settings, *Morbidity and Mortality Weekly Report*, Vol. 37, no. 24, pp. 377–82.

Further reading

Alderton, J. (1984) Administering drugs safely: alone – or in pairs, *Nursing Standard*, Vol. 34, no. 7, p. 5.

Apple, J.L. (1976) The classification of medication errors, *Supervisor Nurse*, Vol. 7, no. 12, pp. 23–9.

Baudhuin, M. *et al.* (1981) *Lithium and the Kidney: A Bibliography*, Lithium Information Centre, Madison.

Bauwens, E. and Clemmons, C. (1978) Foods that foil drugs, *RN*, Vol. 41, no. 9, pp. 79–81.

Brown, C.S., Wright, R.G. and Christensen, D.B. (1987) Association between type of medication instruction and patients' knowledge, side effects and compliance, *Hospital and Community Psychiatry*, Vol. 38, no. 1, pp. 55–60.

Brown, G. (1979) Medication errors: a case study, *Hospitals*, Vol. 52, no. 20, pp. 61–65.

Bryant, W.M. (1981) Common toxic effects of systemic drugs on the eye, *Occupational Health Nursing*, Vol. 33, no. 66, pp. 15–17.

Cahill, C. and Arana, G.W. (1986) Navigating neuroleptic malignant syndrome, *American Journal of Nursing*, Vol. 86, pp. 671–3.

Chalmers, H. (1977) First do no harm, *Nursing Mirror*, Vol. 145, no. 6, pp. i–iv.

Connolly, C.E. (1984) Compliance with outpatient lithium therapy, *Perspectives in Psychiatric Care*, Vol. 22, no. 2, pp. 44–50.

Creagh, T. (1986) Just a little jab?, *Nursing Times*, Vol. 82, no. 49, p. 50.

Creighton, H. (1982) Liability of nurse floated to another unit, *Nursing Management*, Vol. 13, pp. 54–5.

DHSS (1977) *Guide to Misuse of Drugs Act and to Certain Regulations made under the Act*, DHSS, London.

Doller, J.C. (1977) Tardive dyskinesia and changing concepts of antipsychotic drug use: a nursing prospective, *Journal of Psychiatric Nursing*, Vol. 15, no. 11, pp. 23–6.

Duquesne, T. (1983) Focus on drugs, *Nursing Focus*, Vol. 4, no. 5, p. 14.

Fruth, R. (1980) Anaphylaxis and drug reactions. Guidelines for detection and care, *Heart and Lung*, Vol. 9, no. 4, pp. 662–4.

Hogan, T.P., Awad, A.G. and Eastwood, R. (1983) A self-report scale predictive of drug compliance in schizophrenics: reliability and discriminative validity, *Psychological Medicine*, Vol. 13, pp. 177–83.

Hunn, S. *et al.* (1980) Nursing care of patients on lithium, *Perspectives in Psychiatric Care*, Vol. 18, no. 5, pp. 214–20.

Iveson–Iveson, J. (1978) Is your medicine really necessary?, *Nursing Mirror*, Vol. 147, no. 5, p. 9.

Jones, J.W. (1981) Attitudinal correlates of employee theft of drugs and hospital supplies among nursing personnel, *Nursing Research*, Vol. 30, no. 6, pp. 349–51.

Lenz, C.L. (1983) Make your needle selection right to the point, *Nursing*, Vol. 13, no. 2, pp. 50–1.

Long, G. (1982) The effect of medication distribution systems on medication errors, *Nursing Research*, Vol. 31, no. 3, pp. 182–4.

Markowitz, J.S. *et al.* (1981) Nurses, physicians and pharmacists: their knowledge of hazards of medication, *Nursing Research*, Vol. 30, no. 6, pp. 366–70.

Michel, K. and Kolakowska, T. (1981) A survey of prescribing psychotropic drugs in two psychiatric hospitals, *British Journal of Psychiatry*, Vol. 138, pp. 217–21.

Ministry of Health (1965) HM(65)96, *Standard Dangerous Drugs Register for Hospitals,* Ministry of Health, London.

Pierce, M.E. (1984) Reporting and following up on medication errors, *Nursing*, Vol. 14, no. 1, pp. 8–9.

Rettig, F.M. and Soutby, J.R. (1984) Using different positions to reduce discomfort from dorsogluteal injection, in F. Downs (ed.) *A Sourcebook of Nursing Research*, Davis, Philadephia.

Rosenberg, J.M. (1981) Take with meals . . . or not? Quick answers to a pesky question, *RN*, Vol. 44, no. 5, pp. 47–52.

Rosenman, H. *et al.* (1977) Improving control drug distribution through nursing–pharmacy cooperation, *Hospital Topics*, Vol. 55, no. 5, pp. 30–3.

Salzman, C. (1982) A primer on geriatric psychophar-

macology, *American Journal of Psychiatry*, Vol. 139, pp. 67–74.

Sklar, C. (1979) Nursing negligence in the administration of medication . . . could it happen to you?, *Canadian Nurse*, Vol. 75, no. 7, pp. 51–2.

Snyder, S.H. (1986) *Drugs and the Brain*, Scientific American Library, New York.

Vernon, A.W. (1981) Classification of psychotherapeutic drugs, *Journal of Psychosocial Nursing and Mental Health Services*, Vol. 19, no. 11, pp. 15–20.

Wade, B. (1983) Teaching the management of medication, *Nursing Focus*, Vol. 5, no. 1, pp. 9–10.

Wilson, B.S. (1977) Medication error policy, *Supervisor Nurse*, Vol. 8, no. 5, pp. 53–6.

Wolf, M.E. and Brown, P. (1987) Overcoming institutional and community resistance to a tardive dyskinesia management programme, *Hospital and Community Psychiatry*, Vol. 38, no. 1, pp. 65–9.

36

Depot Injections

DEFINITION

A depot injection is a means of administering a drug which is to be absorbed slowly over a period of days or weeks.

DISCUSSION

Nursing research into the use of psychotropic medication has looked at its efficacy in combination or in comparison with other treatments. It is not usually specified in such research whether neuroleptic medication is being given in the form of depots or not, and its effects are not clear. For instance, Slavinsky and Krauss (1982) compared patients attending a medication clinic with patients receiving a social support programme. They found after two years that the patients attending the medication clinic had better outcomes than those attending the support programme. Davidhizar (1982a, 1982b, 1985) has examined patients' attitudes to medication, but whether the drugs were being administered regularly by injection is not stated. She refers to the lack of research in the area, and suggests that individualized treatment plans will be enhanced by better information about clients' attitudes to medication. It is suggested that well-documented casework with patients who receive depot medication will, in its turn, assist future research.

Depot medication tends to be used when there is a problem of compliance with an orally administered drug regimen. Close attention must be paid to patients' rights in terms of their consent to the injections (Turnquist, 1983). Additionally, the patient must be closely monitored in case toxicity develops, which may lead to irreversible effects such as tardive dyskinesia and retinal degeneration. Agranulocytosis and cardiac arrhythmias are uncommon but serious effects. Reversible but still unwanted effects, such as akinesia, akathisia, oculogyric crisis or dysarthria, require immediate medical attention in order to intervene with antiparkinsonian medica-

tion or to reduce the dosage of the depot. Frances and Weiden (1987) suggest that failure to educate patients about side-effects, failure to recognize them when they occur, and delay in treating them are likely to lead to suspicion of and non-compliance with future drug regimens by patients. An extremely useful account of the problems associated with the administration of long-acting neuroleptics is provided by Belanger-Annable (1985). This paper also provides a detailed procedure for repeated injections of depot neuroleptics.

Documentation

To keep close track of all patients receiving depot medication, whether they are inpatients or outpatients, it is advisable to use specific documentation to be used in conjunction with their prescription sheets and nursing process records.

An example of such documentation is a depot injection record sheet, illustrated in Figure 36.1, which bears the record of administration, the patient's details, a copy of the prescription and an *aide-mémoire* of observations to be carried out each time the patient attends for injection. A standard letter, such as that in Figure 36.2, may be completed and sent to the patient's responsible medical officer in case of default or the expiry of the prescription.

Nursing and medical staff share responsibility for ensuring that the patient safely receives the correct medication from an up-to-date prescription and only after a nursing assessment at each visit, and a psychiatric assessment at least every three months. In practice the nursing staff of the ward will be responsible for booking the patient in to see the doctor for his or her psychiatric assessment at least every twelve weeks.

The depot injection record sheets will be kept with the prescription cards. The patient's medical and nursing notes will be kept available for entries to be made on each visit. In this way, a patient's changes and progress or deterioration over time may be monitored.

Name_____ Hospital number_____ Date of birth_____

Address_____

_____

Consultant_____ Telephone_____

Weight and BP record_____

_____

Copy of prescription (to be written by the patient's doctor)

Date	Medication	Dosage	Frequency	Signature	Renewal date

Notes for nurses giving depot injections

A personal knowledge of the patient and interest in his or her complaints, with an occasional direct inquiry about side-effects, is better than asking every patient about every possible side-effect. Do not use the following summary as a checklist. These are possible observations or questions to be borne in mind when assessing individual patients.

1. Excessive drowsiness   2. Excessively dry mouth   3. Excessive constipation   4. Trouble passing water   5. Sexual dysfunction   6. Blurring of vision, which may be associated with painful or red eyes   7. Weight gain   8. Menstrual irregularities   9. Dizziness, especially following sudden postural changes*   10. Pain or spasm in muscles*   11. Development of unusual postures*   12. Development of other abnormal movements   13. Abnormal lack of mobility   14. Irregular involuntary movements of the tongue   15. Difficulty in swallowing or breathing*

* May need immediate medical attention.

Depot injection record sheet

Date due	Date given	Dose given	Signatures of nurse giving and nurse checking	Action taken for non-attendance

Figure 36.1   Example of depot injection record sheet

Depot injection service

From: To:

Ward/Dept: Ward/Dept:

Telephone: Date:

Reference: Hospital number:

Address:
                                         Telephone:

Dear

I am writing to let you know that
*   is due to attend for *his/her three-monthly psychiatric assessment
on   at   . Please would you renew the depot injection prescription at or before this visit.
*   failed to attend for *his/her depot injection which was due on   . *I have/have not contacted
the patient.
*He/she *has/has not agreed to attend to receive the injection on   at   . Please would you let
me know if you wish to see *him/her at this visit.

*   last received a depot injection on   , and has failed to attend the depot injection service for
four weeks. *I have/have not contacted the patient. *He/she *has/has not agreed to attend for a further psychiatric assessment.
Please use this form to give instructions as to the disposal of the current prescription and depot injection record.

Instructions from responsible medical officer

From: To:

Ward/Dept: Ward/Dept:

Telephone: Date:

Reference: Hospital number:

_____

_____

_____(signature)
_____
* Delete as applicable.

Figure 36.2   Example of standard letter to be sent to a patient's responsible medical officer in case of default

It seems to be unavoidable that a certain amount of regular checking takes place in order to ensure that patients receive their injections on time, are carefully monitored and have their medication reviewed by a psychiatrist every three months. Although the calendars and diaries provided by the various drug companies appear attractive, they have limitations which prevent full safety in their use. The main limitation is that they are based on the trade name of the particular medication being promoted. The average ward will be using at least two different types of depot injections, prescribed using their generic names. Moreover, the UKCC Code of

Conduct prohibits nurses from promoting commercial products (Appendix A, p. 301).

Patients receive injections of varying amounts at varying intervals. It is easy to make an error on a calendar which confuses patients' names, their doses and the due dates. If the due date is recorded on each individual depot injection record sheet, the senior registered nurse on duty can, once a week, say at the weekend, check the depot injection records against the patients' treatment cards.

If there are any defaults, omissions or discrepancies, the nurse will use the standard depot injection form to write to the patient's doctor and primary nurse to inform them that the patient has failed to attend, or needs review or requires a new prescription. Standard pre-printed letters could contain a space where the doctor replies by writing instructions to the nurse, as in the example in Figure 36.2. If a person is due to come in for an injection, the nurse also makes sure that any take-away medication is ready, so that the patient does not have to hang around waiting for it to be dispensed.

Objectives

The objectives of this procedure are to ensure that the patient receives the correct medications and assessment, that defaulting patients can be monitored within a week of their failure to come for an injection, and that patients experiencing side-effects of the medication can discuss them with the nurse and doctor as soon as possible.

HIV-positive and hepatitis B antigen-carrying patients

This section is repeated from the main procedure for the administration of medicines, in Chapter 35. Because the human immunodeficiency virus (HIV) and the hepatitis B virus are present in blood and other body fluids, precautions are necessary when depot injections are administered. Provided that nurses know and follow the most recent guidelines for managing contact with HIV-positive individuals or people thought to be HIV-positive, the risks of transmitting infection by the human immunodeficiency virus will be reduced (DHSS, 1986; (US DHSS, 1988). The same is true of hepatitis B (US DHSS, 1988). It is generally recommended that nurses whose own immune responsiveness is lowered for any reason do not come into contact with HIV-positive or hepatitis B antigen-carrying individuals. Because it appears that the human immunodeficiency virus has to travel through the blood-stream to reach the tissues which it infects, as does the hepatitis B virus, nurses who have skin lesions of any kind should either cover them with a waterproof dressing before giving an injection to an HIV-positive or hepatitis B antigen-carrying individual, or refrain from carrying it out at all. Conversely, it must be borne in mind that lesions on the skin of infected individuals are a potential source of infection.

GUIDELINES: ADMINISTERING DEPOT INJECTIONS

Action	Rationale
1 The prescription cards and depot injection record sheets of a ward or unit are filed in a central location such as the clinical room.	To ensure reliably easy access by both nurses and medical staff.
2 Each prescription card and depot injection record has been updated within the last twelve weeks.	To ensure that patients' medication is reviewed at frequent intervals.
3 An 'action file' is used to facilitate the storage, checking and review of prescription cards and depot injection record sheets.	So that a doctor, say, who receives a request to rewrite a prescription can immediately find the relevant records.
4 In- and outpatients' depot injection record sheets are filed together.	To operate two separate files risks confusion between patients whose status alters from, say, inpatient to outpatient.
5 Each depot injection record sheet is completed with the patient's personal details, including hospital number and a copy of the current prescription.	So that if other records are not available, a patient may be contacted if he or she defaults.

6 The charge nurse of the ward or unit designates a day each week when the senior registered nurse on duty checks the documentation of the depot injections and signs as having done so.

(a) So that responsibility for checking may be routinely assigned and accepted.
(b) So that patients who default may be contacted within a week of doing so.

7 The prescription sheets are checked against the depot injection records.

To ensure that there is no discrepancy in dates or dosage.

8 If any defaults, omissions, or discrepancies are found, the nurse reports them in writing using the preprinted standard letter to the patient's RMO and primary nurse.

(a) So that medical staff recognize from ward to ward when the depot injection procedure is being used and can respond correctly.
(b) So that the primary nurse can liaise with the medical staff, especially if the doctor does not know the patient.

9 The primary nurse and the doctor are responsible for deciding what action to take if the patient has defaulted.

The checking nurse's responsibility ends after the necessary information about the default has been communicated and received.

10 The charge nurse is responsible for ensuring that medical and other nursing staff action any communication received concerning any omissions or discrepancies found during the weekly check.

Omissions and discrepancies need to be rectified before the patient concerned next attends for a depot injection or relapses or drops out of treatment.

11 When the patient attends for a depot injection, it is given as soon as possible.

Common courtesy.

12 Before giving the injection a registered nurse who is a permanent member of the ward staff talks with the patient for a while.

(a) To find out how he or she is getting on generally.
(b) To hear any complaints he or she may have.
(c) To observe and listen for evidence of side-effects from the medication.
(d) To assess whether a consultation with the doctor needs to be arranged.

13 The injection is given by the registered nurse who assesses the patient.

In order to retain and reinforce the patient's confidence in the continuity of and attention to his or her care.

14 When the injection has been given, the nurse gives the patient any take-away medication prescribed.

So that it is not forgotten.

15 The nurse confirms with the patient when the next injection is due, and fills in his or her appointment card.

So that he or she will attend on the right day.

16 The nurse completes the entries on the depot injection record and signs them, together with the nurse who witnessed the injection.

(a) To prevent any mistakes when the injection is next due.
(b) To facilitate checking of any queries later.

17 The nurse who carries out the procedure makes a brief entry in the nursing record for that patient.

To record the results of the nursing assessment.

18 If the patient has seen the doctor before attending for the injection, the nurse obtains from the doctor confirmation of the results of the consultation and, in writing, any changes to the prescription.	To ensure that the procedure can be safely carried out.

REFERENCE MATERIAL
References

Belanger-Annable, M.-C. (1985) Long-acting neuroleptics: Technique for intramuscular injection, *Canadian Nurse*, Vol. 81, no. 8, pp. 41–4.

Davidhizar, R. (1982a) Compliance by persons with schizophrenia: a research issue for the nurse, *Issues in Mental Nursing*, Vol. 4, pp. 233–55.

Davidhizar, R. (1982b) Tool development for profiling the attitude of clients with schizophrenia toward their medication, using Fishbein's expectancy-value model, *Issues in Mental Nursing*, Vol. 4, pp. 343–57.

Davidhizar, R. (1985) Can clients with schizophrenia describe feelings and beliefs about taking medication?, *Journal of Advanced Nursing*, Vol. 10, pp. 469–73.

DHSS (1986) *Information and Guidance on AIDS (Acquired Immune Deficiency Syndrome) for Local Authority Staff*, DHSS, London.

Frances, A. and Weiden, P. (1987) Promoting compliance with outpatient drug treatment, *Hospital and Community Psychiatry*, Vol. 38, no. 11, p. 1158–60.

Slavinsky, A.T. and Krauss, J.B. (1982) Two approaches to the management of long-term psychiatric outpatients in the community, *Nursing Research*, Vol. 31, no. 5, pp. 284–9.

Turnquist, A.C. (1983) The issue of informed consent and the use of neuroleptic medications, *International Journal of Nursing Studies*, Vol. 3, pp. 181–6.

US Department of Health and Human Services (1988) Update: Universal precautions for prevention of transmission of human immunodeficiency virus, hepatitis B virus, and other blood borne pathogens in health care settings, *Morbidity and Mortality Weekly Report*, Vol. 37, no. 24, pp. 377–82.

Further reading

Armitage, S. (1980) Non-compliant recipients of health care, *Nursing Times*, Vol. 76, no. 1, pp. 1–3.

Brands, A.J. and Brands, A.B. (1983) Drug therapy and monitoring: a team responsibility, *Family and Community Health*, Vol. 6, no. 3, pp. 63–71.

Brown, C.S., Wright, R.G. and Christensen, D.B. (1987) Association between type of medication instruction and patients' knowledge, side effects and compliance, *Hospital and Community Psychiatry*, Vol. 38, no. 1, pp. 55–60.

Doller, J.C. (1977) Tardive dyskinesia and changing concepts of antipsychotic drug use: a nursing prospective, *Journal of Psychiatric Nursing*, Vol. 15, no. 11, pp. 23–6.

Lader, M. (1980) *Introduction to Psychopharmacology*, Upjohn, Kalamazoo.

Martin, I. (1978) Mirthless merry-go-round, *Nursing Times*, Vol. 74, no. 34, pp. 1426–7.

Rettig, F.M. and Southby, J.R. (1984) Using different positions to reduce discomfort from dorsogluteal injection, in F. Downs (ed.) *A Sourcebook of Nursing Research*, Davis, Philadelphia.

Scott, E., Sharma, J.K. and Temple, K. (1977) Care of the schizophrenic patient, *Nursing Times*, Vol. 73, no. 20, pp. 740–1.

Thomas, B. (1984) Depot drugs in community psychiatry, *Nursing Times*, Vol. 80, no. 3, pp. 43–6.

[Unattributed article] (1982) Giving depot neuroleptic drugs, *Nursing Mirror*, Vol. 154, no. 16, pp. 42–3.

37

Administering an Injection without a Patient's Consent

DISCUSSION

Users of this manual are reminded that procedures involving emergencies may take a good deal longer to read than to implement. It is intended that they are used as the basis for staff training in the issues of consent, statutory requirements, safety and management of disturbed patients. Some of the issues concerning restraint and treatment are recapitulated in this chapter, which is intended to be used in conjunction with Chapters 13 and 14, covering preventing and managing violence, Chapter 10 on consent, Chapter 26 on searching patients' property, Chapter 34 on seclusion and Chapter 42, dealing with the nurse's holding power.

The Mental Health Act provisions

The Mental Health Act 1983 specifies that certain limited forms of 'medical treatment' may be given without consent to patients detained under sections which allow detention for the purposes of treatment. In practice such treatment is limited to administering drugs for a period of time not exceeding three months from the date they were first prescribed. Three months is also the maximum permissible time for administering drugs without consent in any one period of detention. If a section is renewed, it counts as a single period of detention, and so three months remains the maximum permissible period of time for drug treatment of a patient without consent.

The use of tranquillizing medication to control behaviour is a form of restraint in itself, as is the threat to use such medication. If medication is administered to a patient against his or her will, force is required. The issues of the nature of the justification for the use of force and the degree of force that is reasonable in the circumstances are discussed in Chapter 10.

Section 62 sets aside the requirement for the detained patient's consent to treatment. It states that detained as well as informal patients need not consent to 'urgent treatment':

(a) which is immediately necessary to save the patient's life; or
(b) which [not being irreversible] is immediately necessary to prevent a serious deterioration of his condition; or
(c) which [not being irreversible or hazardous] is immediately necessary to alleviate serious suffering by the patient; or
(d) which [not being irreversible or hazardous] is immediately necessary and represents the minimum interference necessary to prevent the patient from behaving violently or being a danger to himself or others.

The decision to medicate without consent

The multidisciplinary clinical team is required to operate and document a clearly defined treatment plan for each detained patient. The use of the nursing process ensures that nurses maintain up-to-date care plans for every patient, whether detained or informal. The nursing assessment will consider whether patients are disturbed enough possibly to need medication without their consent, so that the nursing care plans can anticipate and document the nursing actions that would become necessary in such circumstances. The assessment and plan will also consider that any exercise of authority against a patient's will may actually risk precipitating violence rather than prevent it.

The question whether to inject a patient against his or her will is a decision which is often taken against a background of emotional upheaval and a rapid succession of events, possibly set in train by an act of violence in which injuries have been inflicted. The patient may already have been physically restrained without cessation of the apparent risk of harm.

The emergency team (for example, the duty nurse manager, duty doctor and two other nurses) will have been called. It is usually advisable to summon the patient's doctor and the senior registrar if they are available. It is essential that the discussion of how the patient will be managed is clearly led and that the staff who know him or her and who know the circumstances of the present incident participate. The leader of the discussion will be the senior registered nurse or doctor present. Once a decision has been made, the senior nurse will co-ordinate and identify actions to be taken, designating those who will perform them. The steps in the decision-making process must be clearly identifiable in order that proper documentation and later examination of the incident can take place.

Practical procedure

For the purposes of this procedure it is suggested that six nurses restraining a patient without inflicting pain of any kind is a more reasonable use of force than a smaller number restraining him or her by means of actual or threatened physical pain, such as is involved, say, in certain arm locks or by the use of mechanical restraints. It is suggested that the sixth nurse administers the injection while the patient is immobile, so that it causes the minimum discomfort.

If the injection takes place at a time when the MDCT responsible for the patient is not available (e.g. at weekends and at night), the patient's treatment will need to be reviewed as soon as the team can be assembled. It may be that an outpatient has presented as an emergency and may need to be medicated very quickly before being admitted. A person who has just been admitted as an emergency may not yet be known by the team to which he or she has been allocated. The principle remains that, as soon as is practicable, the team assesses the need for continuing medication in the light of the patient's mental state, social and family circumstances, physical state and any forensic history.

Further actions may include:

1 an application for detention of the patient under section 3 of the Mental Health Act 1983 whereby treatment may be conducted for up to three months;
2 request for a second opinion if the patient has already been detained under section 3 for three months;
3 consideration of the possibility of the use of legal sanctions or the involvement of the police or both.

HIV-positive and hepatitis B antigen-carrying patients

Because the human immunodeficiency virus (HIV) and the hepatitis B virus are present in blood and other body fluids, precautions are necessary when medication is administered by injection. It is generally recommended that nurses whose own immune responsiveness is lowered for any reason do not come into contact with HIV-positive or hepatitis B antigen-carrying individuals (DHSS, 1986; US DHHS, 1988). Because it appears that the human immunodeficiency virus has to travel through the blood-stream to reach the tissues which it infects, as does the hepatitis B virus, nurses who have skin lesions of any kind should either cover them with a waterproof dressing before carrying out an invasive procedure with an HIV-positive or hepatitis B antigen-carrying individual, or refrain from carrying it out at all. Conversely, it must be borne in mind that lesions on the skin of infected individuals are a potential source of infection.

GUIDELINES: ADMINISTERING AN INJECTION WITHOUT A PATIENT'S CONSENT

Action	Rationale
1 If available, the emergency team is summoned, consisting of a clinical nurse manager, a doctor, a trained nurse and another nurse, whether qualified or not.	To provide extra resources in addition to the staff already available in the ward or unit.
2 The nurse in charge of the ward or unit where the patient is to be injected directs the procedure.	So that instructions are clearly given by one person and immediately followed.
3 If there are fewer than eight members of staff present the duty clinical nurse manager will summon help from other wards.	(a) Six people will be required to carry out the injection. (b) At least two nurses, one of whom must be RMN, must be available to look after the rest of the patients in the ward.

4 Away from the clinical area the nurse in charge gives the team a general outline of what is to be done.

It is important that the team which gives the injection is seen to be united and decisive. The preparations for the injection are therefore carried out away from the patient area.

5 The nurse in charge briefly outlines the situation that has led up to the present emergency.

(a) So that the team knows who the patient is;
(b) who the other ward staff are;
(c) who has been brought from other wards to help.
(d) In order to understand the risks.

6 The nurse in charge states the objective of the procedure.

So that team members understand what the risks are.

7 Members of staff remove all personal jewellery, badges and pens.

To prevent accidental injury to the patient or themselves.

8 The nurse in charge assigns to four nurses the task of immobilizing the patient by taking control of his or her limbs, after ascertaining that they have been trained in and have practised the techniques of restraint and immobilization.

So that each nurse understands his or her role in relation to the other staff.

9 Each nurse is responsible individually or jointly for immobilizing a named part of the patient's body.

(a) So that a method will be selected which meets the requirements of the present emergency.
(b) So that nurses know from which side to approach the patient.

10 The nurse in charge nominates two nurses to check and draw up both oral and intramuscular medication.

The oral medication will be offered first to the patient, but the injection is ready to be given immediately if the patient refuses the oral medication.

11 The administering nurse washes his or her hands and draws up the drug, wearing unused protective gloves and plastic apron if necessary.

(a) This is a clean procedure.
(b) The gloves are worn in case of an allergic reaction, as well as in case of infection.

12 The nurse in charge nominates a nurse to fetch any equipment needed, such as mattress, blankets, pillows, sheets.

(a) A mattress or pillow may be used as protection against a knife.
(b) Blankets or sheets may be used to immobilize the patient.
(c) Pillows may be used to protect the patient if he or she is immobilized on the floor.

13 The nurse in charge maintains contact with the nurses observing the patient.

So that the staff know where they are likely to have to restrain the patient.

14 The nurse in charge describes the location where the injection is likely to be carried out.

So that members of the team know where they are expected to be.

15   The nurse in charge co-ordinates the instructions to the members of the team, stating:
   (i)   timings;
   (ii) how the patient will be approached;
   (iii) where the members of the team will position themselves;
   (iv) who will give the injection;
   (v)   any other risks which may be present: for example, an infected patient.

   (a) To ensure that each member of the team is fully briefed about his or her role and responsibilities.
   (b) To ensure that nurses can take the precautions necessary to prevent injury as a result of the risks presented by the patient.

16   The nurse in charge confirms with the duty doctor and the duty clinical nurse manager what their roles will be.

   So that support and help will be available if necessary.

17   The nurse in charge confirms with the remaining nurses in the ward what their roles will be.

   So that the rest of the patients will be safely looked after.

18   The nurse in charge says what his or her words of command to the team will be.

   So that the members of the team know when to act.

19   The nurse in charge confirms that each member of the team understands his or her responsibility.

   The resulting co-ordination will increase confidence in each other.

20   The nurse in charge asks for any questions from team members.

   To confirm finally that the action to be taken is understood by all members of the team.

21   The nurse in charge, carrying oral medication, approaches the patient together with the team, while the nurse responsible for administering the injection follows with the intramuscular medication.

   (a) It must be clear to the patient that the nurse in charge is not threatening him or her but that the patient does not have a choice about accepting medication.
   (b) It is assumed that all other attempts to persuade the patient to take oral medication have failed.

22   The nurse in charge asks the patient to take the oral medication.

   To offer the patient a last chance to take control of his or her behaviour.

23   If the patient refuses, the nurse in charge gives the prearranged command, the team moves quietly to either side and immobilizes the patient as planned. Depending where the patient is this might be on the floor, in a chair or on a bed.

   The patient is immobilized where he or she is in order to prevent injury by unnecessary movement to another location.

24   The nurse in charge remains by the patient's head talking continuously to him or her and restraining it if necessary.

   The effect of one person talking calmly and quietly can be to reduce fear and anger, especially in perplexed patients.

25   When the patient is still, the nurse administering the injection does so through the patient's clothes if necessary; either into the middle third of the outer aspect of the thigh, or the outer upper quadrant of either buttock or both, depending on the size of the injection.

   It may not be possible to remove the patient's clothing in order to expose the injection sites without compromising the team's ability to immobilize him or her.

26 When the injection has been given the team remains in position, the nurse in charge talking to the patient, until it is confirmed that he or she is calm enough to be released.

(a) Because this may take ten to thirty minutes, utmost patience by the team is required.
(b) Psychotic patients are particularly vulnerable to being suddenly released after being immobilized, and may become violent again.

27 If possible the team accompanies the patient to a quiet area of the ward and a nurse who knows him or her takes over from the nurse in charge.

In order to reward the patient's behaviour by remaining nearby and being available to listen and talk.

28 Maximum supervision is implemented by one or two nurses as decided by the nurse in charge.

(a) In case the patient becomes disturbed again.
(b) To monitor the effects of the medication.

29 The team returns to the nursing office to meet with the doctor and the nurse manager and to debrief from the incident.

(a) In order that each staff member can evaluate his or her role in the context of the team's work as a whole.
(b) In order that points for improvement can be noted.
(c) In order to praise individuals for their contribution.
(d) To provide the opportunity for people to talk about their experience of the incident.

30 All debris is disposed into a sharps bin for incineration, using a separate bin labelled High Risk for waste from HIV-positive or hepatitis B antigen-positive patients.

(a) To prevent injury during disposal of the waste.
(b) To prevent any cross-infection.

31 The nurse in charge completes any documentation required by the hospital managers, such as:
(i)   violent incident report form;
(ii) report of treatment without consent.

All such incidents are reviewed by the Mental Health Act Commissioners.

32 The nurse in charge writes an account of the procedure in the patient's nursing record.

To ensure that, if necessary, the incident can be evaluated after the lapse of time.

33 The nurse who administered the medication to the patient records it on the drug administration record.

To comply with the procedure for the administration of medicines.

34 The doctor writes in the medical record an account of the patient's mental state before and after the medication.

So that further prescriptions and assessments can be evaluated against an accurate summary of evidence as to psychopathology and response to treatment.

35 The nurse in charge ensures that any steps required by the Mental Health Act 1983 are begun, such as:
(i)   the obtaining of a second opinion;
(ii)   detaining the patient in hospital for treatment;
(iii) consulting with the Mental Health Act Commissioners.

So that future treatments will continue to comply with the law.

REFERENCE MATERIAL
References

DHSS (1986) *Information and Guidance on AIDS (Acquired Immune Deficiency Syndrome) for Local Authority Staff*, DHSS, London.

Mental Health Act 1983, HMSO, London.

US Department of Health and Human Services (1988) Update: Universal precautions for prevention of transmission of human immunodeficiency virus, hepatitus B virus, and other blood borne pathogens in health care settings, *Morbidity and Mortality Weekly Report*, Vol. 37, no. 24, pp. 377–82.

Further reading

Creighton, H. (1981) Forced medication of mental patients, *Nursing Management*, Vol. 12, no. 9, pp. 72–3.

Hargreaves, W. A. *et al.* (1987) Neuroleptic refusal by involuntary patients: due process protection of the right to refuse, *Psychopharmacology Bulletin*, Vol. 23, no. 3, pp. 526–9.

McGinnis, J. and Foote, K. (1986) Rapid neuroleptization, *Journal of Psychosocial Nursing and Mental Health Services*, Vol. 24, no. 10, pp. 17–22.

Oriol, M. D. and Oriol, R. D. (1986) Involuntary commitment and the right to refuse medication, *Journal of Psychosocial Nursing and Mental Health Services*, Vol. 24, no. 11, pp. 15–20.

Thorner, N. (1976) Nurses violate their patients' rights, *Journal of Psychiatric Nursing*, Vol. 14, no. 1, pp. 7–12.

38

Electroconvulsive Therapy

DEFINITIONS

Electroconvulsive therapy (ECT)
ECT is a treatment which induces a generalized seizure by the application of two electrodes to the temples and passing an electrical stimulus between them.

Bilateral ECT
Bilateral ECT refers to the placing of the electrodes on both temples so that the electrical stimulus passes between them.

Unilateral ECT
Unilateral ECT refers to the placing of an electrode on one temple, and the other on the scalp on the same (non-dominant) side.

DISCUSSION

Electroconvulsive therapy (ECT) is thought to have therapeutic effects on a variety of symptoms by producing a generalized seizure induced by the application of two electrodes and the passing of an electrical stimulus between them. ECT is known to be effective in the treatment of severe depression and puerperal psychosis. It may also be helpful in the management of some other psychotic patients. Responsiveness to ECT varies with age, duration of symptoms, family history and gender. Other variables include the placing of the electrodes and the choice of unilateral or bilateral ECT. Medication regimens may affect responsiveness, as do the drugs administered during a treatment. The frequency, number and duration of treatments have been shown to affect outcomes.

The seizure is modified by the use of a brief general anaesthetic with atropine or similar anticholinergic drug to control secretion and heart rate, intravenous thiopentone sodium or methohexitone sodium to induce anaesthesia, and suxemethonium chloride to produce neuromuscular blockade or paralysis. The duration of apnoea is about five minutes and the patient is artificially ventilated with a mixture of air and oxygen. A rubber bite plate is inserted in the patient's mouth to prevent injury during the seizure, following which an oropharyngeal airway is inserted until the patient is able to maintain his or her own airway.

The effects of ECT

BILATERAL AND UNILATERAL ECT
Evidence conflicts somewhat, but it appears that if both types are carried out with equal care their therapeutic effects are equivalent. However, response to bilateral ECT appears to be quicker than with unilateral; and unilateral ECT appears to produce significantly fewer cognitive deficits.

UNWANTED EFFECTS
Memory deficit has been implicated as a severe effect of ECT. The evidence is difficult to evaluate. The conditions for which ECT is given are often accompanied by cognitive impairment, so that the extent of any additional impairment is hard to evaluate. Some evidence shows that pre-existing deficits have improved following ECT. Because there is a lack of controlled longitudinal studies of large enough populations, it is not possible to say unequivocally what the long-term cognitive effects are.

Immediately after a treatment the effects are unequivocal. The patient may have a headache, may be confused and there may be a retrograde amnesia. Anterograde amnesia interferes with the person's ability to learn and remember new information, but this ability generally returns to normal within weeks of the last treatment. There is some evidence that confusion and headache are worse following bilateral application of the electrodes.

The issues in the ECT debate

Taylor and Carroll (1987) have identified five key issues in the debate about ECT. It is suggested that nurses who are interested in the subject familiarize themselves with the research and make up their minds on the quality of available evidence. The first issue is whether ECT corrects a dysfunctional neurophysiological mechanism or merely causes neurological dysfunction. The second is whether the immediate benefits of ECT that are reliably documented are confirmed in long-term follow-up studies. The third is whether the observable side-effects constitute the only ones, and whether their diminution over time is more apparent than real. The fourth is whether the undoubted life-saving function of ECT could be fulfilled by any other treatment for less cost to the patient's well-being. The fifth is whether present arrangements for obtaining informed consent are sufficient.

Nurses' responsibilities

Aside from debates about the use of ECT, the nurse caring for someone who is having or about to have ECT has seven distinct responsibilities.

ENSURING THAT THE PATIENT IS PROPERLY INFORMED

An acceptable explanation would include the following details.

1 ECT is designed to relieve mental suffering.
2 Although the patient may feel better after one or two treatments, a course of six to ten treatments will be required in order to sustain improvement.
3 A general anaesthetic is administered.
4 The general anaesthetic lasts less than five minutes.
5 An electric current is administered by a doctor while the patient is anaesthetized.
6 The amount of electric current is very small.
7 The duration of the electric current is less than four seconds.
8 The electric current is administered via two electrodes placed on the skin surface of one or both temples.
9 Headaches may be expected following ECT.
10 People may forget the events of the day leading up to ECT.
11 Other apparent disturbances of memory and concentration tend to resolve as the disorder for which ECT is being given resolves.
12 A person is advised not to drive motor vehicles or ride a bicycle on the same day as having a general anaesthetic.
13 After recovery from the anaesthetic a person can eat and drink and participate in the usual ward routine if an inpatient, or go home on public transport with a relative or friend if an outpatient.

The doctor who is responsible for obtaining a person's consent to ECT is responsible for giving the explanation above. It is helpful if the primary nurse is present when the doctor explains the treatment, or at least meets with the doctor afterwards to confirm what has been said.

The primary nurse will continue to ensure that the patient has grasped the explanation, liaising with his or her friends or relatives if necessary.

ENSURING THAT THE PATIENT IS FREE TO CHOOSE

The patient's freedom of choice of treatment exists only if there are no external circumstances forcing him or her to accept treatment: for example, a threat of detention under the Mental Health Act; a promise of discharge from a section of the Mental Health Act. The nurse ensures that no such pressure is applied to a patient.

ENSURING THAT THE PATIENT HAS CONSENTED TO ECT

The patient's primary nurse will liaise with the doctor to confirm the patient's consent before each treatment. This may involve explaining again the nature and effects of ECT, remembering that rumination, perseveration, memory disturbance, gloom about the future, mistrust of other people and anger are aspects of severe depression. (See Chapter 40, p. 264, and Chapter 10, p. 67.) The nurse contributes to the discussion non-directively and, bearing in mind that nurses do not prescribe ECT, he or she will ensure that the patient consults with the RMO.

TREATMENT WITHOUT CONSENT

Consent to treatment is covered by Part 4 of the Mental Health Act. Consent to treatment is required for both informal and detained patients. The circumstances in which ECT can be given without consent to detained patients are limited by sections 58 and 62.

In the case of detained patients, consent must always be obtained for ECT (section 58(1)(b)). Once the patient has consented to ECT the responsible medical officer (RMO) completes Form 38 to say that the patient is capable of understanding the nature, purpose and likely effect of ECT and has consented to it. Additionally the patient signs a standard consent form, agreeing to the administration of a general anaesthetic in order to carry out ECT. The consent form and Form 38 are flagged in the medical notes in order to be readily retrieved. If he or she does not consent a second opinion is sought from a medical practitioner appointed by the Mental Health Act Commission (MHAC). This doctor interviews the patient and consults with the RMO and two other members of the multidisciplinary clinical team caring for the patient, one of whom must be a nurse, the second someone other than a doctor. The doctor appointed by the MHAC will decide that ECT is necessary if 'the patient is not capable of understanding the nature, purpose and likely effects of that treatment' (section 58(3)(b)) and it (ECT) 'will alleviate or prevent a deterioration of his condition'. The doctor completes Form 39, which is retained in the patient's notes, flagged in the same way as Form 38.

The nurse involved in the second opinion will preferably be the patient's primary nurse. He or she will be a first-level nurse and will know the likely cause and outcome of the patient's disorder and the nature and effects of ECT.

ALLEVIATION OF SUFFERING
The nurse's personal beliefs are subordinate to the alleviation of suffering and the prevention of serious harm. Nurses who have strong feelings about ECT have a responsibility to familiarize themselves with the available evidence about its effects and the circumstances which influence its outcome.

SAFETY
The patient is prepared for the general anaesthetic by fasting for at least six hours. Good liaison between nurses on different shifts is necessary to ensure that this in fact happens. Depressed patients may go with the crowd as usual to breakfast or accept a cup of tea, forgetting that they are due for ECT. The nurse who is alert for such circumstances is also alert for the mixed feelings which may underlie forgetfulness, and will offer the patient an opportunity to discuss his or her reservation about treatment. Preferably the primary nurse will be a first-level nurse, so that he or she can check and supervise the patient's medication, record the vital signs before treatment, assist in the treatment area, and recover the patient after treatment.

Each nurse is responsible for checking that resuscitation and other equipment is near to hand and ready for use. A doctor, who is preferably the patient's doctor, is responsible for checking the consent form, placing the electrodes and for administering the electric current. The anaesthetist is responsible for checking and drawing up the anaesthetic agents and for maintaining the anaesthetized patient. Both doctors document their part in the treatment and record in detail their observations.

RECOVERY
The nurse in charge of the recovery phase will have suction and other resuscitation equipment near to hand along with some means of summoning medical help. Before patients are treated, the nurse will have checked all equipment to ensure that it is in good working order.

Nurses in training
A first-level nurse is responsible for devising his or her 'plan of nursing care taking into account the medical prescription', as well as for directing the work of learners and of second-level nurses (Nurses Rules, 1983). Each of the principles outlined in this chapter implies that a first-level nurse will direct the nursing care of patients having ECT. If the organizational model used is primary nursing, the primary nurse will plan and carry out all aspects of the nursing care. It is preferable that the nurse who prepares a patient for ECT is the same nurse who carries out recovery procedures after treatment.

GUIDELINES: ADMINISTERING ELECTROCONVULSIVE THERAPY

Action

1 Ensure that a person for whom ECT may be prescribed has received the following explanation. Do so either by meeting the patient jointly with the doctor or by confirming with the doctor what he or she has told the patient.

(i) ECT is a treatment whose purpose is to alleviate mental suffering.

(ii) In order to carry out ECT a general anaesthetic is given by an anaesthetist.

(iii) The general anaesthetic lasts less than five minutes.

(iv) While the patient is anaesthetized, his or her doctor administers a small amount of electric current lasting less than four seconds via two electrodes placed on the skin surface of one or both temples.

(v) Although the patient may feel better after one or two treatments a course of six to ten treatments will be prescribed in order to achieve sustained improvement in mood.

(vi) After a treatment of ECT a headache and muscle pains may be experienced, relievable by mild analgesia such as paracetamol.

(vii) People may forget the events of a day leading to the general anaesthetic.

(viii) Apparent disturbances of memory and concentration tend to resolve as the disorder for which ECT is being given resolves.

2 Ensure that this explanation is repeated as often as necessary for the patient to understand it, allowing the patient opportunities to express his or her fears about the treatment.

3 When the patient consents to ECT ensure that the responsible medical office (RMO) completes Form 38.

4 Ensure that the RMO has correctly completed with the patient a standard consent form and has prescribed the type, number and frequency of electroconvulsive treatments.

Rationale

(a) Both informal and detained patients must be free to choose whether to have ECT or not.

(b) Both informal and detained patients must give consent before ECT is given.

(c) Real consent involves the patient receiving and understanding a broad explanation of the treatment to be given.

To shift some control to the patient.

In order to confirm that the patient is capable of understanding the nature, purpose and likely effect of ECT and has consented to it.

(a) The patient must agree to administration of a general anaesthetic in order to carry out ECT.

(b) So that the patient agrees specifically to unilateral or bilateral ECT.

(c) So that the patient agrees to a specific number of treatments.

(d) So that the patient agrees to a specific frequency of treatment.

5 The primary nurse participates in any decision to request a second opinion for a patient who refuses to consent to ECT.

(a) The nurse helps to ensure that no patient is treated without consent until a second opinion has been given by a medical practitioner appointed by the MHAC.

(b) As part of his or her assessment this doctor is required to consult with a nurse who has been working with the patient.

6 The primary nurse ensures that the second doctor correctly completes Form 39 if he or she decides that the patient should be treated without consent.

Form 39 is flagged and retained in the patient record as the authority for administering ECT without consent.

7 The primary nurse arranges with the patient's doctor and the nurse in charge of the ECT suite the time that the patient will receive his or her ECT.

(a) In order to give the patient time to prepare: for example, to rearrange an OT programme or reschedule other appointments.

(b) So that the patient and the nurse know from when he or she must fast.

8 Explain to the patient that he or she will be asked to fast for six to eight hours before the general anaesthetic.

(a) To prevent the regurgitation and inhaling of undigested food during the general anaesthetic.

(b) In order to plan when the fasting period will start.

(c) In order to plan the nature of the food and drink taken before the fast begins.

9 Liaise with nurses on other shifts the night before and on the day the patient is due for ECT.

(a) So that the patient and nurses share a plan of care whereby the patient will be safely prepared for ECT.

(b) So that the night nurses can arrange a snack and a drink, if necessary, eight hours before the ECT is due.

10 Meet with the anaesthetist or doctor who examines the patient's physical fitness to undergo a general anaesthetic.

In order to advise the patient appropriately about smoking or premedication and to explain any investigations which may be requested such as chest X-ray.

11 At a time which suits him or her the night before ECT the patient eats an evening meal that is low in fat.

(a) So that the fasting period of six to eight hours is not extended for administrative convenience.

(b) The patient is likely to know the amount and timing of a meal that is tolerable.

(c) A meal that is high in fat remains in the stomach significantly longer and is therefore more likely to be vomited.

12 Check that other patients do not feed the person who is to have ECT.

(a) So that patients will not offer cups of tea and snacks.

(b) The patient who is having ECT may forget about fasting.

13 Check with the patient whether there is any property that he or she would like to deposit into safe-keeping. For example, necklaces, chains, or rings that fit loosely.

Because of the likely amnesia for the morning's events it is possible for patients to lose track of valuable items unless they deposit them in exchange for a receipt.

14 Ensure that a female patient does not use make-up or nail varnish on the day she is due for ECT.

So that changes in skin colour which indicate the patient's cardiovascular state remain visible.

15 Ensure that the patient visits the lavatory and empties his or her bladder before having ECT.

To prevent involuntary micturition during the general anaesthetic.

16 Ensure that the patient removes any hair ornaments.

To prevent abrasion, or contact with the electrodes.

17	Measure and record the patient's vital signs.	To provide baselines in case of any changes after ECT.
18	When accompanying the patient to the ECT suite, take the case notes, chest X-ray and electrocardiogram if relevant, ensuring that Forms 38 or 39 are flagged and visible.	For use by the anaesthetist and the doctor giving the ECT.
19	Ensure that the primary nurse accompanies the patient to ECT.	The same nurse who prepared the patient for ECT accompanies him or her for treatment and recovers him or her afterwards.
20	Ensure privacy for individual patients.	(a) To maintain personal dignity. (b) To avoid alarming other patients who may be unfamiliar with the procedures.
21	Check that the resuscitation equipment is near to hand, in working order and ready for use.	Each nurse is responsible for ensuring the safety of the patient.
22	Ensure that the treatment area is warm enough for the patient to be in bare feet and light, loose-fitting clothing.	(a) So that skin colour is easily visible. (b) So that the minimal signs of a seizure are easily visible. (c) So that in an emergency resuscitation will be unimpeded.
23	Accompany the patient into the treatment area when asked by the anaesthetist or the nurse in charge of the ECT suite.	The anaesthetist will ask for the next patient when satisfied that the preceding one is stable.
24	Introduce the patient to the anaesthetist and doctor if necessary and hand over the notes ensuring that they are placed apart from any other patient's records.	To confirm the identity of the patient.
25	The patient takes off his or her footwear and top layer of clothing such as cardigan or jacket.	(a) To facilitate observation of the seizure. (b) To facilitate assessment of the patient's cardiovascular state. (c) To facilitate administration of the anaesthetic.
26	Under the direction of the anaesthetist the patient removes any false teeth, which are placed in a clean individual container.	(a) So that they can be replaced after the patient has recovered from the anaesthetic. (b) A mouth gag will be used during the general anaesthetic. (c) An oropharyngeal airway is used during the recovery phase.
27	During the treatment phase the nurse works under the direction of the anaesthetist.	(a) The anaesthetist is responsible for the patient while the anaesthetic is in progress. (b) Patient care becomes ineffective if the patient is subjected to simultaneous interventions from different members of staff.

28 Ensure that the patient is lying comfortably flat on his or her back before the administration of the anaesthetic.

(a) So that joints and limbs are in a relaxed and natural position, in case the seizure is less well modified.
(b) To facilitate ventilation of the patient while he or she is unconscious and paralysed.
(c) To facilitate observation of the patient's whole body.
(d) To facilitate resuscitation if it becomes necessary.

29 All members of staff ensure that they speak discreetly while the patient is anaesthetized.

It is possible for the patient to be able to listen while appearing to be unconscious.

30 Once the patient is anaesthetized and oxygenated the anaesthetist gives the go-ahead for the application of electric current.

The rapid action and short duration (five minutes) of the muscle relaxant (usually suxemethonium chloride) and the intravenous anaesthetic (thiopentone sodium or methohexitone sodium) require accurate timing which balances enough artificial ventilation with the necessary paralysis to modify the seizure.

31 If it is the patient's first treatment firmly immobilize his or her limbs at the major joints: for example, shoulders, elbows, hips and knees.

Although the muscle relaxation induced by suxemethonium chloride is rapid and predictable, the dosage required to achieve complete paralysis varies with each patient, so that it is possible for generalized twitching of the limbs to occur during the clonic phase of the seizure. Immobilizing the limbs prevents injury resulting from the spasms.

32 When the doctor places the electrodes and applies the electric current, observe the patient's fingers and toes carefully.

If the seizure is well modified by the muscle relaxant, the only evidence may be slight rhythmic twitching of the big toe.

33 When the twitching stops, the anaesthetist removes the mouth gag and ventilates the patient with a high concentration of oxygen until spontaneous breathing starts again.

The muscle relaxant causes apnoea.

34 When the patient is breathing spontaneously the anaesthetist inserts an oropharyngeal airway.

Recovery from the intravenous anaesthetic, though spontaneous, is not so rapid as for the muscle relaxant, so that the patient remains unconscious.

35 Turn the patient carefully into the recovery position and cover him or her with a light blanket.

(a) To maintain the airway.
(b) To retain body warmth.

36 Wheel the bed or trolley into the recovery area, taking the patient's clothes and shoes.

Thereby ensuring that the three stages of ECT (waiting, treatment and recovery) are kept physically separate.

37 Ensure that the anaesthetist remains easily available until the patient is recovered.

In case of emergency.

38 Remain with the patient on the side of the trolley facing him or her.

(a) To facilitate observation.
(b) So that the patient will see a familiar face on waking up.

39 Measure and record pulse and blood-pressure.

To check the cardiovascular state of the patient.

40 As the patient wakes up, address him or her by name and say who you are.

To begin orientating the patient.

41 Say where the patient is, that he or she has just had ECT and is recovering.

To reduce confusion and bewilderment, especially as the patient is likely to be amnesic for that morning.

42 Repeat 39 to 41 as often as necessary.

Recovery from the anaesthetic will follow a fluctuating course for about fifteen minutes.

43 If the patient is struggling with the oropharyngeal airway ask him or her to hand it to you.

To confirm that the patient is alert enough to protect his or her own airway.

44 Measure and record the pulse and blood pressure until they are stable in lying, sitting and standing positions.

(a) To determine when the patient is ready to leave the recovery area.
(b) To prevent ataxia or loss of consciousness as a result of postural hypotension.

45 If facilities are available in the recovery area accompany the patient to have a warm or soft drink. Otherwise, make a drink in the ward.

The patient's mouth will be dry as a result of the anaesthetic.

46 Arrange for the patient to have a light snack if he or she wishes.

(a) Although the patient may be hungry a heavy meal may result in vomiting.
(b) If the patient is returning home he or she should eat before undertaking the journey.

47 Accompany an inpatient back to the ward.

In order to continue the current nursing care plan.

48 Ensure that an outpatient has a friend or relative or other person with whom to go home.

(a) In case there are unforeseen effects from the anaesthetic.
(b) A patient having ECT by definition is low in mood and should be accompanied because of the risk of suicide.

49 Return the patient's notes to the ward, ensuring that the record of treatment has been completed by the anaesthetist and the doctor who gave the ECT.

(a) For use by anyone assessing the patient's mental state later.
(b) In case the doctors giving ECT next are different.

50 Offer the patient analgesia for any headache or muscle pain.

(a) Headache is common following ECT.
(b) Muscle pains are common following the administration of suxemethonium chloride.

51 Arrange to meet with the patient later in the day.

(a) To provide an opportunity for the patient to describe his or her response to ECT.
(b) To provide information if necessary for patients who have become disorientated or amnesic.
(c) To assess the patient's mood.

52 Advise the patient to refrain from drinking alcohol that day.

The intravenous anaesthetics used in ECT are metabolized slowly and are potentiated by alcohol.

53 Write a detailed account in the nursing record of the treatment and the patient's response.

(a) To evaluate the nursing care plan.
(b) To record any observations which might influence the doctor's prescription of ECT.
(c) To maintain and communicate alertness for any suicidal thoughts or intentions.

REFERENCE MATERIAL
References

Mental Health Act (1983) HMSO, London.

The Nurses, Midwives and Health Visitors Rules Approval Order (S.I. 1983/873), HMSO, London.

Taylor, J.R. and Carroll, J.L. (1987) Current issues in electroconvulsive therapy, *Psychological Reports*, Vol. 60, pp. 747–58.

Further reading

Ahern, L. (1981) Electroconvulsive therapy: an effective treatment, *AORN Journal*, Vol. 34, no. 3, pp. 463–70.

Beardshaw, V. (1982) A question of conscience, *Nursing Times*, Vol. 78, no. 9, pp. 349–51.

Berrios, G.E. and Sage, G. (1986) Patients who break their fast before ECT, *British Journal of Psychiatry*, Vol. 149, pp. 294–5.

Black, D.W., Winokur, G. and Nasrallah, A. (1987) Treatment of mania: a naturalistic study of electroconvulsive therapy versus lithium in 438 patients, *Journal of Clinical Psychiatry*, Vol. 48, no. 4, pp. 132–9.

Blaine, J.D. and Clark, S.M. (eds.) (1986) Report of the NIMH–NIH consensus development conference on electroconvulsive therapy, *Psychopharmacology Bulletin*, Vol. 22, no. 2, pp. 445–502.

Clare, A.W. (1980) *Psychiatry in Dissent: Controversial Issues in Thought and Practice*, Tavistock, London.

Cochran, C.C. (1984) A change of mind about ECT, *American Journal of Nursing*, Vol. 84, pp. 1004–5.

Cohen, R. (1971) EST + group therapy = improved care, *American Journal of Nursing*, Vol. 71, pp. 1195–8.

Fine, M. and Jenike, M.A. (1985) Electroshock: exploding the myth, *RN*, Vol. 48, no. 9, pp. 58–66.

Lerer, B. *et al.* (1986) Pharmacological manipulation of ECT-induced seizure duration, *Clinical Neuropharmacology*, Vol. 9, no. 4, pp. 453–5.

Lindsay, M. (1983) The ogre of treatment, *Nursing Mirror*, Vol. 156, no. 10, pp. iii–vi.

Mawson, D. (1985) Shock waves, *Nursing Times*, Vol. 81, no. 44, pp. 42–3.

Mitchell, R. and Whyte, L. (1983) Electroconvulsive therapy, *Nursing Mirror*, Vol. 156, no. 20, pp. i–viii.

Mulaik, J.S. (1979) Nurses' questions about electroconvulsive therapy, *Journal of Psychiatric Nursing*, Vol. 17, no. 2, pp. 14–19.

Packham, H. (1984) A shocking business, *Nursing Mirror*, Vol. 159, no. 4, pp. 19–23.

Royal College of Nurses (1982) *Nursing Guidelines for ECT*, RCN, London.

Sands, D. *et al.* (1987) Understanding ECT, *Journal of Psychosocial Nursing and Mental Health Services*, Vol. 25, no. 8, pp. 27–30.

Shimamura, A.P. and Squire, L.R. (1987) A neuropsychological study of fact memory and source amnesia, *Journal of Experimental Psychology: Learning, Memory and Cognition*, Vol. 13, no. 3, pp. 464–73.

Small, I.F. *et al.* (1986) Electroconvulsive treatment–indications, benefits and limitations, *American Journal of Psychotherapy*, Vol. 40, no. 3, p. 343.

Talbot, K. (1986) ECT: exploring myths, examining attitudes, *Journal of Psychosocial Nursing and Mental Health Services*, Vol. 24, no. 3, pp. 6–11.

Thomas, S.P. (1978) Uses and abuses of electric convulsive shock therapy, *Journal of Psychiatric Nursing*, Vol. 16, no. 11, pp. 17–23.

Wells, D. (1976) Electroplexy, *Nursing Times*, Vol. 72, no. 22, pp. 848–9.

39

Gastric Lavage

DEFINITIONS

Gastric lavage
A treatment designed to prevent absorption of an ingested poison other than corrosives or petroleum distillates by washing out the stomach within four to twelve hours of ingestion of the poison.

Poisoning
1 Ingestion of more than the maximum therapeutic dose of one or more drugs.
2 Ingestion of a preparation designed for agricultural, household, industrial, mechanical or horticultural use.
3 Ingestion of a plant or fungus resulting in injury to physiological function.
4 Inhalation of a gas resulting in injury to physiological function.

Obviously only the first three are relevant to gastric lavage.

DISCUSSION
Little systematic research by nurses into gastric lavage is to be found. The experience of units such as the Regional Poisoning Centre, Edinburgh, in treating acutely poisoned patients is not being taken up (Johnstone, 1986). Present methods of management of self-poisoning patients are doing nothing to slow or stop the increase in first-time and repeated self-poisoning (Report of a Working Group, 1982). Gastric lavage is often performed as a tiresome, irritating procedure (O'Brien and Stoll, 1977) with little hope for a therapeutic outcome.

One recommendation for the management of self-poisoning patients is that they are cared for by the same staff from first appearance in the accident and emergency department (Wright, 1979).

These factors imply that the procedure of gastric lavage cannot be carried out independently of a thorough assessment of the precipitants for the poisoning attempt. The procedure which follows is understood to be in the context of such an overall assessment of the self-poisoning patient by trained personnel (Meredith and Vale, 1978).

General guideline and its exceptions
Despite the arguments which exist, based on a dearth of reliable research, a reasonable guideline is that the procedure of gastric lavage is carried out when the risk of the poison ingested outweighs the risk of lavage (Yates and Redmond, 1985). The exceptions are as follows (Matthew et al., 1966; Arena, 1978; Blake, Bramble and Evans, 1978; Meredith and Vale, 1978; Rutherford et al., 1980; Yates and Redmond, 1985):
1 for poisoning by petroleum distillates where the risk is of inhalation;
2 for poisoning by corrosives where the risk is of perforation of the gastro-intestinal tract;
3 for poisoning by convulsion-producing drugs like strychnine;
4 when a specific antidote for the ingested poison exists;
5 when the patient is unconscious but cannot be intubated.

Lavage is also contraindicated in (Graham, 1962)
1 the very young;
2 the frail elderly person;
3 those who have had gastric or oesophageal surgery;
4 those having or suspected of having oesophageal varices.

Available advice
Reliable advice as to the likely risk of any poison likely to be used by patients can be obtained from a regional poisons information centre, where a twenty-four-hour service is available (Graham and Hitchens, 1977; Volans et al 1981). Locations and telephone numbers are:

Belfast: Royal Victoria Hospital – 0232 40503

Cardiff: Royal Infirmary – 0222 492233
Dublin: Jervis Street Hospital – 0001 745588
Edinburgh: Royal Infirmary – 031 229 2477
Leeds: General Infirmary – 0533 32799
London: Guys Hospital – 01–955 5000.

Available research

A summary of available research in the *British Medical Journal* in 1977 indicated that 'gastric lavage remains the treatment of choice' (Editorial, 1977, p. 977) in adults compared with the use of emetics. Salt is positively contraindicated as an emetic because of the risk of hypernatraemia. Apomorphine may potentiate any other drug acting on the central nervous system (Graham and Hitchens, 1977). The efficacy of pharyngeal stimulation (sticking two fingers down the throat) in inducing vomiting of the poison is limited in result (Vale and Meredith, 1981). Use of copper sulphate may result in copper toxicity and it is slow to act (Matthew and Lawson, 1979). Deaths have been reported from the use of ipecacuanha fluid extract instead of ipecacuanha syrup, which is in any case toxic in large quantities (Editorial, 1977; Rutherford *et al.*, 1980; Gossel and Wuest, 1981). Similar contraindications to the inducing of vomiting as to the use of lavage exist (Gossel and Wuest, 1981).

If vomiting is to be induced the patient must be fully conscious (Joint Formulary Committee, 1988), not merely with a cough reflex present, because inhalation of stomach contents cannot be so readily prevented as in gastric lavage. Syrup of ipecacuanha 10–20 ml (ten to twenty millilitres) followed by 100–200 ml of water will stimulate emesis (Wilson and Park, 1980). There is an early stage (within twenty to thirty minutes) and a late stage (after thirty minutes) of vomiting (Gossel and Wuest, 1981). The efficacy of ipecacuanha syrup relative to gastric lavage in actually removing poison from the stomach remains problematic, and the choice of method remains a clinical one based on the best assessment and advice available (Editorial, 1977).

When to use gastric lavage

There is now general agreement that gastric lavage is most effective performed within four hours of ingestion of the poison. It is not to be performed 'when the cough reflex is absent and a cuffed endotracheal tube cannot be inserted' (Meredith and Vale, 1978, p. i–iv).

It may be performed at any time after salicylate poisoning because of the likelihood of concretions of tablets remaining in the stomach. It may be performed up to eight hours after ingestion of tricyclics because of the slowing of gastric motility that they cause (Matthew and Lawson, 1979). Other drugs which slow gastric motility and extend the time within which to carry out lavage are diphenoxylate hydrochloride and the opiates. Ingestion of enteric coated tablets also extends the time available to carry out lavage. The regional poisons information centres will give advice on likely drug actions.

GUIDELINES: ADMINISTERING A GASTRIC LAVAGE

Equipment

Resuscitation equipment including the means to ventilate the patient artificially and to intubate the patient.
Suction aparatus.
Oxygen.
Trolley or bed which tilts, can be locked and has side rails.
Wide-bore stomach catheter (1 cm).
50-ml catheter-tip syringe.
Water-soluble lubricating jelly.
5 litres lavage solution, 38–40°C (usually water).
Funnel with tube and connector to fit stomach catheter.
Clean bucket with graduated markings to measure contents.
500-ml graduated measuring jug.
At least two universal specimen containers.
Swabs and wipes.
Tubing clamp.
Large polythene sheets.
Draw sheets.
Safety pins.
Plastic aprons.

Action	Rationale
1 Remove food, vomit, dentures and secretions from the patient's mouth and prevent his or her tongue from falling back.	In order to establish and safeguard the patient's airway.
2 If the patient is unconscious place him or her in the left lateral position.	(a) To facilitate maintenance of the airway. (b) To prevent inhalation of stomach contents.
3 Identify whether gag and cough reflexes are present.	If the cough reflex is absent the patient must be intubated with cuffed endotracheal tube and an anaesthetist must be present during the procedure of lavage.
4 Determine the level of consciousness.	(a) Baseline data. (b) To assist in making a decision about intubation.
5 Measure and record vital signs of pulse, blood pressure and temperature.	(a) Baseline data. (b) Barbiturates are examples of drugs which cause hypothermia. (c) The patient may have been exposed to cold. (d) Phenothiazines and barbiturates are examples of drugs which cause hypotension. (e) Monoamine oxidase inhibitors (MAOIs) and tricyclics are examples of drugs which cause hypertension. (f) Beta-blockers are examples of drugs which cause bradycardia. (g) Amphetamines are examples of drugs which cause tachycardia.
6 Obtain a baseline chest X-ray if inhalation is suspected to have occurred already.	(a) To safeguard the patient. (b) To safeguard the person carrying out the procedure of lavage in case there is a question later as to when inhalation occurred.
7 Start a fluid balance chart.	Dehydration is likely to be present if vomiting has already occurred and as an effect of certain drugs.
8 Identify any contamination of skin or clothing that has occurred from the poisonous substance, and wear gloves to remove the patient's clothing.	Organo-phosphorus pesticides act in small quantities through the skin and must be washed off.
9 Remove the patient's contact lenses or glasses.	To prevent corneal abrasion or other eye injury.
10 Note any steroid or MAOI cards or jewellery giving information about, for example, treatment for diabetes.	(a) To identify a likely poison. (b) To note possible interactions with the poison ingested.
11 Ask the patient what, when and how much of the poison he or she ingested.	To complete the assessment, bearing in mind that the answer is unlikely to be accurate.
12 Allocate a nurse to the patient.	To provide consistency and continuity of care.

13 If the allocated nurse is authorized by the hospital to carry out lavage, allocate another nurse to help.

(a) So that attention is paid to the patient in addition to that needed to carry out the procedure.
(b) Therefore, if a doctor carries out the lavage, the allocated nurse remains with the patient at all times.
(c) Otherwise the second nurse stays with the patient at all times.

14 The two objectives are:
  (i) supportive measures (keeping the patient warm etc.);
  (ii) prevention of absorption of the poison.

There is little point in removing the poison and putting the patient at risk in other ways.

15 Obtain the patient's permission to carry out gastric lavage.

Lavage may be carried out without the patient's consent only if:
(a) his or her life is in danger;
(b) not doing so would result in serious deterioration of his or her health greater than that which would result from performing lavage.

16 Explain slowly, privately and without pressure the procedure to the patient.

If the patient trusts the staff he or she is more likely to go along with the treatment.

17 Lock the trolley wheels.

To avoid injury if the trolley moves during the procedure.

18 Cover the patient with the draw sheets and polythene sheeting, securing them with safety pins of the lockable type.

Fluid and vomit slides about on polythene.

19 Have the resuscitation equipment ready nearby.

So that the patient can be ventilated and given emergency drugs if inhalation of stomach contents occurs.

20 Have the suction apparatus ready nearby.

(a) In case of vomiting as the stomach catheter passes into the oesophagus.
(b) To remove debris at the end of the procedure.

21 Have the oxygen turned on and near to hand.

To assist in ventilation in case of inhalation of stomach contents.

22 Insert a cuffed endotracheal tube.

If cough and gag reflexes are absent (see 3 above).

23 Stop the procedure if the endotracheal tube cannot be inserted.

Inhalation of stomach contents is bound to occur otherwise.

24 Position the patient in the left lateral position with the foot of the trolley elevated and his or her head tilted down.

To drain the stomach contents away from the lungs.

25 Fasten the safety strap.

To stop the patient sliding off the trolley.

26 Pad the side rails.

To prevent injury if the patient struggles or slides.

27 The second nurse talks to the patient, explaining what is happening and holding him or her gently.

This will not restrain a determinedly hostile and angry patient, but may help him or her to calm down.

28	Measure the distance on the stomach catheter from the tip of the patient's nose to the tip of the xiphoid process.	In order to know how much catheter to pass.
29	Mark the catheter proximally to the rounded end with holes.	(a) Guesswork is likely to be inaccurate. (b) It is possible to perforate the stomach if too much catheter is passed.
30	Pass the tube into the patient's mouth, asking him or her to swallow frequently.	If the patient can be persuaded to swallow often and vigorously enough, the catheter will pass the pharynx without stimulating vomiting.
31	When the mark on the catheter is reached, stop.	In order not to pass beyond the pylorus.
32	Aspirate gently with the 50-ml syringe.	To empty as much of the stomach contents as possible.
33	With litmus, test what is withdrawn.	To ensure that the catheter is in the stomach and not in the lungs.
34	If nothing is aspirated, listen with a stethoscope to the stomach while introducing a small amount of air with the syringe.	Bubbling will be heard if the catheter is in the stomach.
35	If in doubt, do not instil water but withdraw the catheter and start again.	It is essential to protect the patient's lungs.
36	Run in through the 50-ml syringe 100 ml of lavage solution, leave for two or three minutes, and aspirate.	To remove as much of the stomach contents as possible.
37	Attach the funnel and tubing to the end of the catheter and run in up to 300 ml of lavage solution under gravity.	To suspend the stomach contents ready for removal.
38	Avoid running in the solution too fast or too forcibly.	(a) To avoid pushing the contents of the stomach into the small intestine. (b) To avoid causing distension and acute discomfort.
39	Raise the funnel.	To speed up the flow.
40	Lower the funnel.	To slow down the flow.
41	Before the last of the solution has left the funnel clamp the catheter.	To prevent air entry.
42	Lower the funnel to below the level of the patient and over the bucket.	To siphon out the solution and the stomach contents.
43	Release pressure on the catheter.	Allowing the lavage solution and stomach contents to flow into the bucket until they stop.
44	Repeat until the solution comes back clear.	(a) Up to 12 litres may be used. (b) To ensure complete emptying of the stomach contents.
45	The second nurse remains with the patient.	To retain his or her co-operation.

46 Measure the fluid that has been returned.

To ensure that all fluid put in has come back, thereby preventing water intoxication.

47 Warn the patient that you are about to withdraw the catheter.

Some friction will be inevitable and potentially distressing.

48 Clamp the catheter.

(a) To prevent air entry.
(b) To prevent inhalation of the stomach contents as it is withdrawn.

49 The second nurse suctions the mouth and cheek areas of the patient.

(a) To clear residual vomit or secretions.
(b) To prevent inhalation of such debris.

50 The second nurse remains with the patient.

(a) To prevent further self-injury.
(b) To maintain continuity of care.

51 Retain samples of the stomach contents from the beginning and end of the lavage.

For toxicological analysis if necessary.

52 Confirm that the patient's airway is patent.

Sudden deterioration is possible because of absorption that has already take place.

53 Ensure that the patient remains in the left lateral position.

As for 52.

54 Measure and record the patient's level of consciousness.

As for 52.

55 Measure and record the patient's vital signs.

As for 52.

56 Fill in the fluid balance chart.

For an exact record of the fluid instilled and returned.

57 Write an account of the procedure.

Nursing process documentation is the means by which responsibility is accounted for.

58 Label the patient's property.

The patient is unlikely to be in a state where he or she is able to look after it without assistance.

59 Arrange transfer to the intensive care unit, short-stay ward, medical ward, or psychiatric ward as decided with the medical staff.

So that the patient is not left in limbo.

60 Inform the patient's next of kin or close friend.

As agreed with the patient.

61 Remain with the patient at all times.

(a) To maintain supportive (physiological) measures.
(b) To prevent further self-injury.

REFERENCE MATERIAL

References

Arena, J.M. (1978) The treatment of poisoning, *Clinical Symposia*, Vol. 30, no. 2, pp. 3–47.

Blake, D.R., Bramble, M.G. and Evans, J.G. (1978) Is there excessive use of gastric lavage in the treatment of self-poisoning?, *Lancet*, Vol. 2, no. 23, pp. 1362–4.

Editorial (1977) Emetics for acute poisoning – treatment or hazard?, *British Medical Journal*, Vol. 2, pp. 977.

Gossel, T.A. and Wuest, J.R. (1981) The right first aid for poisoning, *RN*, Vol. 44, no. 3, pp. 73–5.

Graham, J.D.P. (1962) *The Diagnosis and Treatment of Acute Poisoning*, Oxford University Press, London.

Graham, J.D.P. and Hitchens, R.A.N. (1977) The National Poisons Information Service and hospital admissions for children: the experience in Wales of the Cardiff centre, *British Medical Journal*, Vol. 2, pp. 1339–40.

Johnstone, F. (1986) Acute poisoning, *Nursing Standard*, 13 March, p. 5.

Joint Formulary Committee 1987–1988 of the British Medical Association and the Pharmaceutical Society of Great Britain (1988) *British National Formulary Number 16*, BMA and Pharmaceutical Press, London.

Matthew, H. and Lawson, A.H. (1979) *Treatment of Common Acute Poisonings*, Churchill Livingstone, Edinburgh.

Matthew, H. *et al.* (1966) Gastric aspiration and lavage in acute poisoning, *British Medical Journal*, Vol. 2, pp. 1333–7.

Meredith, T. and Vale, A. (1978) Poisons 1: acute poisoning, *Nursing Mirror*, Vol. 147, no. 15, pp. i–iv.

O'Brien, S.E.M. and Stoll, K.A. (1977) Attitudes of medical and nursing staff towards self-poisoning patients in a London hospital, *International Journal of Nursing Studies*, Vol. 14, pp. 29–35.

Report of a Working Group (1982) *Changing Patterns in Suicide Behaviour*, WHO, Copenhagen.

Rutherford, W.H. *et al.* (1980) *Accident and Emergency Medicine*, Pitman, London.

Vale, J.A. and Meredith, T.J. (1981) *Poisoning: Diagnosis and Treatment*, Update Books, London.

Volans, G.N. *et al.* (1981) National Poisons Information Service: report and comment, *British Medical Journal*, Vol. 282, no. 1, pp. 1613–15.

Wilson, F. and Park, W.G. (1980) *Basic Resuscitation and Primary Care*, MTP Press.

Wright, R.I. (1979) Overdose: self-poisoning trends and management, *Nursing Times*, Vol. 75, no. 46, pp. 1966–8.

Yates, D.W. and Redmond, A.D. (1985) *Lecture Notes on Accident and Emergency Medicine*, Blackwell, Oxford.

Further Reading

Barrett, J. (1980) Bandaging techniques and treatment for other minor injuries, *Nursing Times*, Vol. 76, no. 26, pp. 1127–32.

Blair, F. *et al.* (1982) Primary nursing in the emergency department: nurse and patient satisfaction, *Journal of Emergency Nursing*, Vol. 8, no. 4, pp. 181–6.

Carter, D.A. (1980) A method of gastric lavage, *Nursing Times*, Vol. 76, no. 33, p. 1437.

Catalan, J. *et al.* (1980) The role of the nurses in the management of deliberate self-poisoning in the general hospital, *International Journal of Nursing Studies*, Vol. 17, no. 4, pp. 275–82.

Catalan, J. *et al.* (1980) Comparison of doctors and nurses in the assessment of deliberate self-poisoning patients, *Psychological Medicine*, Vol. 10, no. 3, pp. 483–91.

Cowley, S.A. (1978) We may need the bed, *Nursing Times*, Vol. 74, no. 6, p. 248.

Erb, H.L. (1979) Emergency treatment of drug overdose, *Canadian Nurse*, Vol. 75, no. 5, pp. 30–5.

Jensen, S. (1977) The initial management of acute poisoning, *Journal of Emergency Nursing*, Vol. 3, no. 4, pp. 13–16.

Knepil, J. (1983) Biochemistry at your service, *Nursing Mirror*, Vol. 156, no. 13, pp. 46–7.

Lanros, N.E. (1978) *Assessment and Intervention in Emergency Nursing*, Robert J Brady, Bowie, MD.

Leading article (1977) Emetics for acute poisoning – treatment or hazard, *British Medical Journal*, Vol. 2, p. 977.

Matthew, H. (1971) Acute poisoning: some myths and misconceptions, *British Medical Journal*, Vol. 1, pp. 519–22.

May, H.L. (ed.) (1984) *Emergency Medical Procedures*, Wiley, New York.

McCall, P. and O'Sullivan, P.S. (1982) Vital sign documentation and primary nursing in the emergency department, *Journal of Emergency Nursing*, Vol. 8, no. 4, pp. 187–90.

Mennear, J.H. (1977) The poisoning emergency, *American Journal of Nursing*, Vol. 77, pp. 842–4.

Miller, M. (1981) Emergency management of the unconscious patient, *Nursing Clinics of North America*, Vol. 16, no. 1, pp. 59–73.

Ramon, S. (1980) Attitudes of doctors and nurses to self-poisoning patients, *Social Science and Medicine*, Vol. 14A, pp. 317–24.

Resnik, H.L.P. and Hathorne, B.C. (1974) *Teaching Outlines in Suicide Studies and Intervention*, Charles Press, Maryland.

Robinson, R. and Stott, R. (1983) *Medical Emergencies Diagnosis and Management*, Heinemann, London.

Thomas, S. (1979) Passing tubes and catheters, *Nursing Mirror*, Vol. 148, no. 13, pp. 32–4.

Vale, A., Meredith, T. and Buckley, B. (1984) Eliminating poisons, *British Medical Journal*, Vol. 289, no. 6441, pp. 366–9.

Part Six

Ethical and Legal Aspects of Nursing Practice

40

Ethical Issues

DEFINITION
Ethics is the study of morals, the principles of good and evil, right and wrong. Moral philosophers are concerned with ethics and how human actions are judged to be good.

DISCUSSION
Problems in psychiatric nursing tend to be defined as ethical once they have reached a point where staff are in conflict about the rights and wrongs of a course of action. By then such problems are rarely matters purely of ethics. The relationship of law and justice to moral beliefs, and the relationship of the logical status of arguments to the nature of empirical evidence ensure that few such problems can be simply assigned to the field of ethics. If psychiatric nurses look more closely at apparently trivial decisions, the ways in which they talk and the social, cultural and political contexts of the problems which they encounter, the everyday necessity for moral choice becomes apparent.

Ethics concerns helping people find out how to know what they ought to do. In non-religious ethics, such a decision must be made in the absence of a belief 'in the existence of a God or several gods' (Parfit, 1985, p. 453). How ethical decisions are arrived at and described does not need to be studied in the context of a single philosophical system, but philosophical systems exist and provide very different world views: for example, the view that the function of a human being is self-fulfilment, or that it is self-awareness.

Faced with an apparently ethical problem the nurse wishes to know how to:
1 identify and describe its components;
2 decide on his or her course of action;
3 give advice;
4 evaluate advice;
A practical skill for the nurse to acquire is an ability to evaluate arguments and to discriminate between kinds of reasons given for moral choice.

Different classifications of ethical theories have been attempted to try to convey to non-philosophers the nature of the concepts of moral philosophy. While being informative, ethical theories are not based on empirical data and so are not predictive in the way that scientific theories are. It is all too easy to over-simplify the complex and difficult bases of rules of conduct, as well as to identify a deceptively clear boundary between the fairly narrow field of ethics and other fields of inquiry. Such subjects include political philosophy, which is concerned with how social institutions are judged to be just; logic, which is concerned with how arguments are judged to be valid; or epistemology, which is concerned with theories of knowledge. Some philosophers doubt whether moral philosophy and therefore ethics can be taught unless the student has already grasped some of the other subjects of philosophy such as logic or the philosophy of mind (Warnock, 1966; Mabbot, 1966; Pettit, 1980). Moreover it is not easy to distinguish between ethical and other issues in psychiatric nursing practice without a familiarity with that practice.

Three examples will be used in different ways: one to examine whether people mean what they say; the second to examine the kinds of choices that are possible in an apparent dilemma; the third to examine the effects of apparently insignificant decisions.

EXAMPLE 1
An eighty-four-year-old woman who is depressed will start a course of ECT tomorrow. She has signed the consent form. It is recalled that she ceased to be depressed after two previous courses of ECT when she was aged sixty-three and seventy-six. The anaesthetist says she is fit to have the treatment. This evening she asks the nurse, 'Ought I have ECT tomorrow?'

Nurse One may reply, 'Yes, you ought to have ECT tomorrow.' Nurse Two may reply, 'No, you ought not have ECT tomorrow.' Nurse Three may reply, 'Do *you* think you ought to have ECT tomorrow?'

Analysis: do people mean what they say?

ECT is an example of a treatment about which many nurses have reservations. There is a tendency to think that ECT is good or bad in itself, and to feel that one's actions in relation to ECT are thereby good or bad, as it were, by infection. That is, it is morally right to advise a person to have ECT because ECT is a good thing; or it is morally right to advise a person not to have ECT because ECT is a bad thing; or it is wrong to advise a person to have ECT because ECT is a bad thing; or it is morally right to withhold advice when one cannot make a decision whether ECT is a good or bad thing. This represents a confusion. The result of the confusion is that the issue of ECT is treated as if it is a matter on which the individual nurse may judge only privately and that this private judgement is inaccessible to reason. However, it will be argued that statements like 'You ought [or ought not] to have ECT' do not necessarily follow from the idea that ECT is a good or bad thing.

The patient has asked the nurse for advice and has received three different kinds of answer:

1 Nurse One, who says, 'You ought to have ECT', may be reasoning as follows: 'People like you have been helped by ECT'. (This is a statement which may be true or false.) 'You are likely to be helped by ECT.' (This is a prediction which may turn out to be true or false.)

2 Nurse Two, who says, 'You ought not have ECT', may be reasoning as follows: 'People like you have not been helped by ECT.' (This is a statement which may be true or false.) 'It is not known how ECT works.' (This is true.) 'There is a risk in undergoing a treatment whose mode of action is unknown.' (This is true.) 'The nature of the risk of ECT is such that potential and as yet unmeasured harm may exceed any immediate and measurable benefits.' (This is a prediction which may turn out to be true or false.) 'The short-term benefits of a course of ECT are outweighed by the long-term benefits of taking anti-depressant medicine and of talking to nurses and doctors.' (This is a prediction which may turn out to be true or false.)

3 Nurse Three, who says, 'Do *you* think you ought to have ECT?', may be reasoning that the patient wishes to tell more of how she thinks and so implies, 'Tell me more about what *you* think.' (The nurse refrains from true or false statements or predictions in favour of eliciting from the patient a description of the nature of the problem which prompts the question, 'Ought I to have ECT tomorrow?')

Nurse One may be telling the truth by saying, 'People like you have been helped by ECT', but may predict falsely because on the day of the treatment the machine fails to deliver the necessary current. Whether or not Nurse One knows that the machine is defective the advice to have ECT misleads the patient. If Nurse One knows about the defective machine, he or she knowingly acts on a false belief. If Nurse One does not know about the defective machine, although he or she does not knowingly act on a false belief, he or she does not ensure that the equipment is in the same working order as that which achieves beneficial results for other depressed patients. Nurse One holds a belief which he or she does not attempt to verify and so misleads the patient.

Nurse Two may be telling the truth by saying, 'People like you have been helped by ECT', and, 'It is not known how ECT works', and, 'There is a risk in undergoing a treatment whose mode of action is unknown', and, 'There is a potential as yet unknown risk which may exceed the benefits.' But Nurse Two may predict falsely because he or she does not know the strength of this patient's dislike of taking medicines of any kind, and the strength of her preference for her cats' company than for talking to people. In advising this person not to have ECT, Nurse Two does not attempt to verify his or her beliefs about the situation, and so misleads the patient.

Nurse Three behaves as if he or she believes that the patient is responsible for deciding whether to have ECT or not. However, unless the patient is given the necessary information with which to make a decision, the nurse merely evades the choice required by the patient's question. Moreover, by withholding information such as, 'People of type *p* have been helped by ECT, while people of type *q* have not', or, 'The risks of ECT are *a*, *b* and *c*, and the benefits of ECT are *x*, *y* and *z*', the nurse maintains control over the patient's ability to choose a course of action, even if he or she elicits from the patient a full description of the problem. Nurse Three also misleads the patient.

Moreover, none of the nurses has said to the patient, 'You made your decision, which seemed right at the time. Tell me why you find it difficult to stick to it', thus suggesting to the patient that she is responsible for the decision.

If Nurses One, Two and Three had talked about their attitudes and beliefs with other staff it is possible that some of the confusion might have been sorted out. In this example the psychiatric nurses each behave as if they are on their own in relation to the eighty-four-year-old lady's question. By sharing information and knowledge, participating in discussion, listening to other people and being prepared to examine one's beliefs, it may be possible to establish a different view. The acid test is whether the nurse not only feels in his or her deepest conscience that the patient's best interests are served by a particular course of action, but that this feeling is accompanied by knowing that the nurse has used reason and judgement to evaluate the best knowledge and advice that is available. In other words, any individual can at best have only an imperfect knowledge what is in a patient's best interests. A profesional person's conscience requires him or her to act in accordance with his or her professional knowledge, experience and judgement, and to accept professional guidance when his or her knowledge or skills may be insufficient.

EXAMPLE 2

A white male student nurse in the last six months of training to become a registered mental nurse has read that the number of young black men diagnosed as schizophrenic, detained under the Mental Health Act and medicated without consent is disproportionately greater than the number of white men of the same age. A young unemployed black man is admitted to the ward where the student nurse works. He is discovered in the act of asphyxiating another patient who, he says, is the Devil. The procedure to detain the black patient under a section of the Mental Health Act 1983 is started, and the student nurse is asked to take part in the administration of an injection without the patient's consent. The alternative seems to be that the patient will carry out his threat to exterminate the Devil.

At first sight it appears that the UKCC Code of Conduct's seventh rule provides justification for the student nurse to object to taking part in the treatment on the ground of conscience. Conscientious objection is 'non-compliance with a more or less direct legal injunction or administrative order' (Rawls, 1972, p. 368). However, the white female charge nurse of the ward knows the patient, who has been admitted for short periods twice before. During the previous admissions he attacked members of his family and other patients, accusing them of being the Devil. After being detained under the Mental Health Act and medicated without consent he stopped being violent and denied that the dangerous attacks had taken place: 'It wasn't me, man.' He denied any interest let alone belief in the Devil. He was loving towards his baby daughter and joked with people towards whom he had been hostile and aggressive. He was discharged home from hospital after three or four weeks. He has a place at art college for the beginning of the next academic year.

Analysis: the types of choice possible

A dilemma necessitates choosing a course of action which is repugnant. It is tempting to deal with dilemmas by making them matters of conscience, framing the problem simply in terms of ethics: a question of right or wrong, good or better. It is sometimes felt that the authority of conscience overrides all other authority. However, conscience is not infallible. The conscience of an anti-Semite does not give him or her the authority to deal unjustly with a Jew.

The student nurse could tell the charge nurse that in the case of this patient the hospital is abusing its power by acting as an agent of an unjust state which has institutionalized racism. The student nurse refuses to take part in giving the injection as a protest against this abuse.

Rawls (1972) argues in favour of civil disobedience as a means of opposing unjust social institutions in a democratic society, provided certain conditions apply: first, that the majority of those in the society, including the dissenters, have in common and are guided by a sense of justice; second, that each dissenter does not act according to 'personal interest' or to 'political allegiances narrowly construed', but according 'to the political principles that underlie and guide the interpretation of the constitution' (p. 389). The dissenter acts conscientiously after assessing 'how these principles should be applied to the existing circumstances' (p. 389).

In the case of this patient two principles appear to conflict. One is that no one should be discriminated against on the grounds of their sex or race. The student nurse takes the view that psychiatry is one of society's more powerful ways of labelling and dealing with deviance. Where the law prevents sexist or racist practices, psychiatry is able to make sex or race an aspect of deviance called mental illness, which it is empowered by society to treat, if necessary, against the will of the patient. The student nurse feels that to take part in injecting this patient would be to acquiesce in an unjust and illegitimate use of psychiatry.

The other principle is that people have a right to be prevented from harming themselves or another person when they are not competent to judge the consequences of their actions. The charge nurse takes the view that the behaviour is out of character and that in a different frame of mind the patient expressed quite different kinds of hopes and fears for himself.

If one nurse's view of what is good for a particular patient is merely a 'better' or 'worse' ethical position than that of another nurse, it could be argued that they are both in the position of attempting to persuade each other to act differently on the basis that one moral belief is superior to another. This resembles Toulmin's description of 'two algebraists arguing as to whether $x = 2$ or $x = 3$ is the real solution of $x^2 - 5x + 6 = 0$' (Toulmin, 1960, p. 190).

Such a view would make it immaterial what action either of them took since they were each acting according to their consciences. However, Rawls (1972, p. 373) argues that to be justifiable civil disobedience is used when 'legal means of redress have proved to no avail'. This fits with the practical advice given to nurses who think of being whistleblowers (Beardshaw, 1981).

Alternatives to be considered before a stand-off occurs between the student and the charge nurse include the following.

1 The student or another nurse persuades the patient to take oral medication.
2 The patient is reported to the police and charged.
3 Before any other action is taken the student nurse talks to the patient at length and writes in detail in the nursing record an account of this interview and of his reservations about the patient's treatment. (The Mental Health Act Commissioners have the right to examine any of the patient's records.)
4 As soon as the patient is sectioned or medicated or both, arrangements are made for him to appeal to the Mental Health Act Commissioners.
5 The student nurse meets with the rest of the nursing team and with the other members of the multi-disciplinary clinical team, in particular the social worker and the consultant, and discusses in detail the treatment of the patient and his reservations about it.
6 The student nurse consults with his personal tutor who is, if worried about the educational environment in the ward, obliged take appropriate action.
7 The charge nurse and the student nurse consult with the immediate nurse manager.
8 The multidisciplinary team including the charge nurse and the student nurse consults with the hospital chaplain or other representative of the hospital ethics committee.
9 Finally, the charge nurse ensures that the patient's primary nurse liaises with the social worker and the patient's doctor and together they consult with his family and friends, in particular the nearest relative.

Moral decisions are not identifiable by their magnitude. The student nurse who waits until asked to take part in an injection before conscientously objecting may have made a series of decisions: for example, taking another patient for a walk at the time of a management round when the violent black patient is to be discussed, ringing the chaplain once and not trying again when the number is engaged, starting a grievance procedure instead of having his objections out with the rest of the staff. The charge nurse may make such decisions: for example,

ignoring the student's growing discomfort, asking the student to give the injection without discussing the patient's treatment, deciding to start disciplinary action against the student instead of finding out what was behind his refusal. The alternatives above represent moral choices which themselves incorporate other moral decisions.

EXAMPLE 3

The third example is based on what Parfit (1985) calls 'moral mathematics': looking at the apparently trivial decisions that appear morally insignificant because their consequences if one person acts on them appear small or imperceptible. An example is maintaining ward stocks of supplies such as dressings, syringes and needles. A charge nurse could argue that in the context of his or her available time the priority given to reordering is neces-sarily low. The important thing is that stocks are main-tained at a level where enough is available to carry out necessary work. If this means reordering infrequently and keeping an extra store of surplus equipment in the linen room in case stocks run out it is preferable to the risk of running out on a Sunday afternoon. The charge nurse argues that a couple of extra boxes of needles, say, in a 400-bed hospital are insignificant in comparison to the total amount of supplies used in a day.

This may be seen as a question of how probabilities are assigned: the probability of running out at an incon-venient moment versus the risk that other people elsewhere in the hospital are themselves more likely to run out of supplies as a result of one's hoarding.

Parfit (1985, p. 70) suggests, 'Even if an act harms no one, this act may be wrong because it is one of a set of acts that *together* harm other people. Similarly, even if some act benefits no one, it can be what someone ought to do, because it is one of a set of acts that together benefit other people.' The charge nurse claims that overstocking benefits his or her ward and does not harm anyone else. This claim looks very different if it is found that half the charge nurses in the hospital hoard sup-plies, and that each hospital in the district, area, region and the country contains a proportion of charge nurses who hoard supplies.

'Moral philosophy cannot decide whether particular acts are moral but only under what conditions they would be moral' (Mabbot, 1966, pp. 147, 149).

REFERENCE MATERIAL
References

Beardshaw, V. (1981) *Conscientious Objectors at Work*, Social Audit, London.

Mabbot, J.D. (1966) *An Introduction to Ethics*, Hutchinson, London.

Parfit, D. (1985) *Reasons and Persons*, Oxford University Press.

Pettit, P. (1980) *Judging Justice*, Routledge & Kegan Paul, London.

Rawls, J. (1972) *A Theory of Justice*, Oxford University Press.

Toulmin, S.E. (1960) *An Examination of the Place of Reason in Ethics*, Cambridge University Press.

Warnock, M. (1966) *Ethics Since 1900*, Oxford University Press.

Further reading

Ashworth, P. (1984) Accounting for ethics, *Nursing Mirror*, Vol. 158, no. 10, p. 134–6.

Barker, P. (1980) Ethics, nursing and behaviour modification, *Nursing Times*, Vol. 76, no. 22, pp. 976–8.

Bergman, R. (1976) Evolving ethical concepts for nursing, *International Nursing Review*, Vol. 23, no. 4, pp. 116–17.

Bernzweig, E.P. (1980) When in doubt – speak out, *American Journal of Nursing*, Vol. 80, pp. 1175–6.

Bloch, S. and Chodoff, P. (eds.) (1981) *Psychiatric Ethics*, Oxford University Press.

Bok, S. (1980) *Lying: Moral Choice in Public and Private Life*, Quartet, London.

Boyd, K. (1977) The nature of ethics, *Nursing Mirror*, Vol. 145, no. 3, pp. 14–16.

Carper, B.A. (1979) The ethics of caring, *Advances in Nursing Science*, Vol. 1, no, 3, pp. 11–19.

Chalmers, H. (1977) Ethics, *Nursing Mirror*, Vol. 145, no. 5, pp. i–iv.

Clare, A.W. (1978) Treatment or torture, *Midwife Health Visitor Community Nurse*, Vol. 14, no. 7, pp. 205–6.

Cowart, M.E. and Allen, R.F. (1982) Moral development of health care professionals begins with sensitizing: thirty-three sample encounters, *Journal of Nursing Education*, Vol. 21, no. 5, pp. 4–7.

Cronenwett, L.R. (1983) Helping and nursing models, *Nursing Research*, Vol. 32, no. 6, pp. 342–6.

Curtin, L. and Flaherty, M.J. (1982) *Nursing Ethics: Theories and Pragmatics*, Robert J. Brady, Bowie, MD.

Downie, R. (1982) Three aspects to the job, *Nursing Mirror*, Vol. 155, no. 21, p. 30.

Flanagan, L. (1986) A question of ethics, *Nursing Times*, Vol. 82, no. 35, pp. 39–41.

Fry, S.T. (1985) Individual vs aggregate good: ethical tension in nursing practice, *International Journal of Nursing Studies*, Vol. 22, no. 4, pp. 303–10.

Gortner, S.R. (1985) Ethical inquiry, *Annual Review of Nursing Research*, Vol. 3, pp. 193–214.

Hanvey, C. (1983) At the centre of moral problems, *Nursing Mirror*, Vol. 157, no. 5, pp. 35–6.

Hockey, I. (ed.) (1981) *Current Issues in Nursing*, Churchill Livingstone, Edinburgh.

Kellmer, D.M. (1982) The teaching of ethical decision-making in schools of nursing, *Nursing Leadership*, Vol. 5, no. 2, pp. 20–6.

Ketefian, S. (1985) Professional and bureaucratic role conceptions and moral behaviour among nurses, *Nursing Research*, Vol. 34, no. 4, pp. 248–53.

Kratz, C. (1977) The ethics of research, *Nursing Mirror*, Vol. 145, no. 3, pp. 17–20.

Kurtines, W.M. (1986) Moral behaviour as rule governed behaviour: person and situation effects on moral decision making, *Journal of Personality and Social Psychology*, Vol. 50, no. 4, pp. 784–91.

Lawrence, J. and Crisham, P. (1984) Making a choice, *Nursing Times*, Vol. 80, no. 29, pp. 57–8.

Lawrence, J. and Crisham, P. (1984) A study in resolutions, *Nursing Times*, Vol. 80, no. 30, pp. 53–5.

Levine, M.E. *et al.* (1977) A special AJN feature: ethics, *American Journal of Nursing*, Vol. 77, pp. 845–76.

Mayberry, M.A. (1986) Ethical decision-making: a response of hospital nurses, *Nursing Administration Quarterly*, Vol. 10, no. 3, pp. 75–81.

Norton, D. (1975) The research ethic, *Nursing Times*, Vol. 71, no. 52, p. 2048–9.

Pyne, R. (1987) A duty to shout, *Nursing Times*, Vol. 83, no. 42, pp. 30–1.

Rea, K. (1983) Where law and ethics meet, *Nursing Mirror*, Vol. 156, no. 8, p. 14.

Rouslin, S. (1976) Commenting on professional ethics, *Perspectives in Psychiatric Nursing Care*, Vol. 14, no. 1, pp. 12–13.

Scrivenger, M. (1987) Ethics, etiquette and the law, *Nursing Times*, Vol. 83, no. 42, pp. 28–9.

Sheehan, J. (1985) Ethical considerations in nursing practice, *Journal of Advanced Nursing*, Vol. 10, pp. 331–6.

Smith, J.P. (1983) First international congress on nursing law and ethics, *Journal of Advanced Nursing*, Vol. 8, pp. 263–5.

Smith, S.J. and Davis, A.J. (1980) Ethical dilemmas: conflict among rights, duties and obligations, *American Journal of Nursing*, Vol. 80, pp. 1463–6.

Swider, S.M., McElmurry, B.J. and Yarling, R.R. (1985) Ethical decision-making in a bureaucratic context by senior nursing students, *Nursing Research*, Vol. 34, pp. 108–12.

Tschudin, V. (1986) *Ethics in Nursing*, Heinemann, London.

UKCC (1986) *Code of Conduct*, UKCC, London.

[Unattributed article] (1978) World Psychiatric Association adopts ethical guidelines, *International Nursing Review*, Vol. 25, p. 40.

Wootton, B. (1980) Psychiatry, ethics and the criminal law, *British Journal of Psychiatry*, Vol. 136, pp. 525–32.

Yarling, R.R. and McElmurry, B.J. (1986) The moral foundation of nursing, *Advances in Nursing Science*, Vol. 8, no. 2, pp. 63–73.

Yeaworth, R.C. (1985) The ANA Code: a comparative perspective, *Image*, Vol. 17, no. 3, pp. 94–8.

41

Appearing in Court

DISCUSSION

Nurses are likely to be asked to appear in the following types of court:

1 the coroner's court;
2 a civil court;
3 a magistrates' or other criminal court,

and in the quasi-judicial setting of administrative tribunals, such as industrial or mental health review tribunals.

The circumstances in which a nurse may appear in court may be related to his or her nursing duties or not. An example of the latter would be after an assault in the hospital grounds by a person who was not a patient in the hospital.

The common law

The structure of the justice system in the UK is quite complex. There are two main categories of law: the civil law and the criminal law. The ways in which 'the law' is formulated are by case law and by legislation. Case law makes up the body of the common law and consists of judicial precedents or decisions formulated by judges in courts since the eleventh century. The common law is especially relevant to nurses because the law of tort (see 'Civil law', below), as well as the law of contract, derives mainly from case law. Standards of professional practice are set by the nursing profession itself, and are tested in court against actual cases of alleged negligence.

Civil law

The distinction between the civil and criminal law rests on the difference in purpose. The primary purpose of the civil law is to provide compensation for individuals who suffer a wrong in one of the areas it covers, whereas the primary purpose of the criminal law is to punish the wrongdoer.

A wrongdoing under civil law may be known as a tort, a word derived from the French word for wrong. The law

of tort broadly encompasses the following issues:

1 owing a professional duty of care;
2 trespass to the person (assault, battery and false imprisonment);
3 vicarious liability (master and servant relationship);
4 defamation.

Apart from the law of tort, the civil law includes contract law, property law, family law and the law of succession. The civil law is administered by the civil courts whose structure is shown in Figure 41.1.

Figure 41.1 Structure of civil courts

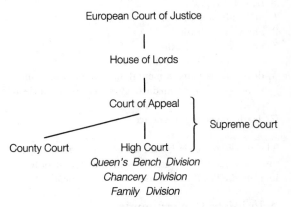

European Court of Justice

House of Lords

Court of Appeal

County Court   High Court
Queen's Bench Division
Chancery Division
Family Division

Supreme Court

The nurse may be asked to appear in a civil court as an expert witness, or as a defendant in a civil action. An example of a case where the nurse may be an expert witness would be in a case where custody of children is disputed in a divorce case being heard by the Family Division of the High Court (Rea, 1982). An example of a case where a nurse may be a defendant in a civil action would be one heard in the High Court where a patient was suing the nurse or the hospital or both for negligence.

Criminal law

A wrong under criminal law is one against the state, in the person of the Queen (Regina), and is termed a crime. A crime is 'an act of disobedience of the law forbidden under pain of punishment' (Padfield and Barker, 1981, p. 313). The purpose of the criminal court is the prosecution and punishment of crimes committed by offenders who are brought before the courts by the police.

The criminal law is administered by the criminal courts whose structure is shown in Figure 41.2. The nurse is likely to be asked to appear in a criminal court as a material witness of fact, or as a defendant.

Figure 41.2   Structure of criminal courts

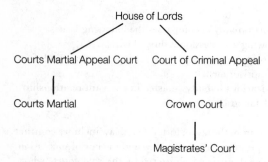

Coroner's court

Although the coroner is empowered to investigate any death, his or her duties are to investigate (Padfield and Barker, 1981, p. 63):

1 any sudden death;
2 any violent death;
3 any unnatural death;
4 deaths of prisoners while in custody;
5 deaths of patients in mental institutions where there is no satisfactory medical evidence as to cause of death;
6 deaths involving the police.

The investigation is by means of a post-mortem and formal inquest, if necessary, with a jury, in order to identify the dead person and the cause of death.

Administrative tribunals

Administrative tribunals include the Mental Health Review Tribunal, industrial tribunals, social security tribunals, immigration adjudication tribunals and rent tribunals. Nurses may be involved in industrial tribunals, an example of whose structure is shown in Figure 41.3.

A tribunal is a specialized body set up under the Tribunals and Inquiries Act 1971 to deal with grievances. A Council on Tribunals, set up by the 1971 Act, makes an annual report. Appeals to the High Court can

Figure 41.3   Example of industrial tribunal structure

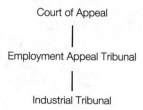

be made from tribunal decisions. There is evidence that people being heard by tribunals have a better chance of success if they are represented (Blake, 1986, p. 42).

Mental health review tribunals

The Mental Health Act 1959 introduced mental health review tribunals. There is one for each regional health authority in England, one for Wales and one for N. Ireland (S.I. 1986). In Scotland detained patients may appeal to the Mental Welfare Commission. Each tribunal has three members: a lawyer, a doctor (usually a psychiatrist) and a lay member. The legal member is the chairman. Patients who are detained in hospital or subject to guardianship under the Mental Health Act 1983 are entitled to appeal to a mental health review tribunal within the periods specified in the Act. Patients who appeal to a tribunal are entitled to legal aid to pay a solicitor to advise and assist them. If they need to be represented at a hearing, the solicitor applies for assistance by way of representation (ABWOR), which is an extension of legal aid and ensures that patients without money can have legal representation (Gostin, Rassaby and Buchan, 1984). ABWOR also pays for any independent psychiatric or social inquiry reports (Gostin, 1983).

A patient who wishes to appeal to a mental health review tribunal must apply in writing, either in person or by authorizing someone else to write for him or her. No special form is required. Gostin, Rassaby and Buchan (1984) supply a model application whose format can be copied. The application is sent to the tribunal office of the region in which the patient is detained. The hospital manager who is responsible for the administration of the Mental Health Act 1983 will have the address of the tribunal, and it may be necessary for a nurse to help the patient obtain it. Hospital managers are required under the Mental Health Act 1983 to refer certain patients automatically to the mental health review tribunal. Gostin (1983) gives details of the periods of entitlement for application to a mental health review tribunal.

Although a patient may withdraw an application at any time, he or she must do so in writing, and will be interviewed by someone from the tribunal office to ensure that no pressure is being applied. The tribunal can refuse to accept the withdrawal and conduct a hearing if it is thought to be in the patient's interests. If a patient does withdraw an application, doing so does not affect his or her ability to apply again within the same period of entitlement (Gostin, Rassaby and Buchan, 1984).

The hospital managers supply to the tribunal the medical and nursing records of patients who have applied. The tribunal is empowered to disclose these to applicants or their authorized representatives.

The atmosphere of tribunal hearings is kept as informal as possible. However, in extreme circumstances a tribunal can subpoena a member of staff who otherwise refuses to give information to it; and the tribunal procedures are strictly laid down. Patients may request that hearings are held in public, although the tribunal has discretion over who may be admitted to hearings. Patients or their representatives may call and question their own witnesses and question other witnesses.

Health Service Commissioner

The Health Service Commissioner or 'Ombudsman' (from a Swedish word introduced in the UK in 1965 to describe a person who is appointed to investigate complaints against government departments (*OED*)) is an official whose job in the National Health Service was created in 1973. The Commissioner is empowered to investigate complaints by or on behalf of individuals against health authorities (see Chapter 8). He or she delegates the investigation itself to other officials who interview the person making the complaint and the staff concerned. Rarely the Commissioner will conduct the investigation personally, interviewing individuals under oath. Although the procedures of the Commissioner's department are deliberately non-legalistic, anyone obstructing an inquiry may be charged with contempt of court (Clothier, 1982).

Summary and indictable offences

Indictable offences are those crimes which may be tried in the Crown Court. Summary offences are those which may be tried by magistrates. Some offences may be tried either in the magistrates' courts or in the Crown Court. In such cases, at the preliminary hearing, the magistrate gives the accused person the choice of proceeding to the Crown Court or consenting to summary trial. The magistrate may make the decision that an offence must be heard in the Crown Court.

Juvenile courts

The age range for juvenile cases is sixteen and below. A young person is defined as over fourteen and under seventeen; a child is defined as under fourteen. All juvenile cases are tried summarily, except where the charge is murder or the young person or child is charged

with another person who is over seventeen. Up to the age of ten a child cannot be guilty of any crime. Between ten and fourteen the child can be found guilty only if it is shown that he or she knew that the action was wrong.

Professional misconduct

The UKCC Working Group on Professional Conduct distinguished the disciplinary role of the employer from that of the statutory bodies. It is possible for a nurse to incur disciplinary action in his or her employment, while not incurring it by the UKCC. However, the Working Group recommended that, if necessary, both the employer and UKCC should conduct investigations concurrently but independently.

The UKCC Professional Conduct Committee consists of five representative members who meet in public to investigate alleged misconduct brought to its attention by the courts after a conviction, or by a complainant. Respondents are represented or represent themselves and must expect to be cross-examined. The Health Committee deals with cases thought by the Preliminary Committee to involve misconduct resulting from illness or other disability. The committees deal with qualified nurses. Learners are the responsibility of the student conduct committees of the national boards. Hearings are held in camera, that is, not open to the public or the media.

Adversarial system

In the civil and criminal courts the system of justice is adversarial. The prosecution in a criminal case and the plaintiff in a civil case must prove their case to the satisfaction of a magistrate or bench of magistrates, or a judge and jury in the Crown Court, or the judge in the county court or High Court, or the group of judges in the Court of Appeal and the House of Lords. This means that witnesses may be called and questioned by both sides. It is worth visiting a variety of such courts in order to be prepared for the possibility in the future of being called to appear in court. Role-play and rehearsal are also useful tools for the preparation of a prospective witness, in order that he or she will remember and adhere to facts when answering questions. Chapters 8 and 40 discuss further the professional and legal responsibilities of nurses.

Confidentiality

Martin writes:

> Many health authorities will not allow their staff to attend court as witnesses until they have been served with [a subpoena or a witness summons]. Once in it all questions must be answered. The fact that the answer will involve disclosing confidential information is irrelevant, and to

refuse to answer is a contempt of court which can land the witness in prison.

(Martin, 1978, p. 503)

In the event of a case being brought to court, the nurse should seek legal advice beforehand as to the status of any documents or other evidence.

GUIDELINES: APPEARING IN COURT

Action

1 A nurse who is asked to appear in court as a witness, or to assist in an investigation of any kind, takes advice from his or her immediate nurse manager or trade union or professional organization representative or both.

2 If the questions relate to patient care the nurse reads in full any relevant nursing records whether he or she wrote them or not.

3 If the nurse cannot remember details and written records are not available, he or she will say so.

4 A nurse who is notified that a claim of negligence or other civil wrong is to be made against him or her will consult a solicitor.

5 If the nurse wishes to contest the action, his or her lawyers will enter a 'pleading' on his or her behalf within fourteen days of being served with a writ.

6 The master will name the court and date for the action.

7 The nurse attends with his or her lawyers on the date fixed.

8 The plaintiff's case is heard first, consisting of an opening speech and an examination of witnesses.

9 The defendant's lawyer examines the defendant's witnesses.

10 Whether the nurse is called as an expert witness by the plaintiff or the defendant he or she will be asked for his or her professional opinion on the case being heard.

11 The defendant's lawyer sums up the defendant's case.

12 The plaintiff's lawyer replies.

Rationale

(a) In order that the nurse can receive reliable advice as to the best course of action.
(b) In order to negotiate time off and any expenses to which the nurse may be entitled.
(c) In order to debrief after any court appearance, adhering to the guidelines for confidentiality.

In order to provide accurate details of the nursing care that was provided to the patient in question.

An inaccurate account which cannot be verified would be damaging to the nurse's credibility as a witness.

(a) In order to arrange and carry out the necessary legal procedures and to brief a barrister.
(b) If the nurse belongs to a professional organization it will provide the necessary legal representation.

(a) The plaintiff will then reply to the defendant's pleading.
(b) The 'master' (or registrar or judge) will decide how the case will continue.
(c) The master will decide whether the trial will be by judge alone or by judge and jury.

So that both parties know when to attend.

Assuming there has been no adjournment.

The defendant's lawyer may cross-examine the plaintiff's witnesses.

(a) To make the case for the defendant.
(b) The plaintiff's lawyer may cross-examine the defendant's witnesses.

In order for the judge or the judge and jury to evaluate the case against what the nurse tells them is good professional practice.

Asking for judgement in the defendant's favour.

Asking for judgement in the plaintiff's favour.

13 The jury, if there is one, decides on the verdict and the damages.

(a) After the judge directs the jury.
(b) The judge decides costs.
(c) If there is no jury the judge will decide the verdict, damages and costs.

14 Criminal cases in the Crown Court are tried by jury.

The jury delivers its verdict after the adversaries have presented their cases.

15 The defendant may be examined, cross-examined and re-examined during the trial, but has the right to refuse.

It is thought that if a person refuses, his or her defence is less convincing.

16 Nurses who are required to appear as witnesses in criminal cases in the Crown Court will need to be well prepared and might like to be accompanied by a friend on the days on which they attend court.

As in the civil court a witness may be examined, cross-examined and possibly re-examined.

17 In the magistrates' court a case proceeds in a similar way.

Solicitors not barristers often conduct the cases: examining, cross-examining and re-examining.

18 It is advisable to dress 'neatly and conventionally' (Klimon, 1985, p. 99).

In order to present a neutral appearance which cannot be used to your disadvantage.

19 When questioned in court by a lawyer the nurse looks at the judge or magistrate.

(a) The judge is in charge of the proceedings.
(b) In order that the nurse's answers can be clearly heard.

20 The nurse replies only to questions asked.

(a) Extra details could compromise the case of the lawyer who has called the nurse.
(b) Non-verbal communication may be misunderstood or used to the nurse's disadvantage.

REFERENCE MATERIAL

References

Blake, C. G. (1986) *Issues of Law*, BBC, London.

Clothier, C. (1982) The work of the Health Service Commissioner, *Nursing*, Vol. 1, no. 36, pp. 1549–50.

Gostin, L. (1983) *A Practical Guide to Mental Health Law*, National Association for Mental Health, London.

Gostin, L., Rassaby, E. and Buchan, A. (1984) *Mental Health: Tribunal Procedure*, Longman, London.

Klimon, E. L. (1985) Do you swear to tell the truth?, *Nursing Economics*, Vol. 3, pp. 98–102.

Martin, A. (1978) Confidentiality – its nature in law, *Nursing Times*, Vol. 74, no. 2, pp. 503–4.

Padfield, C. F. and Barker, D. L. A. (1981) *Law*, Heinemann, London.

Rea, K. (1982) Appearing in court, *Nursing*, Vol. 1, no. 36, p. 1550–1.

S.I. (1986) *Mental Health (Northern Ireland) Order, SI1986/595(NI4)*, HMSO, London.

Tribunals and Inquiries Act 1971, HMSO, London.

Further reading

Bernzweig, E. P. (1980) When in doubt speak out, *American Journal of Nursing*, Vol. 80, pp. 1175–6.

Cust, K. (1986) Assault: just part of the job?, *Canadian Nurse*, Vol. 82, no. 6, pp. 19–20.

Finch, J. (1980) When are you liable for negligence?, *Nursing Mirror*, Vol. 151, no. 10, pp. 22–4.

Finch, J. (1981) When is a learner not a learner?, *Nursing Mirror*, Vol. 152, no. 26, p. 8.

Finch, J. (1984) Professional expectations, *Nursing Mirror*, Vol. 158, no. 5, p. 37.

Grounds, A. (1985) The psychiatrist in court, *British Journal of Hospital Medicine*, Vol. 34, no. 1, pp. 55–8.

Hargreaves, M. (1979) *Practical Law for Nurses*, Pitman Medical, Tunbridge Wells.

Joint Committee of the General Council of the Bar of England and Wales, the Law Society and the BMA (1965) *Medical Evidence in Courts of Law*, BMA, London.

Lee, S. (1986) *Law and Morals*, Oxford University Press.

Martin, A. J. (1976) The liability of nurses for professional negligence, *Nursing Mirror*, Vol. 142, no. 20, pp. 69–71.

Martin, A. J. (1978) [Indemnity insurance], *Nursing Mirror*, Vol. 148, no. 23, p. 10.

Martin, A. (1979) Employment law – 4, *Nursing Times*, Vol. 75, no. 2, p. 83.

Napier, B. (1980) *Law at Work: Discipline*, Sweet & Maxwell, London.

Northrop, C. (1987) Judicial Perspectives on nursing, *Nursing Outlook*, Vol. 35, no. 3, p. 150.

Rea, K. (1984) So you think you are insured? *Nursing Mirror*, Vol. 158, no. 19, pp. 12–13.

Rea, K. (1987) The UK legal system, *Nursing*, Vol. 3, no. 14, pp. 537–9.

Rowden, R. (1987) Employment law and nurses, *Nursing*, Vol. 3, no. 14, pp. 530–2.

Rowe, P. (1980) *Law at Work: Health and Safety*, Sweet & Maxwell, London.

Schwarz, C. J. and Greenfield, G. P. (1978) Charging a patient with assault of a nurse on a psychiatric unit, *Canadian Psychiatric Association Journal*, Vol. 23, no. 4, pp. 197–200.

Scrivenger, M. (1987) Ethics, etiquette and the law, *Nursing Times*, Vol. 83, no. 42, pp. 28–9.

Segal, M. (1984) A cautionary tale, *Nursing Mirror*, Vol. 158, no. 21, pp. 20–1.

Sheffield, R. (1978) Complex medicolegal issues surrounding modern nursing practice, *Hospitals*, Vol. 52, no. 9, pp. 105–10.

[Unattributed article] [Delegation to nurses by doctors] *Nursing Mirror*, Vol. 147, no. 21, p. 12.

Whincup, M. H. (1978) *Legal Aspects of Medical and Nursing Service*, Ravenswood, Beckenham.

Williams, B. (1977) *Occupiers' Liability Act 1957 and the Liability of Hospitals*, Ravenswood, Beckenham.

[anon] (1982) *Health Commissioner for England*, Office of the Health Commissioner for England, London.

Young, A.P. (1989) *Legal Problems in Nursing Practice 2nd edn.* Harper & Row, London.

42

The Nurse's Holding Power

DEFINITION

The nurse's holding power is defined as the power of 'a nurse of the prescribed class' to detain a person 'who is receiving treatment for mental disorder as an in-patient in a hospital . . . for a period of six hours from the time when that fact is so recorded', or until a registered medical practitioner arrives, whichever is sooner (Mental Health Act, 1983). A nurse 'of the prescribed class is a first level nurse trained in nursing people suffering from mental illness or mental handicap.' (DHSS, 1987, p. 12).

DISCUSSION

The Mental Health Act 1983 consolidated the Mental Health (Amendment) Act 1982, which substantially amended the Mental Health Act 1959. Because the 1983 Act gives little guidance to nurses concerning specific kinds of nursing management problems, much of what is said here is inferred from the provisions of the Act itself, and from interpretation by lawyers of their implications. (See Chapter 10 concerning consent to treatment.)

Section 5(4) of the 1983 Act

Section 5(4), which became known as the nurse's holding power, was introduced in the 1983 Act and formally recognized the concept of professional judgement by psychiatric nurses. The nurse exercising the judgement required to detain patients must be a first-level nurse trained as RMN or RNMH.

The nurse cannot be directed to use or not to use the power, and is liable for the consequences of his or her decision to use it or not. A nurse who invokes the power of section 5(4) and restrains a patient from leaving hospital must be prepared to have the steps leading to the decision closely examined by the Mental Health Act Commissioners or a court if necessary. A decision not to invoke the power would be subject to the same scrutiny.

It is also implied that nurses performing duties related to the provisions of the 1983 Act must have been instructed and found competent to do so. That is, they are registered mental nurses (RMN) or registered nurses for the mentally handicapped (RNMH), and they carry out specifically nursing duties as defined in the 1983 Act or Mental Health Act Commission (MHAC) Code of Practice and agreed by the management team of officers of their health authority.

Section 5(4) states that the nurse may use the holding power when it appears to him or her:

(a) that the patient is suffering from mental disorder to such a degree that it is necessary for his health or safety or for the protection of others for him to be immediately restrained from leaving the hospital; and

(b) that it is not practicable to secure the immediate attendance of a practitioner for the purpose of furnishing a report under subsection (2) above [i.e. a doctor is not available to assess and detain, if necessary, the patient under section 5(2)].

Restraint

As stated in Chapter 10, restraint of patients is permissible in very limited circumstances. They are repeated here.

1 When consent has been given (for instance, to a treatment programme involving restraint as a response to specific behaviours). This consent must be written, and may be withdrawn at any time. (Clearly, if a patient was consenting to remain in hospital, while refusing other forms of restraint, the nurse would not need to use the holding power.)

2 To *prevent*, by using 'reasonable' force, a crime as defined in section 3(1) of the Criminal Law Act 1967.

3 To *prevent*, by using 'reasonable' force, a breach of the peace. The definition of a breach of the peace involves the threat of violence which is likely to harm another person or his or her property.

4 In self-defence, defence of the employer's property, or defence of another person.
5 *Prevention*, by the use of 'reasonable' force, of harm to a person who appears to be so mentally disordered as not to be competent to keep him- or herself safe or who appears likely to cause harm to others, or both.

The use of the holding power

The use of the holding power is an emergency procedure that hinges on the nurse's professional judgement of the circumstances. By definition, if a doctor were present, the nurse would be relieved of the responsibility for deciding whether or not to detain a patient. However, a doctor may not telephone the nurse and instruct him or her to detain the patient until the doctor arrives. In the emergency the nurse must make and record the decision, detain the patient and inform immediately the doctor and the nurse manager responsible for the ward or department.

Restraining a person against his or her will without authority or lawful justification is false imprisonment. It is a criminal offence and also makes the restrainer subject to a civil action. The nurse's holding power is therefore a power to be used with great discretion. Section 5(4) of the 1983 Act empowers the RMN or RNMH to detain a patient in hospital if a doctor is not available to assess him or her in order to decide whether detention is the correct management. In itself, the use of or threat to use the section is a form of restraint. The nurse must be aware that each step taken to detain a patient effectively increases the amount of restraint used.

THE MATTERS TO CONSIDER

As with all matters of restraint two issues must be considered: the justification for its use; and the degree of restraint that is reasonable in the circumstances. The question of what is reasonable tends to be considered in the light of what resources are available to the nurse.

The amount of restraint applied will be the minimum required to achieve the objective of detaining the patient in hospital.

A nurse alone or with one other nurse in the ward will be able to do little more than lock the ward door, record that the patient is detained and telephone for a doctor to come and assess the patient. A patient who is running out of a ward where there are, say, six nurses, may be caught and detained (see Chapter 14) under the direction of the senior registered nurse on duty, who must document the detention and summon the doctor immediately.

In practice, the nurse will also summon help from nursing colleagues and from the nurse manager responsible for the ward or unit. Once help has arrived, any further action will depend on the patient's behaviour, of which a fresh assessment must be made. Use of section 5(4) is not in itself a justification in any sense for physical restraint or for giving any treatment. It is an emergency procedure designed to buy time until the patient can be assessed by a medical practitioner. The initiation or continuing of physical or chemical restraints depends on further assessment of the patient once he or she has been detained.

GUIDELINES: NURSE'S HOLDING POWER

Action	Rationale
1 A registered mental nurse may detain a patient in a ward or department of the hospital under these circumstances: (i) If he or she judges that the patient is so mentally disordered that it is necessary to detain him or her in hospital in order to prevent harm to the patient or other people. (ii) If a doctor cannot practicably be obtained to assess and, if necessary, detain the patient under section 5(2), which lasts for seventy-two hours. (iii) In order to prevent a crime as defined in section 3(1) of the Criminal Law Act 1967. (iv) In self-defence or defence of the nurse's employer's property. (v) In order to prevent harm to a person who appears to be so mentally disordered as not to be competent to keep him- or herself safe and who appears likely to cause harm to others. (vi) In order to prevent the threat of violence which is likely to harm another person or his or her property.	Essentially the nurse's holding power is intended to prevent harm and injury in an emergency and to detain a patient long enough for detailed assessment of the risk to be carried out by a doctor, who may not be immediately available.
2 The RMN wishing to detain a patient completes Form 13, following which the patient may be detained for six hours.	Form 13 is the 'Record for the purposes of the MHA 1983, section 5(4)'.
3 The RMN detains the patient by locking the ward door.	(a) Physical restraint is likely to be impossible because of lack of numbers of nurses. (b) Seclusion is positively not advised.
4 If available, an emergency team is summoned, consisting, say, of a clinical nurse manager (representing the hospital managers), the duty doctor, another trained nurse, and another nurse, whether qualified or not.	Because by definition, what is happening is an emergency, the nurse who implements the holding power will need additional resources as soon as possible.
5 The senior registered nurse on duty will implement maximum supervision of the patient by at least one trained or senior student nurse.	To ensure that no harm comes to the patient, other patients or staff.
6 As soon as is practicable, if not immediately, the nurse who detained the patient, or another RMN, gives to the patient Leaflet 1 (MHA 1983, section 5(4)), and explains its contents.	In order to inform the patient of his or her rights.
7 As soon as possible after the nurse manager arrives in the ward, the nurse who detained the patient gives the immediate manager Form 13 and an oral report.	The immediate manager is authorized to receive such reports on behalf of the hospital managers.

8 If within one hour a doctor authorized to make a report under section 5(2) has not made the decision whether to do so or not, the nurse detaining the patient, or another RMN, informs the nurse manager responsible for the ward or department.

Although section 5(4) remains in force for six hours or until a doctor authorized to make a report under section 5(2) has seen the patient and decided to make the report or not, the situation is necessarily a psychiatric emergency and a decision by a doctor may be expected within an hour of it occurring.

9 As soon as the doctor decides whether or not to make a report under section 5(2), the nurse who detained the patient, or another RMN, completes Form 16 (record of time at which power to detain under section 5(4) elapsed).

(a) If the doctor decides to make a report under section 5(2) the time elapsed under section 5(4) counts as part of the seventy-two hours.
(b) As soon as the six hours under section 5(4) have expired or the authorized doctor has decided not to make a report under section 5(2), the patient must be released from detention.

10 Form 16 is delivered by hand to the medical records department as soon as possible during office hours, or kept in an envelope in the ward or department medical notes cupboard for delivery at the earliest possible time.

The hospital managers must be informed as soon as possible of both the use and duration of use of section 5(4)

11 The nurse who detained the patient writes a full account in the patient's nursing record of what led up to the detention and of what happened after section 5(4) was used. A summary is also written in the day or night report.

In order that subsequent evaluation will have the necessary material to determine the outcomes of the procedure and to identify the processes which led to the outcomes.

REFERENCE MATERIAL
References

DHSS (1987) *Mental Health Act 1983: Memorandum on Parts I to VI, VIII and X*, HMSO, London.
Mental Health Act, 1983, HMSO, London.

Further reading

Brooking, J. (1984) The art of applying the Act, *Nursing Mirror*, Vol. 159, no. 10, pp. i–viii.
Cooke, E. (1984) Holding on to the patient, *Nursing Times*, Vol. 80, no. 46, pp. 46–7.
Dimond, B. (1983) Powers of detention, *Nursing Mirror*, Vol. 157, no. 13, p. 35.
Dimond, B. (1983) The right to be consulted, *Nursing Mirror*, Vol. 157, no. 13, pp. 34–5.

Finch, J. (1984) The six-hour deadline, *Nursing Mirror*, Vol. 159, no. 10, p. 26.
Gostin, L. (1986) *Mental Health Services – Law and Practice*, Shaw, London.
Jones, R. (ed.) (1985) *Mental Health Act Manual*, Sweet & Maxwell, London.
Kilpack, V. (1984) Ethical issues and procedural dilemmas in measuring patient competence, *Advances in Nursing Science*, Vol. 6, no. 4, pp. 22–33.
Snell, H. (1986) *Representation before the Mental Health Review Tribunal*, King Edward's Hospital Fund, London.

43

The Media

DISCUSSION

Three aspects of nurses' dealings with the media will be emphasized in this discussion. The first is the general view of nurses held by the different media. The second is the response to be made by an individual nurse to representatives of the press who get in touch with him or her. The third is the responsibility of the nurse to the organization within which he or she works.

The media view of nurses

Even the so-called quality newspapers and journals are sometimes confused about basic issues such as the distinction between mental nurses and mental handicap nurses, which has led to deficiencies in their reporting of matters of public concern such as ill-treatment of patients. A nurse from the USA observes that the public image of nurses often differs greatly from the way nurses perceive themselves and is often inaccurate (Curran, 1985, p. 840).

However, it is not possible or necessarily desirable to control what the media write about nurses. Local and national newspapers report and interpret news according to their editorial priorities. They depend for their existence on their circulation. The image of nursing may sometimes be objectionable to nurses, but rejecting the paper which portrays such images is unlikely to achieve an improvement. Instead nurses may regard the media as potential recipients of information which they can provide. The task of nurses is to make their information attractive enough to claim a space in newspapers on its own merits. The professional organizations have tackled this task by spending a good deal of money on public relations and on maintaining press departments. The press departments keep a register of interested and interesting nurses with television and journalistic skills as well as proven expertise in their specialities, so that an inquiry from a journalist can be redirected to them if necessary. The procedure is designed to ensure that the

media receive factual and accurate information on which to base their research for articles.

Confidentiality is basic to the practice of both journalists and nurses. Journalists often wish to maintain exclusive rights over information they have obtained, and in the process may guarantee the confidentiality of their sources. Careful planning by nurses is necessary in order to ensure that their work with the press remains ethical as well as of mutual benefit.

The same principles apply to relations with television companies. However, there is much greater pressure on a television journalist in terms of the need to predict and react swiftly to events, and to compress information in a way not necessarily required by a newspaper or magazine. Similarly, a radio journalist is often working towards providing easily assimilable short items of news interspersed with entertainment. Nurses must plan carefully the information they wish to provide for radio programmes in order to avoid distortions due to pressure of time and competition from other news.

The nurse's responsibility to his or her employer

The last part of this discussion focuses on the psychiatric nurse's responsibility to his or her employing authority and, consequently, the correct response to media approaches. The guidelines themselves will be confined to these aspects.

All contact with representatives of the media must be made within the context of the health authority's policies for public relations, procedures for confidentiality, professional relationships, grievances, consultation and discipline. Where there is a public relations officer (PRO) it is easier to comply with the hospital's requirements by consulting with him or her before meeting a journalist. Although it is unfortunately true that many of the major scandals of ill-treatment of patients were disclosed by nurses to the press, and had, in some cases, been festering for years, the nurse's first action in pursuing a grievance will not usefully be to get in touch with a journalist. Beardshaw (1981) advises the stages of action for would-be whistle-blowers, involving exhaustive pursuit of issues through existing channels, and personal conduct of the highest standard.

Even when the issues are apparently uncontroversial, it is necessary to consult the PRO in case there could be consequences unforeseen by the nurse providing the press with information. A nurse's professional organization is helpful since it has representatives on the joint staff consultative committees who can take up issues if necessary. Its press department can give advice on ways to approach hospital managers, or alternative courses of action.

DIRECT MEDIA APPROACHES

It is possible that individual nurses will be approached by press representatives in connection with stories which could be seen as making an adverse impression if published. Such stories may be as various as the admission to hospital of a well-known person, injury or death resulting from staff negligence or cuts in services. It is essential that the nurse refers the journalist or inquirer to the senior manager in the health authority responsible for public relations. The nurse is likely to be asked for explanations or information or both. The nurse will behave at the time of the inquiry as if confidentiality is the primary measure to be upheld and will arrange for the journalist to speak to the PRO. It is possible that the PRO will authorize an individual nurse to make a statement to the press in such circumstances. But it is more likely that he or she would be asked for as much information as possible in order for the PRO to conduct negotiations with the press.

If the nurse is not happy with the outcome he or she may choose a number of different steps, such as to consult with a trade union or professional organization representative, a nurse manager, or the hospital ethics committee. To be guided by their advice is likely to be of more benefit to the nurse and the organization than to go it alone.

GUIDELINES: HANDLING THE MEDIA

Action

1   If approached by a member of the press the nurse considers the following criteria for determining his or her next step. Will contact with the press affect:
    (i)   his or her own good name;
    (ii) the good name of the hospital;
    (iii) confidentiality of patient care?

2   If in any doubt, the nurse asks the journalist to make his or her request in writing to the hospital manager responsible for public relations.

3   If the journalist is on the telephone and wishes an immediate reply, transfer the call to the relevant hospital manager, explaining that you will try to arrange for his or her request to be suitably met.

4   If the journalist is in the ward or department show him or her to one of the ward offices away from the patient areas and immediately telephone for the relevant hospital manager to come to the ward.

Rationale

Careful consideration is necessary to ensure that the nurse is fully aware of and takes full responsibility for the consequences of his or her actions.

(a) In order to clarify the journalist's intentions.
(b) So that the hospital manager can reach an agreement with the journalist on the nature of the material to be published.

Even if you decide to speak to the journalist yourself, the hospital administration will wish to be involved in any discussions before an interview.

(a) As for 3 above.
(b) To ensure that only patients who have consented are seen by journalists.

5 If a journalist approaches you with a suggestion for a news story or interview, explain the following conditions regarding patient confidentiality:
   (i)   patient confidentiality must be preserved;
   (ii) in the absence of such confidentiality, the patient's consent in writing is obtained;
   (iii) if the patient wishes, his or her responsible medical officer will monitor and countersign any consent.

So that undue pressure will not be put on any patient by a journalist who may be unaware of the effect of a person's mental state on what he or she might say.

6 Explain that a representative of the health authority will wish to see and negotiate, if necessary, amendments to the finished item.

So that the journalist is aware of potential constraints that the health authority may wish to exercise.

7 In the case of film or videotape, the patient must see the finished piece and give a second written consent to its showing or distribution or both.

The finished version may be unacceptable to the patient.

8 Even if the nurse is confident that his or her contact with the press is free from doubt, it is wise to check with the hospital manager responsible for public relations.

In case there are relevant issues of which the nurse is unaware.

9 Before first contact with a representative of each medium of the press obtain guidance from your local representative or the press department of your professional organization or trade union or both.

In order to be aware of the constraints on journalists and possible pitfalls for the nurse.

REFERENCE MATERIAL
References

Beardshaw, V. (1981) *Conscientious Objectors at Work*, Social Audit, London.

Curran, (1985) Effective utilization of the media, in J.C. McCloskey and H.K. Grace (eds.) *Current Issues in Nursing*, Blackwell, Oxford.

Further reading

Best, G., Dennis, J. and Draper, P. (1977) *Health, the Mass Media and the National Health Service*, Unit for the Study of Health Policy, London.

Bland, M. (1979) *You're on next! How to Survive on Television and Radio*, Kogan Page, London.

Campbell, C. (1985) A chance to air your views, *Nursing Mirror*, Vol. 160, no. 25, pp. 36–8.

Campbell, C. (1986) Tips of the TV trade, *Nursing Mirror*, Vol. 160, no. 24, pp. 18–22.

Hodge, J. (1986) *Face the Press*, Management Update, London.

Kalisch, P. A. and Kalisch, B. J. (1984) Psychiatric nurses and the press: a troubled relationship, *Perspectives in Psychiatric Care*, Vol. 22, no. 1, pp. 5–15.

Kalisch, P. A. and Kalisch, B. J. (1986) A comparative analysis of nurse and physician characters in the entertainment media, *Journal of Advanced Nursing*, Vol. 11, pp. 179–95.

Kratz, C. (1982) Nursing and journalism – legal and ethical considerations, *Nursing Times*, Vol. 78, no. 47, pp. 135–6.

Ministry of Health (1956) HM(56)58, *Information to the Press about the Condition of Patients*, Ministry of Health, London.

Mitchell, K. and Taylor, W. (1983) *You may Quote me: A Guide to Press and Public Relations in the National Health Service*, Institute of Health Service Administrators, London.

Sadler, C. (1985) Trust, respect and use, *Nursing Mirror*, Vol. 160, no. 25, p. 59.

Silver, R. (ed.) (1985) *Health Service Public Relations: A Guide to Good Practice*, King Edward's Hospital Fund, London.

Welch, L. B. and Welch, C. W. (1979) Making press interviews work for you, *Journal of Nursing Administration*, Vol. 9, no. 5, pp. 48–51.

Part Seven

Supervision and Appraisal

44

Supervision

DEFINITIONS

A supervisor has a variety of roles: administrative, supportive, consultative, educative. Stanford *et al.* (1957, p. 4) define supervisory activities as those which are 'concerned with the overall management and operation of one or more nursing units and the growth and development of unit personnel for the attainment of optimum effective patient care'. Implicit in this definition is the idea that nursing activities must be operationalized, their skills analysed for effective supervision to occur. According to this view the purpose of supervision is to increase the independence of trainees and supervisees so that they can be accountable for specific tasks. It is necessary for both supervisor and supervisee to be thoroughly familiar with the components of the supervisee's work.

Yuill (1968) specifically defines supervisors as first-line managers, citing charge nurses as an example. Supervision is the means by which the charge nurse of a ward or department ensures that the staff of that unit acquire and practise the attitudes, knowledge and skills necessary to carry out their jobs effectively. Supervision organised by a charge nurse can therefore also be defined as training which is carried out in the ward or unit itself (Smith and Delahaye, 1987; DuBrin, 1988).

DISCUSSION

Supervision is closely tied to the hierarchical system of a ward or department, ensuring that only appropriate delegation of responsibility for tasks and procedures takes place. That is, work is delegated only to students or trained nurses possessing the necessary competence as defined in the Nurses Rules (S.I. 1983/873) to carry it out. Supervision ensures that members of the nursing team who are lower in the hierarchy can participate in the work of the multidisciplinary clinical team (MDCT) alongside its other members.

In the context of Smith and Delahaye's (1987) defini-

tion of supervision as training (see above), in order to be effective that training will fulfil a number of conditions:
1 it will be skill-based;
2 the supervisor and supervisee work one-to-one;
3 a supervisor works with the same supervisee(s) for the duration of their placement;
4 the skills taught are relevant to the supervisee's work;
5 the supervisor rewards desired accomplishments according to a rational schedule;
6 supervision takes place in the context of regular documented appraisal;
7 supervision is directed towards the acquisition of accurate self-appraisal by the supervisee;
8 the supervision system of the ward or department is documented in its professional operating procedures.

Ward-based and classroom-based supervision

To some extent the supervisor can break down each task or procedure into its component skills and select an appropriate method whereby the supervisee can learn and practise the skills. The supervisor also practises to a standard necessary for the supervisee to model his or her own practice on. But given that procedures are skills ordered in such a way as to reach a specific goal and professional operating procedures detail the activities that nurses are required to carry out in a ward or department, the ward-based supervisor has less scope for selecting skills to teach than the classroom-based tutor.

Skills-based supervision attempts to identify the skills involved in professional relationships and to use a variety of educational and training methods for trainees to acquire and practise the attitudes, knowledge and behaviour necessary for each skill. Each skill ranges from basic psychomotor skills such as speaking or listening to complex diagnostic skills such as defining problems in ways that are acceptable to patients and on which patients can act.

Whereas in a school of nursing trainees can watch, imitate and practise new skills in a comparatively safe setting, their responsibilities in a ward are more complex and unpredictable, requiring them to assess unfamiliar situations and select appropriate skills in order to intervene effectively. Psychiatric nurses are required to learn techniques for intervening successfully with angry, distressed, deluded or hallucinating patients. The responsibilities of the ward-based supervisor involve enabling students to practise new skills safely.

A ward supervision programme arises from the integration and development of a charge nurse's management and clinical skills. It enhances patient care by clarifying the ways in which authority is delegated. The use of 'live' supervision ensures that charge nurses maintain their involvement in direct nursing care.

Mentor and preceptor roles

Many writers in the USA identify certain kinds of supervision with the development of relationships between nurses and mentors and nurses and preceptors. The mentor relationship is one where a usually older and more experienced nurse undertakes to guide another (Pilette, 1980). It has arisen in the USA where the influence of feminism on nursing has been stronger than in the UK. Writers disagree quite fundamentally about definitions of the mentor relationship, but a predominant characteristic is its informal origins, unlike the supervisor or preceptor relationship which arises from a more senior nurse's management responsibilities for more junior nurses' work.

The effort to establish mentor and preceptor relationships can be seen as a way of tackling the more traditional views of how to organize training and line management. Roch (1980) identified the importance of educative methods of establishing nurses in their professional role, and Menzies (1960) identified how the social organization of a nursing service can oblige nurses to perform their roles in dysfunctional ways. It may be said that the charge nurse's ward supervision programme ensures that nurses learn in an environment that is safe both psychologically and physically.

Types of supervision and supervisors

The clinical nurse specialist can play a valuable part in supervision. As an experienced clinician who is not required to administer a ward or unit, he or she can relieve ward-based supervisors of some of the burden of teaching where the material requires step-by-step introduction and practice before nurses work directly with patients.

Supervision may be conducted by a supervisor one-to-one (the supervision dyad), one-to-two (supervision triad), or one-to-a-group (group supervision). Peer supervision is conducted between colleagues occupying the same grade and depends on a stable working environment and long experience of working together. Simulation activities can be helpful, especially in group supervision.

It is essential that primary nurses receive supervision of their work with individual patients based on their documentation in the nursing record, especially on written process recordings of interactions. Similarly, it is a necessary condition that all nurses who attend therapeutic groups receive supervision by a group therapist whose training qualifies him or her to conduct such supervision.

In general, a ward or department will have a mixture of student and trained nurses. The charge nurse is therefore responsible for devising a supervision programme whereby the trained nurses supervise the students and he or she supervises the trained nurses. In this way the charge nurse monitors the standards of safety as well as of practice.

The supervisor's responsibilities

The supervisor is accountable to patients, colleagues in the nursing and multidisciplinary teams, managers and the director of nurse education, who is tasked by the National Boards to provide satisfactory clinical experience for students of nursing. The supervision of student nurses provides the opportunity to integrate the relationship between hospital departments and the school of nursing. Since a student nurse's line management is in the school of nursing, the supervisor is well advised to liaise with tutors, so that the steps necessary to resolve problems may be taken as soon as possible.

Part of the work of the supervisor is to sort out which problems belong to paients and which to nurses. In one-to-one supervision it can be tempting to drift into discussion of the supervisee's personal problems. This tendency may be a product of the supervisor regarding the supervisee as requiring direction and protection rather than as being responsible for his or her own learning. Sometimes a supervisee's attempt to discuss personal problems can be handled by discussing similar problems presented in material related to patients with whom the supervisee has difficulty. It is essential that at the beginning of an evaluation period the supervisor and supervisee negotiate a plan which specifies the goals towards which they both work so that personal problems, if they occur, can be practically dealt with.

GUIDELINES: SUPERVISING STAFF

Action	**Rationale**

1 The charge nurse of a ward or unit is responsible for arranging systematic supervision for the permanent and student nurses.

(a) So that each person receives formal supervision of his or her work.
(b) The charge nurse works in a system of supervision which is geared to the appraisal cycles of the different nurses.

2 The charge nurse ensures that students preparing for Parts 1, 3, 5 and 8 of the register are supervised by nurses qualified in those parts.

In accordance with the Nurses Rules (S.I. 1983/873).

3 The charge nurse ensures that nurses who are qualified in Parts 2, 4, 6 or 8 of the register are supervised by nurses who are qualified in Parts 1, 3, 5 or 8.

In accordance with the Nurses Rules.

4 The charge nurse bases supervision on the guidelines laid down in the nursing service policy manual.

Although charge nurses are free to develop some of the criteria for supervision and evaluation, the nursing service policy manual determines the specific components of each job description.

5 The charge nurse delegates to each first-level nurse the supervision of the student nurses in the ward or department.

(a) The charge nurse is responsible for supervising the first-level nurses.
(b) The charge nurse's supervision of the first-level nurses includes formal and regular monitoring of their work with the untrained staff in the ward.

6 The charge nurse agrees with each first-level nurse his or her plans for supervision.

The plans provide individually based criteria for supervising nurses.

7 The charge nurse conducts regular meetings of all ward supervisors.

To monitor progress and development of nurses who are not supervised individually by the charge nurse.

8 Each supervisor agrees with individual supervisees a timetable for supervisions and appraisal interviews.

(a) So that performance may be continuously monitored.
(b) So that objectives can be set within the agreed time frame.

9 Each supervisor arranges the time of a supervision session at least a week in advance, preferably at the end of each supervision.

(a) So that the duty rota can be arranged.
(b) So that both the supervisor and the supervisee can make necessary preparations.

10 The intervals between each supervision are agreed between the supervisor and supervisee at the beginning of a placement or appraisal period.

It is important that the supervisions are run according to a rational plan, especially if the teaching methods used are relatively unstructured and require the supervisee to take responsibility.

11 Each supervisor uses the following criteria when planning supervisions:
  (i)   the appraisal requirements of the hospital nursing service or the school of nursing;
  (ii) supervisee's personal objectives as agreed with the supervisor;
  (iii) the UKCC Code of Conduct;
  (iv) special requirements of the ward or department;
  (v)   ward policies, procedures and objectives.

It is essential that there are externally validated statements of duties and responsibilities to which the supervisor can refer.

12 When the supervision is booked both supervisor and supervisee agree to spend at least forty-five minutes on whatever agenda they negotiate.

In order to allow enough time for introducing, working in and evaluating the session.

13 If the supervisor is concerned about the performance of a supervisee he or she takes advice from the charge nurse or another nurse manager before finding out the staff member's view of his or her performance and communicating to him or her the perceived deficits in his or her performance.

(a) A formal evaluation of poor performance can be made only if the individual has had an opportunity to know and correct any deficits.
(b) Since it may be necessary to discipline a person if his or her work continues to be poor, it is essential that the supervisor has gone over in detail with and instructed him or her in the areas where performance may be improved.

14 The supervisor identifies and communicates the areas in which he or she finds such a person's work satisfactory.

(a) In order to provide a sense of proportion between satisfactory and unsatisfactory performance.
(b) In order to reward and encourage desirable standards of work.

15 The supervisor confirms after such a supervision that both participants agree about what has taken place, the objectives for the next assessment period, the duration of the next assessment period and the nature of any action to be taken if the poor performance continues.

So that there is as complete agreement as possible about the outcome of the supervision, and the timing of the next.

16 The supervisor keeps a confidential record of all supervisions.

An up-to-date record is more useful for any subsequent appraisal of the supervisee because of the 'halo effect' which results from partly remembered and subjective impressions.

17 The supervisor is responsible for conducting appraisals of his or her supervisees.

(a) In order that appraisals are conducted by first-level nurses who have worked closely with student nurses.
(b) In order that the charge nurse retains accountability through his or her supervision of the first-level nurses for the entire supervision and appraisal processes.

18 The supervisor uses observable and measurable behaviours rather than personality traits and emotional factors as the basis for supervision.

Judgements about emotions and attitudes are inferences about behaviour.

19 The supervisor identifies and communicates the areas in which a supervisee's performance is seen to be satisfactory or of a high standard.

In order to reward desirable achievements.

20 When supervising a nurse's work with individual patients the supervisor first ensures that the nurse's documentation in the nursing record reaches the standards specified in the procedures for the nursing process.

(a) In order for a nurse's accountability for his or her work to be monitored the evidence of what has been done must be available.

(b) The nursing record is the means by which nurses render account for work which has been delegated to them.

(c) Unless the supervisor has the necessary documentation available, supervision is likely to be based on vague and partial memories.

21 The shift rota is compiled in such a way that supervisee and supervisor work shifts together.

(a) It is helpful if the supervisor can model nursing skills.

(b) Later on the supervisor can observe a supervisee's practice.

22 Group supervisions and supervision of groups are timetabled so that all nurses are able to attend.

Nurses who do not receive supervision of their work in groups are likely to respond in ways that they do not understand to group processes and thereby to jeopardize the safety of patients and colleagues.

23 Staffing levels are regulated so that supervision is not compromised by staff shortages.

The Nurses Rules place a legal obligation on nurse managers to ensure that students and nurses qualified in Parts 2, 4, 6 or 7 of the register are directed by nurses qualified in Parts 1, 3, 5 or 8 of the register.

REFERENCE MATERIAL
References

DuBrin, A. J. (1988) *Human Relations: A Job Oriented Approach*, Prentice-Hall, New Jersey.

Nurses, Midwives and Health Visitors Rules Approval Order (1983) SI, 1983/873, HMSO, London.

Menzies, I. (1960) *The Functioning of Social Systems as a Defence Against Anxiety*, Tavistock, London.

Pilette, P. C. (1980) Mentoring: An encounter of the leadership kind, *Nursing Leadership*, Vol. 3, no. 2, pp. 22–6.

Roch, J. (1980) The uses and limits of the concept of role for nurse education, *Nursing Times*, Vol. 76, no. 19, p. 839.

Smith, B. J. and Delahaye, B. L. (1987) *How To Be An Effective Trainer*, Wiley, New York.

Standford, E. *et al.* (1957) *How to Study Supervision Activities*, US Government Printing Office, Washington DC.

Yuill, B. (1968) *Supervision: Principles and Techniques*, George Allan and Unwin, London.

Further reading

Authier, J. and Gustafson, K. (1976) Application of supervised and unsupervised microcounselling paradigms in the training of registered and licensed practical nurses, *Journal of Consulting and Clinical Psychology*, Vol. 44, no. 5, pp. 704–9.

Barile, L. A. (1982) A model for teaching management of disturbed behaviour, *Journal of Psychosocial Nursing and Mental Health Services*, Vol. 20, no. 11, pp. 9–11.

Bergman, R. (1977) Interpersonal relations in health care delivery, *International Nursing Review*, Vol. 24, pp. 104–7.

Block, B. (1976) Preparing students for physical restraints, *Journal of Psychiatric Nursing*, Vol. 14, no. 10, pp. 9–10.

Buccheri, R. C. (1986) Nursing supervision: a new look at an old role, *Nursing Administration Quarterly*, Vol. 11, no. 1, pp. 11–25.

Burke, R. J. (1982) Personality self-image and informal helping processes in work settings, *Psychological Reports*, Vol. 50, no. 3, pp. 1295–1302.

Choppin, R. G. (1983) *The Role of the Ward Sister*, King Edward's Hospital Fund, London.

Dimarco, N. and Kuehl, C. (1976) Predictors of management training effectiveness for nursing supervisors, *Journal of Continuing Education in Nursing*, Vol. 7, no. 4, pp. 38–46.

Farnish, S. (1983) *Ward Sister Preparation: A Survey in Three*

Districts, Nursing Education Research Unit, Chelsea College, London.

Fretwell, J. (1980) An inquiry into the ward learning environment, *Nursing Times*, Vol. 76, no. 16, pp. 69–73.

Fretwell, J. E. (1982) *Ward Teaching and Learning*, RCN, London.

Gregg, D. E., Bregg, E. A. and Spring, F. E. (1976) Individual supervision: a method of teaching psychiatric concepts in nursing education, *Perspectives in Psychiatric Nursing Care*, Vol. 14, no. 3, pp. 115–29.

Hagerty, B. K. (1986) A competency based orientation program for psychiatric nursing, *Journal of Continuing Education in Nursing*, Vol. 17, no. 5, pp. 157–62.

Hardin, S. B., Stratton, K. and Benton, D. (1983) The video connection: group dynamics onscreen, *Journal of Psychosocial Nursing and Mental Health Services*, Vol. 21, no. 11, pp. 12–21.

Hersey, P., Blanchard, K. and LaMonica, E. (1976) A situational approach to supervision: leadership theory and the supervising nurse, *Supervisor Nurse*, Vol. 7, no. 5, pp. 17–20.

Hughes, C. M. (1985) Supervising clinical practice in psychosocial nursing, *Journal of Psychosocial Nursing and Mental Health Services*, Vol. 23, no. 2, pp. 27–32.

Jackson, S. E. (1983) Participation in decision-making as a strategy for reducing job-related strain, *Journal of Applied Psychology*, Vol. 68, no. 1, pp. 3–19.

Johnson, J. and Luciana, K. (1983) Managing by behaviour and results linking supervisory accountability to effective organizational control, *Journal of Nursing Administration*, Vol. 13, no. 12, pp. 19–28.

Keyzer, D. M. (1985) Learning contracts, *Nursing Research Abstracts*, Vol. 7, no. 4, p. 9.

Krikorian, D. A. and Paulanka, B. J. (1984) Students' perception of learning and change in the psychiatric clinical setting, *Perspectives in Psychiatric Nursing Care*, Vol. 22, no. 3, pp. 118–24.

Lamonica, E. *et al.* (1977) Empathy training, *Nursing Mirror*, Vol. 145, no. 8, pp. 22–5.

Lathlean, J. (1988) *Research in Action: Developing the Role of the Ward Sister*, King Edward's Hospital Fund, London.

Limon, S., Bargagliotti, L. A. and Spencer, J. B. (1982) Providing preceptors for nursing students: what questions you should ask, *Journal of Nursing Administration*, Vol. 12, no. 6, pp. 16–19.

Park, C. L. (1982) A clinical instruction observation tool, *Nursing Papers*, Vol. 14, no. 3, pp. 7–16.

Parsons, V. (1972) Contact vs contract: the process of taming, *Journal of Psychiatric Nursing*, Vol. 10, no. 3, pp. 18–20.

Pettes, D. E. (1979) *Staff and Student Supervision*, Allen & Unwin, London.

Pozgar, G. D. (1983) Perceptive communication, *Health Care Supervisor*, Vol. 1, no. 4, pp. 1–13.

Schroder, P. J. (1985) Recognising transference and countertransference, *Journal of Psychosocial Nursing and Mental Health Services*, Vol. 23, no. 2, pp. 21–6.

Stull, M. K. (1986) Staff nurse performance: effects of goal-setting and performance feedback, *Journal of Nursing Administration*, Vol. 16, no. 7, 8, pp. 26–30.

Topf, M. and Dambacher, B. (1981) Teaching interpersonal skills: a model for facilitating optimal interpersonal relations, *Journal of Psychosocial Nursing and Mental Health Services*, Vol. 19, no. 12, pp. 29–33.

Wessel, F. (1985) Communication: getting the most from your staff, *Hospital and Healthcare*, Vol. 16, no. 4, pp. 8–10.

Wong, S. and Wong, J. (1980) The effectiveness of clinical teaching: a model for self-evaluation, *Journal of Advanced Nursing*, Vol. 5, pp. 531–7.

45

Appraisal

DEFINITION

Appraisal is a key activity of anyone who is responsible for supervising other people's work. It is both a means of assessing the performance of individuals and of defining the nature of the work they are expected to carry out. Supervision is the process by which a person over time monitors and directs the other people's work for which he or she is responsible. Appraisal is the process whereby the supervisor meets with a supervisee at specific times, usually laid down by the organization within which they work, in order to record an assessment of his or her performance in a way which allows them both to make what amounts to a position statement. That is, where the supervisee is now, what has brought him or her to this point, and where he or she sees him- or herself moving over the next appraisal period.

DISCUSSION

Huckaby (1979) tested different appraisal systems to establish whether learning by graduate nursing students was enhanced by the use of graded as opposed to ungraded tests. She found that achieving grades did not motivate students to take responsibility for their learning, and possibly hindered them from taking satisfaction in learning for its own sake. Uphold (1983) used such findings to recommend that gradings should not be used in appraisal, and that students should be required to devise their own self-evaluation strategies in the context of a limited number of behavioural competencies. Usually the organization provides a standardized form for recording the appraisal.

As a result of the reorganization of nursing management which followed the Report of the Committee on Senior Nursing Staff Structure (Report, 1966), appraisal was conceived as being integral to the system of line management, where the nurse was appraised by his or her immediate manager, and the appraisal was reviewed by the next nurse in line.

It was thought that career counselling and develop-

ment could be facilitated by identifying aspects of the nurse's performance which could be improved either by personal change or training, and by using the appraisal to provide a reliable source for references. Stated categories would combine evaluation of personality attributes with attempts to quantify specific components of the person's job. However, without stating specifically the expected behaviours by a job-holder, it is difficult for appraisers to measure accurately the degree to which a person discharges his or her responsibilities. There is now considerable doubt about the validity of using assessments of traits and attributes. Appraisal must therefore be linked closely to the setting and evaluation of nursing standards, and the drafting and implementation of policies and procedures. It cannot be performed in isolation from the evaluation of the standards of nursing care and management generally.

A typical system of job and performance review develops with the objectives of improving performance, providing information for staff about their role in the organization and developing the potential of staff to carry out their present work as well as think about future jobs. Factual recording of qualifications, previous appointments and education, and professional qualifications and training is accompanied by performance targets negotiated by the appraiser and the job-holder. An appraisal is often countersigned by the manager next in line to the appraiser.

Two principles can be identified: encouraging the person being appraised to make personal objectives for his or her work; and valuing appraisal as a step towards enhanced career prospects. The same principles apply to the appraisal of student nurses. The first part of the guidelines will deal with the appraisal of the permanent nurses in a ward or department, the second will deal with the appraisal of student nurses.

The importance of properly conducted appraisal for student nurses is that it helps in assessing their potential to achieve competence as registered nurses.

GUIDELINES: APPRAISING STAFF

Action

Rationale

1 The senior charge nurse is responsible for systematically evaluating the work of the permanent nurses in a ward or unit once a year. He or she will be working in a cycle of assessment programmes because staff will have joined at different times in a given year.

So that each person receives formal assessment of his or her work every twelve months.

2 The charge nurse bases his or her evaluation on the guidelines laid down in the nursing service policy manual.

Although charge nurses are free to develop some of the criteria for evaluating performance, the nursing service policy manual determines the specific components of each job description.

3 The charge nurse makes clear to ward staff his or her criteria for evaluation at the beginning of each person's assessment year.

(a) Each evaluation of a subordinate's performance is also an evaluation of that of the charge nurse.
(b) So that nurses know the standards they must achieve.
(c) So that problems may be dealt with as they arise and not left until the appraisal.

4 The charge nurse agrees with each staff member a plan for the coming year.

To provide individually based criteria by which performance can be evaluated.

5 The charge nurse agrees with individual subordinates a time scale for assessment and evaluation.

(a) It is essential that both the charge nurse and the staff member are aware of the need to monitor performance continuously.
(b) Appraisal interviews concerning poor performance are extremely difficult to conduct if a person's attention has not been drawn to the quality of his or her work before.
(c) So that objectives can be set within the agreed time frame.

6 The charge nurse arranges the time of an appraisal interview at least a week in advance.

(a) So that the duty rota can be arranged.
(b) So that other commitments can be rearranged if necessary.
(c) So that both the supervisor and the person to be appraised can prepare for the interview.

7 The charge nurse evaluates the performance of subordinates against the following criteria:
   (i) any formal ratings required by the hospital;
   (ii) subordinates' personal objectives as agreed with the charge nurse at the start of the evaluation period;
   (iii) the UKCC Code of Conduct;
   (iv) special requirements of the ward or department;
   (v) ward policies, procedures and objectives;
   (vi) observable and measurable behaviour.

(a) It is essential that there are externally validated statements of duties and responsibilities to which the charge nurse can refer for evidence of standards for particular evaluations.
(b) To provide a counterbalance to the charge nurse's subjective judgements.

8 When the appraisal interview is booked an agenda and a time limit for its duration are stated.

(a) In order that the necessary business can be effectively carried out in the time available.
(b) Objectives for the interview will be different depending on the performance of the individual member of staff.

9 When the charge nurse is formally evaluating poor performance his or her objectives in the appraisal interview will be to:
(i)   learn the staff member's view of his or her performance;
(ii) communicate to the staff member the deficits in his or her performance;
(iii) state the objectives he or she must achieve in order to improve.
This depends on the charge nurse having already made the person concerned aware of concern about his or her performance.

(a) A formal evaluation of poor performance can be made only if the individual has had an opportunity to know and correct any deficits.
(b) Since it may be necessary to discipline a person if his or her work continues to be poor, it is essential that the charge nurse has gone over in detail with and instructed him or her in the areas where performance may be improved.

10 The charge nurse identifies and communicates the areas in which he or she finds the person's work satisfactory.

(a) In order to provide a sense of proportion between satisfactory and unsatisfactory performance.
(b) In order to finish the interview by encouraging the person concerned.

11 When formally evaluating average to good performance the charge nurse's objective in the appraisal interview will be to:
(i)   negotiate ratings;
(ii) negotiate objectives for the next assessment period.

(a) Such an interview will require the person being assessed to take the initiative.
(b) By encouraging the other person to state opinions frankly the charge nurse hopes that the initiative for constructive change will be taken by him or her.

12 Before the appraisal interview both the charge nurse and the subordinate complete in pencil any formal rating schedule required by the health authority.

(a) In order to negotiate corrections of over- or under-rating by either participant.
(b) In order to develop mutuality and co-operation in the task.

13 The charge nurse listens to any criticisms made by the person being appraised.

In order to convey the idea that the person being appraised on good performance takes the initiative in the appraisal process.

14 The charge nurse completes the final ratings with the person being appraised.

The charge nurse is prepared to change ratings as a result of discussion.

15 The charge nurse discusses observable and measurable behaviours rather than personality traits and emotional factors.

Judgements about emotions and attitudes are inferences about behaviour.

16 The charge nurse identifies and communicates the areas in which the person's performance is seen to be satisfactory or of a high standard.

In order to reward desirable achievements.

17 The charge nurse discusses with the person being appraised any plans he or she has for career development.

(a) So that promotion opportunities can be anticipated and planned for.
(b) So that the charge nurse can plan with all nurses how further educational or training opportunities can be fairly distributed.
(c) So that the charge nurse can advise the line manager who can make the necessary recommendations to the relevant committee.

18 The charge nurse finishes the interview by confirming that both participants agree about what has taken place, the objectives for the next assessment period, the duration of the next assessment period.

So that there is as complete agreement as possible about the outcome of the interview, and the timing of the next.

19 The charge nurse keeps a detailed, confidential record of the interview.

A complete record kept up to date is more likely to be fair to the person being assessed because of the 'halo effect' which results from partly remembered and subjective impressions.

20 The charge nurse sends to his or her immediate manager a copy of the assessments, ratings and action plans.

(a) The immediate manager routinely reads the assessments and interviews the staff being appraised.
(b) In this way standards are monitored and compared throughout the nursing service.
(c) The charge nurse's performance as a supervisor is being assessed each time he or she appraises a member of staff.

Procedure for appraising student nurses

21 The charge nurse is responsible for ensuring that each nurse in training for Parts 1, 3, 5 and 8 of the register is supervised by a first-level nurse qualified in the same part of the register for which the student is preparing.

To comply with the Nurses Rules (S.I. 1983/873).

22 The first-level nurse supervising the student is called the supervisor.

To emphasize the training as well as managerial aspects of appraising students.

23 The supervisor is responsible for systematically evaluating the work of student nurse supervisees in accordance with the directions of the school of nursing. The supervisor will be working in a cycle of appraisals because of the different rates of student allocation.

So that each student receives formal assessment of his or her work at the times specified by the school of nursing.

24 The supervisor bases his or her evaluation on the guidelines laid down by the nursing service policy manual and the school of nursing.

(a) Although charge nurses are free to develop some of the criteria for evaluating performance the nursing service policy manual determines the specific components of each job description.
(b) The school of nursing specifies the responsibilities of student nurses in relation to the nursing service policy manual.

25   The supervisor agrees with each student for whom he or she is responsible a plan for the period leading to the first appraisal.

(a) Each appraisal of a student nurse's performance is an evaluation of the supervisor's performance.
(b) So that students agree the standards they must achieve.
(c) So that problems are dealt with as they arise and not left until the appraisal.

26   The supervisor arranges the date of the first appraisal when he or she first has a supervision with the student.

(a) So that the duty rota can be arranged well in advance.
(b) So that the student knows the time frame for objectives.

27   The supervisor evaluates the performance of students against the following criteria:
(i) any formal ratings required by the school of nursing;
(ii) students' personal objectives as agreed with the supervisor at the start of the evaluation period;
(iii) the UKCC Code of Conduct;
(iv) special requirements of the ward or department;
(v) ward policies, procedures and objectives;
(vi) observable and measurable behaviour.

(a) It is essential that there are externally validated statements of duties and responsibilities to which the supervisor can refer for evidence of standards for particular evaluations.
(b) Such criteria provide a counterbalance to the supervisor's subjective judgements.

28   When the appraisal interview is booked an agenda and a time limit for its duration are stated.

(a) In order that the necessary business can be effectively carried out in the time available.
(b) Objectives for the interview will be different depending on the performance of the individual student.

29   When the supervisor is formally evaluating poor performance his or her objectives in the appraisal interview will be to:
(i) learn the student's view of his or her performance;
(ii) communicate to the student the deficits in his or her performance;
(iii) state the objectives he or she must achieve in order to improve.
This depends on the supervisor having already made the student aware of concern about his or her performance.

(a) A formal evaluation of poor performance can be made only if the student has had an opportunity to know and correct any deficits.
(b) Since it may be necessary to discipline a student if his or her work continues to be poor, it is essential that the supervisor has gone over in detail with and instructed him or her in the areas where performance may be improved.

30   The supervisor identifies and communicates the areas in which he or she finds the student's work satisfactory.

(a) In order to provide a sense of proportion between satisfactory and unsatisfactory performance.
(b) In order to finish the interview by encouraging the student.

31   The supervisor consults with the charge nurse about any appraisal of apparently poor performance.

(a) So that the charge nurse can liaise with other members of staff if necessary to help the student correct poor performance.
(b) So that the charge nurse can consult with the student and his or her personal tutor in the school of nursing.
(c) The charge nurse rings the tutor even if the staff nurse is the appraiser.

32   If the charge nurse is the appraiser he or she consults with the line manager or a tutor or both.

In order to ensure that the student has the best chance to correct poor performance.

33 When formally evaluating average to good performance the supervisor's objective in the appraisal interview will be to:
(i) negotiate ratings;
(ii) negotiate objectives for the next assessment period.

(a) Such an interview will require the student being assessed to take the initiative.
(b) By encouraging the student to state opinions frankly the supervisor hopes that the initiative for constructive change will be taken by him or her.

34 Before the appraisal interview both the supervisor and the student complete in pencil any formal rating schedule required by the school of nursing.

(a) In order to negotiate corrections of over- or under-rating by either participant.
(b) In order to develop mutuality and co-operation in the task.

35 The supervisor listens to any criticisms made by the student being appraised.

In order to convey the idea that the student being appraised on good performance takes the initiative in the appraisal process.

36 The supervisor completes the final ratings with the student being appraised.

The supervisor is prepared to change ratings as a result of discussion.

37 The supervisor discusses observable and measurable behaviours rather than personality traits and emotional factors.

Judgements about emotions and attitudes are inferences about behaviour.

38 The supervisor identifies and communicates the area in which the student's performance is seen to be satisfactory or of a high standard.

In order to reward desirable achievements.

39 The supervisor finishes the interview by confirming that both participants agree about what has taken place, the objectives for the next assessment period, the duration of the next assessment period.

So that there is as complete agreement as possible about the outcome of the interview, and the timing of the next.

40 The supervisor keeps a detailed, confidential record of the interview.

A complete record kept up to date is more likely to be fair to the person being assessed because of the 'halo effect' which results from partly remembered and subjective impressions.

41 The student writes on the appraisal form any comments he or she thinks are relevant.

The student may want to dissent entirely from the appraisal, and this is recorded on the form when it is sent to the immediate line manager and the school of nursing.

42 The charge nurse reads, underwrites and countersigns all appraisals before they are sent to the immediate line manager and the school of nursing.

(a) The charge nurse is responsible for all the supervision in the ward or department.
(b) So that the charge nurse is thoroughly in touch with the progress of all students in the ward.

REFERENCE MATERIAL

References

Huckabay, L. M. D. (1979) Cognitive-affective consequences of grading versus nongrading of formative evaluations, *Nursing Research*, Vol. 28, no. 3, pp. 173–8.

Report (1966) *Report of the Committee on Senior Nursing Staff Structure* (the Salmon Report), Ministry of Health, London.

Uphold, C. R. (1983) Using an individualized clinical evaluation strategy to motivate the RN student, *Journal of Nursing Education*, Vol. 22, no. 9, pp. 397–400.

Further reading

Breeden, S. A. (1978) Participative employee evaluation, *Journal of Nursing Administration*, Vol. 8, no. 5, pp. 13–19.

Brief, A. P., Aldag, R. J. and Van Sell, M. (1977) Moderators of the relationship between self and superior evaluations of job performance, *Journal of Occupational Psychology*, Vol. 50, pp. 129–34.

Corton, B. (1986) Sorting out standards, *Health Service Journal*, Vol. 96, no. 5011, p. 1051.

Cunningham, C. V. (1981) Performance appraisal tests for staff nurses, *Nursing Times*, Vol. 77, no. 16, pp. 61–3.

Dieterle, J. A. (1983) Clinical validation of psychiatric nursing skills, *Journal of Nursing Education*, Vol. 22, no. 9, pp. 392–6.

Finch, J. (1982) The importance of being frank, *Nursing Mirror*, Vol. 154, no. 26, pp. 25–6.

Gourlay, J. R. (1986) Staff appraisal, *Health Services Manpower Review*, Vol. 2, no. 2, pp. 16–24.

Gourlay, R. (1986) Performance appraisal – a systematic approach, *Health Care Management*, Vol. 1, no. 1, pp. 32–5.

Grantham, M. A. *et al.* (1986) Development and evaluation of nurses giving direct patient care, in S. M. Stinson *et al.* (eds.) *New Frontiers of Nursing Research*, University of Alberta, Edmonton.

Haar, L. P. and Hicks, J. R. (1976) Performance appraisal: derivation of effective assessment tools, *Journal of Nursing Administration*, Vol. 6, no. 9, pp. 20–9.

Johnson, J. and Luciano, K. (1983) Managing by behaviour and results – linking supervisory accountability to effective organizational control, *Journal of Nursing Administration*, Vol. 13, no. 12, pp. 19–28.

King Edward's Hospital Fund (1982) *Assessment: A Guide for the Completion of Progress Reports on Nurses in Training*, KEHF, London.

Lees, M. (1986) A study of staff appraisal of sisters and charge nurses in the medical and surgical wards of four general hospitals, *Nursing Research Abstracts*, Vol. 8, no. 1, p. 4.

Long, P. (1976) Judging and reporting on student nurse clinical performance: some problems for the ward sister, *International Journal of Nursing Studies*, Vol. 13, pp. 115–21.

McKenzie, I. (1985) Being objective about appraisal, *Nursing Times*, Vol. 81, no. 51, pp. 25–6.

Megel, M. A. (1983) Establishing a criterion-based performance appraisal for a department of nursing, *Nursing Clinics of North America*, Vol. 18, no. 3, pp. 449–56.

Miller, A. (1985) Head hunting, *Nursing Times*, Vol. 81, no. 26, pp. 38–40.

Mitchell, W. (1976) Assessments in psychiatric nursing, *Nursing Times*, Vol. 72, no. 9, pp. 350–2.

National Association of Health Authorities (1985) *NHS Handbook*, NAHA, Birmingham.

South East Thames Regional Health Authority (1978) *Management Job and Performance Review*, SETRHA, Bexhill.

Squier, R. W. (1981) The reliability and validity of rating scales in assessing the clinical progress of psychiatric nursing students, *International Journal of Nursing Studies*, Vol. 18, pp. 157–69.

Stone, S. *et al.* (1984) *Management for Nurses*, Mosby, St Louis.

Stull, M. K. (1986) Staff nurse performance: effects of goal-setting and performance feedback, *Journal of Nursing Administration*, Vol. 16, no. 7, 8, pp. 26–30.

Thompson, D. J. C. (1979) Staff development and performance review, *Nursing Times*, Vol. 75, no. 6, pp. 25–8.

Walton, M. (1985) Trying to do better, *Nursing Times*, Vol. 81, no. 28, pp. 30–1.

Young, A. P. (1982) Reports and references, *Nursing*, Vol. 1, no. 36, pp. 1547–8.

Part Eight | Appendices

A

Code of Professional Conduct for the Nurse, Midwife and Health Visitor

Each registered nurse, midwife and health visitor shall act, at all times, in such a manner as to justify public trust and confidence, to uphold and enhance the good standing and reputation of the profession, to serve the interests of society, and above all to safeguard the interests of individual patients and clients.

Each registered nurse, midwife and health visitor is accountable for his or her practice, and, in the exercise of professional accountability shall:

1 Act always in such a way as to promote and safeguard the well being and interests of patients/clients.
2 Ensure that no action or omission on his/her part or within his/her sphere of influence is detrimental to the condition or safety of patients/clients.
3 Take every reasonable opportunity to maintain and improve professional knowledge and competence.
4 Acknowledge any limitations of competence and refuse in such cases to accept delegated functions without first having received instruction in regard to those functions and having been assessed as competent.
5 Work in a collaborative and co-operative manner with other health care professionals and recognise and respect their particular contributions within the health care team.
6 Take account of the customs, values and spiritual beliefs of patients/clients.
7 Make known to an appropriate person or authority any conscientious objection which may be relevant to professional practice.

8 Avoid any abuse of the privileged relationship which exists with patients/clients and of the privileged access allowed to their property, residence or workplace.
9 Respect confidential information obtained in the course of professional practice and refrain from disclosing such information without the consent of the patient/client, or a person entitled to act on his/her behalf, except where disclosure is required by law or by the order of a court or is necessary in the public interest.
10 Have regard to the environment of care and its physical, psychological and social effects on patients/clients, and also the adequacy of resources, and make known to appropriate persons or authorities any circumstances which could place patients/clients in jeopardy or which militate against safe standards of practice.
11 Have regard to the workload of and the pressures on professional colleagues and subordinates and take appropriate action if these are seen to be such as to constitute abuse of the individual practitioner and/or to jeopardise safe standards of practice.
12 In the context of the individual's own knowledge, experience, and sphere of authority, assist peers and subordinates to develop professional competence in accordance with their needs.
13 Refuse to accept any gift, favour or hospitality which might be interpreted as seeking to exert undue influence to obtain preferential consideration.
14 Avoid the use of professional qualifications in the promotion of commercial products in order not to compromise the independence of professional judgement on which patients/clients rely.

B

Advertising

A UKCC Advisory Paper. An elaboration of Clause 14 of the Code of Professional Conduct.

1 Advertising general availability for professional work as a nurse, midwife or health visitor.

A registered nurse, midwife or health visitor may state his/her registration status in any published advertisement for professional employment, provided that any such advertisement:
(a) is not ostentatious, and;
(b) does not make claims that the practitioner is to be preferred over others.

This authority extends to any statement of registration status in business cards, letter headings, or advertisements placed in the press or other places.

2 Advertising availability for a specific type of professional work as a nurse, midwife or health visitor.

A registered nurse, midwife or health visitor who has successfully completed a specific post-basic course and thus obtained specialist knowledge and skills (e.g. in stoma care) may state his/her registration status (and recorded qualification status) in advertising his/her availability for care, advice or teaching in that speciality. The principles stated in 1 above apply.

3 Use of registration status in respect of a business owned or managed by the registered nurse, midwife or health visitor.

A registered nurse, midwife or health visitor may indicate his/her registration status in connection with any business (associated with professional practice) of which he/she is the proprietor or manager. This authority applies to letter headings, business cards, advertisements, wall plates, etc., but the general

principles of clause 1 above again apply.

4 Use of registration status in respect of employment by a person or company in a field related to nursing, midwifery or health visiting.

A registered nurse, midwife or health visitor employed by another person or company in any capacity which requires him/her to correspond with or call on medical practitioners, pharmacists, hospitals, clinics etc. to promote particular products may indicate his/her registration status in association with his/her name on letters, or on business cards of modest size and design.

5. Use of registration status in promotional films or literature.

Any registered nurse, midwife or health visitor who becomes involved in providing advice for, writing for or featuring in any films or other material, a purpose of which is to promote a commercial product or brand name must ensure that, if his/her name appears in any acknowledgements of credits, it should not be accompanied by any indication of registration status.

6 Use of registration status in respect of educational or documentary films or literature.

Publication of an individual registered nurse, midwife or health visitor's registration status in association with his/her name is regarded as acceptable in educational or documentary films or literature provided that the purpose is not and could not be construed as to advertise the practitioner in his/her professional capacity other than as authorised elsewhere in this document.

7 Use of registration status in respect of writing for publication, participation in radio or television

programmes and participation in conferences, seminars etc.

Indication of an individual's registration status with his/her name is regarded as acceptable, provided that the purpose is not and could not be construed as to advertise the practitioner in his/her professional capacity other than as authorised elsewhere in this document.

8   Use of nurse, midwife or health visitor registration status in advertising for professional work outside nursing, midwifery and health visiting.

Advertising for professional work within the province of other professions should not be undertaken by persons on the UKCC register under any circumstances where registered practitioners of the profession in question are not allowed to advertise their services.

A registered nurse, midwife or health visitor who is also a registered practitioner of another profession which does allow advertising, and who wishes, in advertising his/her availability for work in that other profession, to indicate his/her status on the UKCC register should seek permission from the statutory body for that other profession before proceeding.

Some registered nurses, midwives and health visitors obtain non-registerable qualifications in other areas of health care, fully qualified practitioners in which are subject to regulation by registration. Such registered nurses, midwives and health visitors must not, in any circumstances, indicate their status in the UKCC register when advertising for work in another professional sphere on the basis of a non-registerable qualification unless permission has first been obtained from the UKCC.

9   Advertising outside the tolerances indicated in Clauses 1 to 8 above.

The indication of a person's registration status as a nurse, midwife or health visitor outside the above stated tolerances may be regarded as unacceptable and result in charges of misconduct.

Any registered nurse considering using or authorising the use of his/her registration status in ways not referred to in this notice should seek specific advice from the Professional Conduct Division of the UKCC before proceeding.

C

Exercising Accountability

A UKCC Advisory Document. A framework to assist nurses, midwives and health visitors to consider ethical aspects of professional practice.

A. INTRODUCTION

1 The United Kingdom Central Council for Nursing, Midwifery and Health Visiting regulates the nursing, midwifery and health visiting professions in the public interest.

The UKCC was established by the Nurses, Midwives and Health Visitors Act 1979.

Section 2(1) of the Nurses, Midwives and Health Visitors Act 1979 states that '**The principal functions of the Central Council shall be to establish and improve standards of training and professional conduct**'.

Section 2(5) of the same Act moves from the requirement to improve conduct to one of the methods to be employed when it states that '**The powers of the Council shall include that of providing in such manner as it thinks fit, advice for nurses, midwives and health visitors on standards of professional conduct**'.

2 The Code of Professional Conduct for the Nurse, Midwife and Health Visitor is the Council's definitive advice on professional conduct to its practitioners. In this extremely important document practitioners on the UKCC's register find a clear and unequivocal statement as to what their regulatory body expects of them. It therefore also provides the backcloth against which any alleged misconduct on their part will be judged.

The Code of Professional Conduct is considered to be:

a statement to the profession of the primacy of the interests of the patient or client.

a statement of the profession's values.

a portrait of the practitioner which the Council believes to be needed and which the Council wishes to see within the profession.

3 The Council has already published three advisory documents to supplement the Code of Professional Conduct. Practitioners now seek:

(i) elaboration of clauses 10 & 11 of the Code and support for their position when doing as these clauses require. These Clauses state that:

'**Each registered nurse, midwife and health visitor is accountable for his or her practice and, in the exercise of professional accountability, shall:**

10 **Have regard to the environment of care and its physical, psychological and social effects on patients/clients, and also to the adequacy of resources, and make known to appropriate persons or authorities any circumstances which could place patients/clients in jeopardy or which militate against safe standards of practice.**

11 **Have regard to the workload of and the pressures on professional colleagues and subordinates and take appropriate action if these are seen to be such as to constitute abuse of the individual practitioner and/or to jeopardise safe standards of practice**'.

(ii) advice and guidance on issues related to consent and the general subject of truth telling.

(iii) advice and guidance on that part of the practitioner's role which concerns advocacy on behalf of patients and client.

(iv) elaboration of clause 5 of the Code which states that

each registered nurse, midwife and health visitor shall:

5 **'Work in a collaborative and co-operative manner with other health care professionals and recognise and respect their particular contributions within the health care team'.**

(v) advice and guidance on issues related to contentious treatments and conscientious objection.

This document provides a response to those requests, aims to assist professional practitioners to exercise their judgement and reinforces the importance of the Code of Professional Conduct.

B. THE CODE OF PROFESSIONAL CONDUCT AND THE SUBJECT OF ACCOUNTABILITY

1 This new UKCC advisory document has been produced in order to establish more clearly the extent of accountablity of registered nurses, midwives and health visitors and to assist them in the exercise of professional accountability in order to achieve high standards of professional practice.

2 The Code begins with an unequivocal statement: **'Each registered nurse, midwife and health visitor shall act, at all times, in such a manner as to justify public trust and confidence to uphold and enhance the good standing and reputation of the profession, to serve the interests of society, and above all to safeguard the interests of individual patients and clients'.**

This introductory clause indicates that a registered practitioner is accountable for his or her actions as a professional at all times, whether engaged in current practice or not and whether on or off duty.

In situations where the practitioner is employed he or she will be accountable to the employer for providing a service which he or she is employed to provide and for the proper use of the resources made available by the employer for this purpose.

In the circumstances described in the preceding two paragraphs the practitioner has an ultimate accountability to the UKCC for any failure to satisfy the requirements of the introductory paragraph of the Code of Professional Conduct.

The words 'accountable' and 'accountability' each occur only once in the Code, both being found in the stem paragraph out of which the subsequent 14 clauses grow. They do, however, provide its central focus as the Code is built upon the expectation that practitioners will conduct themselves in the manner it describes.

3 Accountablity is an integral part of professional practice, since, in the course of that practice, the practitioner has to make judgements in a wide variety of circumstances and be answerable for those judgements. The Code of Professional Conduct does not seek to state all the circumstances in which the accountability has to be exercised, but to state important principles.

The primacy of the interests of the public and patient or client provide the first theme of the Code and establish the point that, in determining his or her approach to professional practice, the individual nurse, midwife or health visitor should recognise that the interests of public and patient must predominate over those of practitioner and profession. The second major theme is the exercise by each practitioner of personal professional accountablity in such a manner as to respect the primacy of those interests.

4 The Code of Professional Conduct states unequivocally that all practitioners who are registered on the UKCC's register are required to seek to set and achieve high standards and thereby to honour the requirement of **Clause 1 of the Code** which states that each registered nurse, midwife and health visitor shall:

1 **'Act always in such a way as to promote and safeguard the wellbeing and interests of patients and clients'.**

It is recognised that, in many situations in which practitioners practice, there may be a tension between the maintenance of standards and the availability or use of resources. It is essential, however, that the profession, both through its regulatory body (the UKCC) and its individual practitioners, adheres to its desire to enhance standards and to achieve high standards rather than to simply accept minimum standards. Practitioners must seek remedies in those situations where factors in the environment obstruct the achievement of high standards: to start from a compromise position and silently to tolerate poor standards is to act in a manner contrary to the interests of patients or clients, and thus renege on personal professional accountability.

C. CONCERN IN RESPECT OF THE ENVIRONMENT OF CARE

1 The dilemma for practitioners in many settings in respect of the environment of care is very real and has been well documented. If practitioners express concern at the situations which obstruct the achievement of satisfactory standards they risk censure from their employers. On the other hand, failure to make concerns known renders practitioners vulnerable to complaint to their regulatory body (the UKCC) for failing to satisfy its standards and places their registration status in jeopardy.

The sections of the Code of Professional Conduct that are particularly relevant to this issue are the introductory paragraphs and clauses numbered 1,2,3,10 & 11. **These parts of the Code apply to each and every person on the Council's register. Whether engaged in direct care of the patient or client, or further removed but in a position to exert influence over the setting in which that contact exists, the practitioner is subject to the Code and has an accountablity for his or her actions or omissions.**

2   The import of the Sections of the Code referred to is that, having, as part of his or her professional accountability, the responsibility to **'serve the interests of society and above all to safeguard the interests of individual patients and clients'** and to **'act always in such a way as to promote and safeguard the wellbeing and interests of patients/clients'**, the registered nurse, midwife and health visitor must make appropriate representations about the environment of care:

(a) where patients or clients seem likely to be placed in jeopardy and/or standards of practice endangered;

(b) where the staff in such settings are at risk because of the pressure of work and/or inadequacy of resources (which again places patients at risk);

and

(c) where valuable resources are being used inappropriately.

This is an essential part of the communication process that should operate in any facility providing health care, to ensure that those who determine, manage and allocate resources do so with full knowledge of the consequences for the achievement of satisfactory standards. Nurses, midwives and health visitors in management positions should ensure that all relevant information on standards of practice is obtained and communicated with others involved in health policy and management in the interests of standards and safety.

3   Practitioners engaged in direct patient or client care should not be deterred from making representations of their concerns regarding the environment of care simply because they believe that resources are unavailable or that action will not result. The immediate professional manager to whom such information is given, having assessed that information, should ensure that it is communicated to more senior professional managers. This is important in order that, should complaints be made about the practitioners involved in delivering care, the immediate and senior managers will be able to confirm that the perceived inadequacies in the environment of care have been drawn to their attention.

It is clearly wrong for any practitioner to pretend to be coping with the workload, to delude him- or herself into the conviction that things are better than they really are, to aid and abet the abuse and breakdown of a colleague, or to tolerate in silence any matters in his or her work setting that place patients at risk, jeopardise standards of practice, or deny patients privacy and dignity.

In summary, Section C of this document simply restates the UKCC's expectations (set out in the Code of Professional Conduct) that while accepting their responsibilities and doing their best to fulfil them practitioners on its register will ensure that the reality of their clinical environment and practice is made known to and understood by appropriate persons or authorities, doing this as an expression of their personal professional accountability exercised in the public interest. An essential part of this process is the making of contemporaneous and accurate records of the consequences for patients and clients if they have not been given the care they required.

4   **The Code of Professional Conduct applies to all persons on the Council's register irrespective of the post held. Their perspective will vary with their role, but they share the overall responsibilty for care. No practitioner will find support in the Code or from the UKCC for the contention that genuinely held concerns should not be expressed or, if expressed, should attract censure.**

D. CONSENT AND TRUTH

1   It is self-evident that for it to have any meaning consent has to be informed. For the purposes of this document 'informed consent' means that the practitioner involved explains the intended test or procedure to the patient without bias and in as much detail (including detail of possible reactions, complications, side effects and social or personal ramifications) as the patient requires. In the case of an unquestioning patient the practitioner assesses and determines what information the patient needs so that the patient may make an informed decision. The practitioner should impart the information in a sensitive manner, recognising that it might cause distress. The patient must be given time to consider the information before being required to give the consent unless it is an emergency situation.

2   In many instances the practitioner involved in obtaining informed consent would be a registered medical practitioner. In those circumstances it is the medical practitioner who should impart the information and subsequently seek the signed consent. Normally, in

respect of patients in hospital, there are good reasons why the information should be given and the consent sought in the presence of a nurse, midwife or health visitor. Where the procedure or test is to be performed by a nurse, midwife or health visitor the standards described in the preceding paragraph apply to the consent sought.

3 If the nurse, midwife or health visitor does not feel that sufficient information has been given in terms readily understandable to the patient so as to enable her or him to make a truly informed decision, it is for him or her to state this opinion and seek to have the situation remedied. The practitioner might decide not to co-operate with a procedure if convinced that the decision to agree to it being performed was not truly informed. Discussion of such matters between the health professionals concerned should not take place in the presence of patients.

In certain situations and with certain client groups the practitioner's level of responsibility in this respect is greatly increased where he or she stands in 'loco parentis' for a patient or client.

4 There are occasions on which, although the patient has been given information by the medical practitioner about an intended procedure for which she or he has given consent, her or his subsequent statements and questions to a nurse, midwife or health visitor indicate a failure to understand what is to be done, its risks and its ramifications. Where this proves to be the case it is necessary for that practitioner, in the patient's interest, to recall the relevant medical practitioner so that the deficiences can be remedied without delay.

The purpose of this approach is to ensure that all professional practitioners involved in the patient's care respect the primacy of that patient's interests, honour their personal professional accountability and avoid the risk of complaint or charges of assault. The practitioner who properly fulfils his or her responsibilities in this respect should be recognised by medical colleagues as a source of support and information to improve the overall care of the patient.

5 The concept of informed consent and that of truth telling are closely related. If it is to be believed that, on occasions, practitioners withhold information from their patients the damage to public trust and confidence in the profession, on which the introduction to the Code of Professional Conduct places great emphasis, will be enormous.

6 This is yet another area in which judgements have to be made and introduces another facet of the exercise of accountability. If it is accepted that the patient has a

right to information about her or his condition it follows that the professional practitioners involved in her or his care have a duty to provide such information. Recognition of the patient's condition and the likely effect of the information might lead the professionals to be selective about 'what' and 'when' but the responsibility is on them to provide information. There may be occasions on which, after consultaton with the relatives of a patient by the health professionals involved in that patient's care, some information is temporarily withheld. If, however, something less than the whole truth is told at a particular point in time it should never be because the practitioner is unable to cope with the effects of telling the whole truth. Such controlled release of information (i.e. less than the whole truth) should only ever be in the interests of the patient, and the practitioner should be able to justify the action taken.

7 It is recognised that this is an area in which there is the potential for conflict between professionals involved in the care of the same patient or client. The existence of good, trusting relationships between professionals concerned will promote the development of agreed approaches to truth telling. This subject should be discussed between all the professional practitioners involved so that the rights of patients are not affected adversely. This should minimise the number of occasions on which, after a patient or client has been given incomplete information, a nurse, midwife or health visitor is faced with a request for the whole truth. Accountability can never be exercised by ignoring the rights and interests of the patient or client.

E. ADVOCACY ON BEHALF OF PATIENTS AND CLIENTS

1 The introductory paragraphs of the Code of Professional Conduct, together with several of its clauses, indicate clearly the expectation that the practitioner will accept a role as an advocate on behalf of his or her patients/clients. Opinions vary as to what exactly that means. Some tend to want to identify advocacy as a separate and distinct subject. It is not. It is a component of many professional activities of this and other professions. Some of these professional activities are the subject of other sections of this document.

2 **Advocacy is concerned with promoting and safeguarding the wellbeing and interests of patients and clients. It is not concerned with conflict for its own sake.** It is important that this fact is recognised, since some practitioners seem to regard advocacy on behalf of patients or clients as an adversarial activity and feel either attracted to it or not able to accept it for that reason. Dictionaries define an advocate as 'one who

pleads the cause of another' or 'one who recommends or urges something' and indicates that advocacy is a positive, constructive activity.

3   There are occasions on which the practitioner's advocacy role has to be exercised to 'plead the cause of another' where, in the case of any person incapable of making informed decisions, the parents or relatives withhold consent for treatment which the various practitioners involved believe to be in the best interests of the patient. The parents or relatives, from their knowledge of the patient, will also have an opinion as to what constitutes her or his best interests. There have been a limited number of cases in which the courts have taken the view that the parents or relatives have not decided in the patient's best interests. Taking the right of decision away from the parents or relatives should only occur in the rarest of cases. The practitioner's advocacy role in situations of this kind requires knowledge of the patient's condition and prognosis, sensitivity to the feelings of the parents or relatives and considerable empathy.

4   **To fulfil the Council's expectations set out in the Code is, therefore, to be the advocate for the patient or client in this sense. Each practitioner must determine exactly how this aspect of personal professional accountability is satisfied within her particular sphere of practice. This requires the exercise of judgement as to the 'when' and 'how'. The practitioner must be sure that it is in the interests of the patient or client that are being promoted rather than the patient or client being used as a vehicle for the promotion of personal or sectional professional interests. The Code of Professional Conduct envisages the role of patient or client advocate as an integral and essential aspect of good professional practice.**

5   Just as the practice of nursing involves the practitioner in assisting patients with those physical activities which they would do for themelves were they able, so too the exercise of professional accountability involves the practitioner in assisting patients by making such representations on their behalf as they would make themselves if they were able.

F. COLLABORATION AND CO-OPERATION IN CARE

1   Clause 5 of the Code of Professional Conduct requires that **'Each registered nurse, midwife and health visitor, in the exercise of professional accountability shall work in a collaborative and co-operative manner with other health care professionals and recognise and respect their particular contributions within the health care team'.** This clause deliberately emphasises the importance of collaboration and co-operation and, by implication, the importance of the avoidance of dispute and the promotion of good relationships and a spirit of co-operation and mutual respect within the team.

2   It does so because it is clearly impossible for any one profession or agency to possess all the knowledge, skill and resources to be employed in meeting the total health care needs of society. The delivery of full and appropriate care to patients/clients frequently necessitates the participation of professional practitioners from more than one profession, their efforts often being supplemented by other agencies and persons.

The UKCC recognises the complexity of medical and health care and stresses the need to appreciate the complementary contribution of the professions and others involved.

The delivery of care is therefore often a multi-profession and multi-agency activity which, in order to be effective, must be based on mutual understanding, trust, respect and co-operation.

3   It is self-evident that collaborative and co-operative working is essential if patients and clients are to be provided with the care they need and if it is to be of the quality required. It is worthy of note that this concept of teamwork is evident in many situations in which the care of patients and clients is a shared responsibility.

Unfortunately there are exceptions. Experience has demonstrated that such co-operation and collaboration is not always easily achieved if:

(a) individual members of the team have their own specific and separate objectives;
   or
(b) one member of the team seeks to adopt a dominant role to the exclusion of the opinions, knowledge and skill of its other members.

In such circumstances it is important to stress that the interests of the patient or client must remain paramount.

4   The UKCC and the General Medical Council agree that there is a range of issues which calls for co-operation between the professions at both national and local level and wish to encourage this co-operation.

5   In spite of acceptance of the importance of co-operation and collaboration, differences can sometimes occur within the team regarding appropriate care and treatment. Such conflict can become an influence for good if it results in full discussion between members of

the team. It may prove harmful to the care and treatment of patients or clients unless resolved in a manner which recognises the special contribution of each professional group, agency and individual and ensures that the interests and needs of the patient or client remain paramount.

6   Collaboration and co-operation between health care professionals is also necessary in both research and planning related to the provision or improvement of services. This may sometimes give rise to concern where one professional group is requested to pass information (obtained by its members in the course of professional practice) to a member of another professional group to use for a purpose other than that for which it was obtained and recorded. That level of concern will inevitably rise unless it can be seen that the purpose for which the information is required is valid, the information is made available only to persons bound by the same standards of confidentiality and the means of storage of that information is secure.

This should not present a problem where consent can be obtained from the patients or clients to whom the information relates or from relatives who have been provided with the relevant information. In certain fields, such as care of the elderly and persons with mental illness and mental handicap, the information gathering and research geared to the provision of services for these client groups may need to proceed without specific consent. This should only occur where the individuals receiving care are unable to give informed consent and where there is no close contact with relatives. Those who proceed without consent in these particular circumstances must be satisfied that their activities will not affect the current provision of care adversely and that the activity is directed to the provision of appropriate or improved services for future recipients of care.

It is anticipated that disputes will be avoided by relevant inter-professional discussions in advance of submissions of the projects for approval by the appropriate ethical committees. Where a dispute does arise it should be resolved between colleagues and the ethical committee.

Clause 9 of the Code of Professional Conduct and the UKCC's Advisory Paper on *Confidentiality* provide further sources of reference for nurses, midwives and health visitors in respect of this aspect of practice.

G. OBJECTION TO PARTICIPATION IN CARE AND TREATMENT
1   **Clause 7 of the Code of Professional Conduct states:**

'**Make known to an appropriate person or authority any conscientious objection which may be relevant to professional practice.'**

2   The law does not provide a general opportunity for practitioners to register a conscientious objection to participation in care and treatment. That right applies in respect of termination of pregnancy only (not the care of the patient thereafter) under the terms of Section 4 of the Abortion Act 1967.

3   Some practitioners choose not to participate in certain other forms of treatment on the grounds of conscience. Since the law provides no basic right to such a refusal it is imperative that any practitioner should be careful not to accept employment in a post where it is known that a form of treatment to which he or she has a conscientious objection is regularly used. In circumstances where a practitioner finds that a form of treatment to which he or she objects, but which is not usually employed, is to be used he or she must declare that objection with sufficient time for his or her managers to make alternative staffing arrangements and must not refuse to participate in emergency treatment.

Some practitioners may object to participation in certain forms of treatment, such as resuscitative treatment of the elderly, the transfusion of blood, or electroconvulsive therapy. These practitioners must respect clause 7 of the Code and make their position clear to their professional colleagues and managers, and recognise that this may have implications for their contract of employment.

4   Objection to participation in treatment does not only occur as a product of conscience. It is the Council's stated position that, on each and every occasion a prescribed mediation is being administered, the practitioner should ensure that, in his or her view, the patient is not presenting symptoms that contra-indicate its administration. The practitioner who is concerned about the administration of a particular drug in these circumstances might reasonably ask the prescribing doctor to attend the patient and if the prescriber still requires it to be given, to request him or her to administer the medication if not fully reassured. The practitioner involved in such an incident should make a detailed record of the reasons why he or she felt concern and, if so, why, he or she declined to administer prescribed medication.

5   The principle that applies in the previous paragraph can also be applied in appropriate circumstances to substances that are prescribed for topical use including wound dressing. Where the practitioner attending the patient believes (from knowledge, published research evidence or from previous experience) that the pre-

scribed substance may be harmful, or even more so where it is evident that it is actively harmful, he or she should make a record of the condition of the wound or site (where appropriate including a photographic record) and ask the prescribing medical practitioner to attend.

If the prescription stands after medical examination the practitioner, having chosen either to respond to the prescription or not, should make a detailed record of the reasons for his or her expressed concern and subsequent actions.

It is believed that the spirit of co-operation and mutual respect referred to at paragraph F 1 of this document should make such situations exceptional

6   Objections to participation in treatment are not always associated with the nature or form of treatment or its appropriateness in a particular set of circumstances. Some practitioners indicate their wish or active intention to refuse to participate in the delivery of care to patients with certain conditions. Such refusal may be associated particularly with patients suffering from Hepatitis B Infection and those with Acquired Immune Deficiency Syndrome, AIDs Related Complex or who are HIV sero-positive but asymptomatic.

Those who seek the UKCC's support for such actual or intended refusal are informed that the Code of Professional Conduct does not provide a formula for being selective about the categories of patient or client for whom the practitioner will care. To seek to be so selective is to demonstrate unacceptable conduct. The UKCC expects its practitioners to adopt a non-judgemental approach in the exercise of their caring role.

H. SUMMARY OF THE PRINCIPLES AGAINST WHICH TO EXERCISE ACCOUNTABILITY

1   **The interests of the patient or client are paramount.**

2   **Professional accountability must be exercised in such a manner as to ensure that the primacy of the interests of patient or clients is respected and must not be overridden by those of the professions or their practitioners.**

3   **The exercise of accountability requires the practitioner to seek to achieve and maintain high standards.**

4   **Advocacy on behalf of patients or clients is an essential feature of the exercise of accountability by a professional practitioner.**

5   **The role of other persons in the delivery of health care to patients or clients must be recognised and respected, provided that the first principle above is honoured.**

6   **Public trust and confidence in the profession is dependent on its practitioners being seen to exercise their accountability responsibly.**

7   **Each registered nurse, midwife or health visitor must be able to justify any action or decision not to act taken in the course of his or her professional practice.**

D

Confidentiality

A UKCC Advisory Paper. An elaboration of Clause 9 of the Code of Professional Conduct. A framework to assist individual professional judgement.

A. INTRODUCTION

1 *The Code of Professional Conduct for the Nurse, Midwife and Health Visitor* **(Second Edition) published by the United Kingdom Central Council for Nursing, Midwifery and Health Visiting is:**

a statement to the profession of the primacy of the interests of the patient or client;

one of the principal means by which the Council is seeking to comply with Section 2(5) of the Nurses, Midwives and Health Visitors Act 1979 and give advice to its practitioners on standards of professional conduct;

a portrait of the practitioner the Council believes to be needed and wishes to see within the profession.

2 In approving the terms of this edition of the **Code** the Council authorised the publication of key statements on a number of important professional issues.

3 One of these key statements (Clause 9) concerns 'Confidentiality'. It reads:

"Each registered nurse, midwife and health visitor is accountable for his or her practice, and, in the exercise of professional accountability shall:

Respect confidential information obtained in the course of professional practice and refrain from disclosing such information without the consent of the patient/client, or a person entitled to act on his/her behalf, except where disclosure is required by law or by the order of a court or is necessary in the public interest."

4 It can be seen from the general description of the Code of Professional Conduct and the particular contents of Clause 9 that **breaches of confidentiality should be regarded as exceptional,** only occurring after careful consideration and the exercise of personal professional judgement.

5 Any codified statements of this nature need continuous exploration, and on occasions a more detailed and authoritative elaboration. It is for the whole profession to recognise its responsibility to share in such exploration, to use the respective knowledge and skill of practitioners to facilitate it and to recognise the important contribution the professional press makes to this essential debate. The subject of confidentiality has emerged as one on which the profession's practitioners need the relevant clause in the Code of Professional Conduct to be developed more fully by the UKCC. It must be said, however, that **no exploration or elaboration by others alters the fact that the ultimate decision is that of the individual practitioner in the situation.**

The demand for elaboration of Clause 9 of the Code has focused particularly on **determining the difficult boundary that applies in any case between the expectations of patients/clients that information, whether recorded or not, obtained in the course of professional practice will not be disclosed, and the expectations of the public that they will not be put at risk because practitioners unreasonably withhold information.**

It is not the purpose of this document to seek to provide answers to the many dilemmas which practitioners face. It is necessary, however, to provide examples of them since they have been a backcloth against which the discussions culminating in the publication of this document have taken place.

Correspondence on this point has come (for example) from:

a sister in a psychiatric day hospital who found a patient possessed of large quantities of controlled drugs that he cannot have obtained legally;

a medical practitioner concerned that a community midwife reported to her employers the fact that while visiting the wife of a hospital employee in a professional capacity she saw substantial quantities of stolen hospital property;

a health visitor who has been told by one child that another child is being sexually abused;

Accident and Emergency Department nursing staff who found that the unconscious patient they were treating had a gun on his person;

nurses working in the community who have been instructed by their managers (following approval by an ethical committee) to give researchers direct access to confidential information in respect of patients, but who knew that the consent of those patients had not been sought;

psychiatric nurses who fear that information revealed by a patient in a therapeutic group may be passed on by other patients and that the nurses will be held responsible;

occupational health nurses faced with requests from their managers for information about employees;

community psychiatric nurses who were reluctant to comply with the instruction to put full names and addresses of patients visited on their travel expense claims;

a health visitor who had become aware that information she shared with a social worker in a case conference had been given in evidence in a Magistrates' Court;

practitioners who have chosen not to make a record of information given to them by patients in confidence, and who have later been worried about the propriety of their decision;
and

a health authority chairman who asks 'Who is to define the public interest?' and 'How is the nurse to recognise the authenticity of the claim of public interest?'

The Council has been left in no doubt that it has a responsibility to address this important subject in greater depth.

As already stated, the **UKCC is not seeking to provide responses to those dilemmas since a judgement must be made by the individual practitioner concerned. It is instead seeking to provide guidance on disclosure of information:**

(a) to assist development of understanding about the nature and scope of the dilemma which practitioners face, and to encourage those who employ nurses, midwives and health visitors to recognise the difficult and stressful situations encountered by practitioners and to offer support and guidance, stimulate discussion and develop and publicise policies on this important matter;

(b) to state certain principles which it is hoped will assist practitioners to consider situations which they encounter and to make sound professional judgements;

(c) to emphasise that the responsibility of whether or not information should be withheld or disclosed without the consent of the patient/client lies with the practitioner involved at the appropriate time and cannot be delegated;

(d) to stress that those who employ or supervise nurses, midwives and health visitors have an obligation to support these practitioners in discharging their responsibilities in respect of the right to disclose or withhold information using their professional judgement;

(e) to indicate the conditions which should be met before disclosure of information, so that the decision to either disclose or withhold information can be justified.

B. DEFINING TERMS

1   What do we mean when we speak of something being 'Confidential'? Turn to almost any dictionary and you find that the focal word in the definitions of 'confide' 'confidence' or 'confidential' is **'TRUST'**. To trust another person with private and personal information about yourself is a significant matter. **Where the person to whom that information is given is a nurse, midwife or health visitor the patient/client has a right to believe that this information, given in confidence in the expectation that it will be used only for the purposes for which it was given, will not be released to others without the consent of the patient/client.** The death of a patient/client does not absolve the practitioner from this obligation.

2   Clearly it is impractical to obtain the consent of the patient/client every time that health care information needs to be shared with other health professionals, or other staff involved in the health care of that patient/client. Consent in these instances can be implied provided that it is known and understood by the patients/clients that such information needs to be made available to others involved in the delivery of his/her care. Patients/clients have a right to know the standards of confidentiality maintained by those providing their care, and these standards should be made known by the health professional at the first point of contact. These standards of confidentiality can be reinforced by the additional use of leaflets and posters where the health care is being delivered.

3   When an individual practitioner considers that it is necessary to obtain the explicit consent of a patient/client before disclosing specific information, it is the responsibility of the practitioner to ensure that the patient/client can make as informed a response as possible as to whether that information can be disclosed or withheld.

4   It is essential that nurses, midwives and health visitors recognise the fundamental right of their patients or clients to information about them being kept private and secure. This point is sharply reinforced by only brief consideration of the personal, social or legal repercussions which might follow unauthorised disclosure of information concerning a person's health or illness.

5   **Disclosure of information occurs in the following ways:**
(a) with the consent of the patient/client;
(b) without the consent of the patient/client when the disclosure is required by law or order of a court;
(c) by accident;
(d) without the consent of the patient/client when the disclosure is considered necessary in the public interest.
   It is the latter two categories that this Advisory Paper is particularly addressing, for a breach of confidentiality occurs if anyone deliberately or by accident gives information, which has been obtained in the course of professional practice, to a third party without the consent of the patient/client.

6   The public interest, in the context of this Advisory Paper, is taken to mean the interests of an individual, of groups of individuals or society as a whole, and would (for example) encompass matters such as serious crime, child abuse and drug trafficking.

C. OWNERSHIP AND CARE OF CONFIDENTIAL INFORMATION

1   The organisations which employ professional practitioner staff who make records (whether in the National Health Service or in other spheres of practice) are the legal owner of such records, but such ownership does not give them any legal right of access to the information contained in those records. The patient also is involved in the ownership. The ownership of a record is therefore irrelevant to the patient's right of confidentiality and his/her expectation that identifiable personal health information will not be disclosed without consent.

2   In many situations genuine difficulties can be experienced in preventing the leakage of confidential information or its inadvertent spread into management layers leading to possible misuse. There is need for particular caution where a system of shared records is employed, it being incumbent on the author of any particular entry to satisfy himself or herself that other people with access to that shared record will respect the confidentiality of the information and will place neither the patient/client nor the author of the entry at risk by its release without consent.

3   The task with which individual professional practitioners are faced is not limited to that of exercising a judgement as to what information can be or should be disclosed. It also includes that of ensuring or helping to ensure that record keeping systems are not such as to make the release of information possible or likely. Neither technology nor management convenience should be allowed to determine principles. Each practitioner has a responsibility to recognise that risks exist, and to satisfy himself or herself in respect of the system for storage and movement of records operated in the health care setting in which he or she works and to ensure that it is secure. The concern for the environment of care for which each practitioner is held accountable under the terms of clause 10 of the Code of Professional Conduct for the Nurse, Midwife and Health Visitor extends to include this.

4   The practitioner should act so as to ensure that he/she does not become a channel through which confidential information obtained in the course of professional practice is inadvertently released. The dangerous consequences of careless talk in public places cannot be overstated.

5   Where access to the records of patients or clients is necessary so that students may be assisted to achieve the necessary knowledge and competence it must be recognised that the same principles of confidentiality stated earlier in this document extend to them and their

teachers. The same applies to those engaged in research. It is incumbent on the practitioner(s) responsible for the security of the information contained in these records to ensure that access to it is closely supervised, and occurs within the context of the teacher and student undertaking to respect its confidentiality, and in knowledge of the fact that the teacher has accepted responsibility to ensure that students understand the requirement for confidentiality and the need to observe local policies for the handling and storage of records. It is expected that the student or teacher who is active in giving care as a practitioner will apprise the patient of their role, thus enabling the patient who is so capable to control the information flow. Where deemed necessary the recipient of confidential information from a patient/client will advise him/her that the information will be conveyed to the nurse, midwife or health visitor involved in his/her care on a continuing basis.

6   It is advisable that the contracts of employment of all employees not directly involved with patients/clients but who have access to or handle confidential records contain clauses which emphasise the principles of confidentiality and state the disciplinary consequences of breaching them. Paragraph 3.20 of the Report from the Confidentiality Working Group of the DHSS Steering Group on Health Services Information suggests a form of words worthy of consideration as follows:

"In the course of your duties you may have access to confidential material about patients, members of staff or other health service business. On no account must information relating to identifiable patients be divulged to anyone other than authorised persons, for example medical, nursing or other professional staff, as appropriate, who are concerned directly with the care, diagnosis and/or treatment of the patient. If you are in any doubt whatsoever as to the authority of a person or body asking for information of this nature you must seek advice from your superior officer. Similarly, no information of a personal or confidential nature concerning individual members of staff should be divulged to anyone without the proper authority having first been given. Failure to observe these rules will be regarded by your employers as serious misconduct which could result in serious disciplinary action being taken against you, including dismissal."

The circumstances in which a nurse, midwife or health visitor chooses to disclose or withhold confidential information are explored in Section D.

D. DELIBERATE BREACH OF CONFIDENTIALITY IN THE PUBLIC INTEREST OR THAT OF THE INDIVIDUAL PATIENT/CLIENT

1   The examples given in paragraph A5 remind us that we live in a real world, and that sometimes there are a range of interests to consider.

Pressure is often exerted on practitioners to breach the principle of keeping confidential and maintaining the security of information elicited from patients/clients in the privileged circumstances of a professional relationship. This should not be regarded as surprising, since **'Confidentiality' is a rule with certain exceptions. There is no statutory right of confidentiality; but there is also no bar to an aggrieved individual bringing a common law case before a civil court alleging breach of confidentiality and seeking financial recompense.**

It is essential that before determining that a particular set of circumstances constitute such an exception, the practitioner must be satisfied that the best interests of the patient/client are served thereby or the wider public interest necessitates disclosure.

2   The needs of the community can, on occasions, take precedence over the individual's rights as for example in those situations where a Court rules that the administration of justice demands that a professional confidence be broken or the law requires that patient confidence be breached.

3   In many other situations sharing of confidential information occurs by intention. This is the case where information obtained in the course of professional practice is shared with other professionals in the health and social work fields in the belief that to do so is in the interests of the patient/client. Legislation concerned with data protection and its associated codes is not intended to prevent the exchange of information between professional staff who share the care of the patient/client. It is, however, the duty of the practitioner who obtains and holds the information to ensure, as far as is reasonable, before its release that it is being imparted in strict professional confidence and for a specific purpose. The same duty applies where the practitioner is contributing to a shared record. Wherever possible the consent of the patient/client to the sharing of information should first be obtained.

4   The situations that are the most exceptional and problematic for the practitioner are those where the deliberate decision to withhold confidential information or disclose it to a third party can have very serious consequences. The information can have been given to

the practitioner in the strictest confidence or the practitioner may have obtained the information inadvertently in the course of his or her professional practice. The decision as to whether to make a record of such information, like the decisions as to whether or not to disclose, poses many dilemmas, for the situations are invariably complex. In some instances the practitioner can be under pressure to divulge information but it must be emphasised that the responsibility lies with him or her as an individual. This responsibility cannot be delegated.

5   In all cases where the practitioner deliberately discloses or withholds information in what he/she believes the public interest he/she must be able to justify the decision. These situations can be particularly stressful, especially where vulnerable groups are concerned, as disclosure may mean the involvement of a third party as in the case of children or the mentally handicapped. **Practitioners should always take the opportunity to discuss the matter fully with other practitioners** (not only or necessarily fellow nurses, midwives and health visitors), and if appropriate consult with a professional organisation before making a decision. There will often be ramifications and these are best explored before a final decision as to whether to withhold or disclose information is made.

Once having made a decision the practitioner should write down the reasons either in the appropriate record or in a special note that can be kept on file. The practitioner can then justify the action taken should that subsequently become necessary, and can also at a later date review the decision in the light of future developments.

E. SUMMARY OF THE PRINCIPLES ON WHICH TO BASE PROFESSIONAL JUDGEMENT IN MATTERS OF CONFIDENTIALITY

1   That a patient/client has a right to expect that information given in confidence will be used only for the purpose for which it was given and will not be released to others without their consent.

2   That practitioners recognise the fundamental right of their patients/clients to have information about them held in secure and private storage.

3   That, where it is deemed appropriate to share information obtained in the course of professional practice with other health or social work practitioners, the practitioner who obtained the information must ensure, as far as is reasonable, before its release that it is being imparted in strict professional confidence and for a specific purpose.

4   That the responsibility to either disclose or withhold confidential information in the public interest lies with the individual practitioner, that he/she cannot delegate the decision, and that he/she cannot be required by a superior to disclose or withhold information against his/her will.

5   That a practitioner who chooses to breach the basic principle of confidentiality in the belief that it is necessary in the public interest must have considered the matter sufficiently to justify that decision.

6   That deliberate breaches of confidentiality other than with the consent of the patient/client should be exceptional.

E

Administration of Medicines

A UKCC Advisory Paper. A framework to assist individual professional judgement and the development of local policies and guidelines.

INTRODUCTION

1   **The framework which is set out in this document should be considered against the background of the extracts from Statutory Instrument 1983 No. 873 (The Nurses, Midwives and Health Visitor Rules) and the UKCC Code of Professional Conduct for the Nurse, Midwife and Health Visitor which are reproduced for convenience, and of the definitions given for the terms 'professional judgement' and, 'professional responsibility'.**

2   It is intended for practitioners of nursing, midwifery and health visiting wherever they are practising. The main body of the text relates to 'normal' circumstances. Guidelines in respect of exceptional circumstances are set out in an Appendix to the main document.

3   **The relevant primary legislation concerning the administration of medicines is the Medicines Act, 1968, and the Misuse of Drugs Act, 1971.**

4   The term 'medicine' refers to controlled drugs and 'prescription only' medicines as defined in those Acts. It includes 'General Sales List' medicines in those settings where they are normally subject to prescription.

5   **Wherever in this paper the word 'practitioner' is used it refers to a practitioner of nursing, midwifery or health visiting.**

6   This advisory document is released following helpful consultation with the General Medical Council and the Pharmaceutical Society.

BACKGROUND

1   **Rule 18 of Statutory Instrument 1983 No. 873 states:**

Courses leading to a qualification the successful completion of which shall enable an application to be made for admission to Part 1, 3, 5 or 8 of the register shall provide opportunities to enable the student to accept responsibility for his/her personal professional development and to acquire the competencies required to:

(a) advise on the promotion of health and the prevention of illness;

(b) recognise situations that may be detrimental to the health and well-being of the individual;

(c) carry out those activities involved when conducting the comprehensive assessment of a person's nursing requirements;

(d) recognise the significance of the observations made and use these to develop an initial nursing assessment;

(e) devise a plan of nursing care based on the assessment with the co-operation of the patient, to the extent that this is possible, taking into account the medical prescription;

(f) implement the planned programme of nursing care and where appropriate teach and co-ordinate other members of the caring team who may be responsible for implementing specific aspects of the nursing care;

(g) review the effectiveness of the nursing care provided, and where appropriate, initiate any action that may be required;

(h) work in a team with other nurses, and with medical and para-medical staff and social workers;

(i) undertake the management of the care of a group of patients over a period of time and organise the appropriate support services;

related to the care of the particular type of patient with whom he/she is likely to come in contact when registered in that Part of the register for which the student intends to qualify.

Courses leading to a qualification the successful completion of which shall enable an application to be made for admission to Part 2, 4 6 or 7 of the register shall be designed to prepare the student to undertake nursing care under the direction of a person registered in Part 1, 3, 5 or 8 of the register and provide opportunities for the student to develop the competencies required to:

(a) assist in carrying out comprehensive observation of the patient and help in assessing his/her care requirements;

(b) develop skills to enable him/her to assist in the implementation of nursing care under the direction of a person registered in Part 1, 3, 5 or 8 of the register;

(c) accept delegated nursing tasks;

(d) assist in reviewing the effectiveness of the care provided;

(e) work in a team with other nurses, and with medical and para-medical staff and social workers;

related to the care of the particular type of patient with whom he/she is likely to come into contact when registered in that Part of the register for which the student intends to qualify.

The different but quite specifically stated competencies in Rule 18(1) for the nurses whose names appear in the first level parts of the register (i.e. Registered General Nurse, Registered Mental Nurse, Registered Nurse of the Mentally Handicapped, Registered Sick Children's Nurse), and in Rule 18(2) for the nurses whose names appear in the second level parts of the register (i.e. Enrolled Nurse, General; Enrolled Nurse, Mental; Enrolled Nurse, Mental Handicap; Enrolled Nurse) should be noted.

3 In relation to the administration of medicines, the midwife has the same responsibility as the first level nurse.

4 The UKCC Code of Professional Conduct for the Nurse, Midwife and Health Visitor contains the following important statements:

Each registered nurse, midwife and health visitor shall act, at all times, in such a manner as to justify public trust and confidence, to uphold and enhance the good standing and reputation of the profession, to serve the interests of society, and above all to safeguard the interests of individual patients and clients.

Each registered nurse, midwife and health visitor is accountable for his or her practice, and, in the exercise of professional accountability shall:

(i) act always in such a way as to promote and safeguard the well being and interests of patients/clients;

(ii) ensure that no action or omission on his/her part

or within his/her sphere of influence is detrimental to the condition or safety of patients/clients;

(iii) take every reasonable opportunity to maintain and improve professional knowledge and competence;

(iv) acknowledge any limitations of competence and refuse in such cases to accept delegated functions without first having received instruction in regard to those functions and having been assessed as competent;

5 For the purpose of this advisory paper the following definitions are drawn to your attention:

(i) **Professional Judgement in health care is personal judgement based on special knowledge and skill, and always and above all is exercised in the best interests of the patient/client.**

(ii) **Professional Responsibility in health care is personal responsibility based on special knowledge and skill for actions, attitudes and policies always and above all directed to the best interests of the patient/client.**

THE FRAMEWORK

1 *Treatment with medicines*

The treatment of a patient with medicines for therapeutic, diagnostic or preventative purposes is a process which involves prescribing, dispensing, administering and receiving.

The word 'patient' is used since any person receiving a prescribed medicine is the patient of that prescriber at the time of prescription.

2 *Prescribing (the doctor's role)*

(a) This involves obtaining a patient's consent (commonly this is implicit) based on an understanding of the treatment, and issuing a prescription written legibly, indelibly and dated. The prescription must ensure accurate patient identification, specify the preparation to be given and where appropriate its form (e.g. tablets, capsules, suppositories) and strength, the dose, the timing and frequency of administration and the route of administration. In the case of patients for whom a prescription is provided in the Out-Patient or Community setting, the number of dose units or total course must be stated.

(b) In the case of controlled drugs, the dose must be written in words and figures and in the Out-Patient or Community setting the total dose or number of dose units in both words and figures to be supplied, the whole being in the prescriber's own handwriting.

(c) Prescriptions must be signed and dated by the prescribing doctor.

(d) There are certain situations (e.g. in Registered Nursing Homes) where a medicine will have to be administered against a prescription which is no longer available. Unless the prescription was very specific the container will probably bear the instruction to administer 'as directed' only. In such circumstances the prescribing doctor should produce a written order against which medicines can be checked.

(e) Any practitioner faced with a prescription not satisfying the above criteria should withhold administration and request the doctor concerned to write a full and correct prescription. (See paragraph 4(c)).

(f) The administration of medicines on verbal instruction except in emergencies does not satisfy acceptable criteria.

(g) Instruction by telephone to a nurse to administer, even in an emergency situation, a hitherto unprescribed drug cannot be supported. This practice is unreliable and involves a nurse in a procedure which is potentially hazardous to the patient. This paragraph must, however, be read in the context of the supplementary advice set out in the appendix to this document on pages 320 and 321.

(h) Where it is the wish of the doctors that nursing staff be authorized to administer certain medicines such as mild analgesics, laxatives and topical applications a local protocol which satisfies the general criteria of the appendix to this paper should be agreed between the medical, nursing and pharmaceutical professionals involved.

(i) The exemptions for midwives and occupational health nurses under the terms of the Medicines Act 1968 and the Misuse of Drugs Act 1971 and subsequent regulations are referred to in paragraph 4(i) on page 319.

3   Dispensing (the pharmacist's role)

(a) This involves checking that the prescription is written correctly to avoid misunderstanding or error, appropriate in the circumstances, and that any newly prescribed medicine will not dangerously interact with or nullify the effect of any previously prescribed medicines or food.

(b) In addition the pharmacist is involved in determining quality, advising on security and storage conditions, compounding the medicine in a form suitable for administration to the relevant patient, providing relevant additional information on container labels and annotating the prescription to render it accurate.

(c) Still further the pharmacist is involved in monitoring the adverse side effects of medicines, and should therefore be sent any information which the administering practitioner deems relevant.

(d) **It should be noted that amendments to a prescription which are made and signed by the pharmacist after consultation with the prescribing doctor are acceptable.**

(e) When the pharmacist is satisfied on all appropriate points, his/her role further involves clear labelling, insertion into an appropriate container and secure delivery.

4   Administering (the role of the nurse, midwife and health visitor)

(a) **The exercise of professional judgement (which involves the application of his/her knowledge and experience to the situation faced) will lead the practitioner to satisfy himself/herself that he/she is competent to administer the medicine and prepared to be accountable for that action. Once that decision has been made, the practitioner follows a sequence of steps to ensure the safety and well being of the patient, and which must as a prerequisite be based on a sound knowledge of the patient's assessment and the environment in which care is given.**

(b) **Correctness**

This involves interpretation of the prescription and container information in terms of what has been prescribed. Illegibility and lack of clarity of the instruction must be questioned. It also involves ensuring that the medicine is to be administered to the patient for whom it has been prescribed, and in the form and by the method prescribed.

Certain of these points do not usually apply in the context of a patient's home where the patient is receiving medicines from a personalised container. The visiting practitioner does, however, have a responsibility to assist the patient's understanding and help ensure safe administration.

Where a patient is in possession of a range of medicines in containers which are not labelled with precise instructions, and the danger of over or under administration exists, it may be necessary for the practitioner to advise the prescribing doctor so that he/she may consider whether any action is required.

(c) **Appropriateness and the possible need to withhold**

This involves checking the expiry date of the medicine, careful consideration of the dosage and the method, route and timing of administration in the context of the condition of each specific patient. It may be necessary or deemed advisable at the time

when a medicine is due to be administered to withhold it in order to seek further verification from the
prescribing doctor, or confirmation from the responsible senior nurse that it should be given. Where, in
the opinion of the administering nurse or responsible senior nurse (i.e. the nurse on duty to whom the
administering nurse is in line responsibility at the
time), contra-indications to the administration of
the medicine are observed the prescribing doctor
should be contacted without delay. (In respect of
this point and that at (b) above the advice of the
relevant pharmacist will often be helpful in those
situations where the prescribing doctor or an appropriate alternative doctor cannot be contacted.)

(d) **Reinforcement**
The positive effect of treatment may need to be
reinforced by the nurse. Every occasion on which a
medicine is administered is an opportunity for such
reinforcement and for reassurance. In the community particularly it is also an opportunity to help
ensure avoidance of misuse of self-medication, and
the misuse of the prescribed drugs by others who
reside in or are visiting the household.

(e) **Recording/Reporting**
As part of the ongoing process (not solely at the
times of administration of medicines) the effects and
side-effects of the treatment should be noted. Taking
appropriate action in relation to side-effects is essential. Positive and negative effects should be reported
to the appropriate doctor and recorded.

(f) **Record of administration**
Where a practitioner is involved in the administration of medicines thorough and accurate records of
the administration must be maintained. In hospital
settings this will normally be achieved by initialling
the appropriate box on a treatment record at the
time of administration. Otherwise the date and time
of administration, together with the administering
practitioner's signature are essential minimum requirements, and all must be legibly written. If (as a
result of consideration as in 'c' above) a medicine is
not administered a record to that effect should be
made.

(g) The UKCC is of the view that practitioners
whose names are on the first level parts of the
register, and midwives, should be seen as competent to administer medicines on their own,
and responsible for their actions in so doing.
The involvement of a second person in the
administration of medicines with a first level
practitioner need only occur where that practitioner is instructing a learner or the patient's
condition makes it necessary or in such other
circumstances as are locally determined. Where

two persons are involved responsibility still
attaches to the senior person.

(h) The UKCC is totally opposed to the involvement of personnel who are not professionally
registered such as nursing auxiliaries or assistants in the administration of medicines since it
gives a false sense of security, undermines true
responsibility, and fails to satisfy points (c) and
(d) of this section.

(i) Given the wording of Rule 18(2) of Statutory
Instrument 1983 No. 873, the UKCC is opposed
to the use of a second level practitioner for the
administration of medicines other than under
the direction of a first level nurse. It is recommended that employers adopt the same stance
unless:
(1) they have provided additional instruction
relevant to the medicines likely to be encountered in a particular setting;
(2) they have undertaken an assessment of the
individual's knowledge and competence to perform the task; and
(3) they are prepared to accept the responsibility for any errors that are consequential
upon using a second level practitioner beyond
the role for which training prepared him/her.
(See BACKGROUND 1 and 2 of this paper).

(j) The principles enunciated in this section are
equally applicable to a medicine round or to the
administration of medicines within individual
care.

(k) The responsibility of the nurse varies in the
setting of a patient's home, where he/she needs to
be cognizant of the 'freedom' of the patient in his/her
own setting, and the implications of self-medication
and the possession of 'over the counter' medicines.
Where a nurse working in the community becomes
involved in obtaining prescribed medicines for patients he/she must recognise his/her responsibility
for their safe transit and correct delivery.

(l) In accordance with the requirements of the Medicines Act 1968 and the Misuse of Drugs Act 1971
and subsequent regulations there are specific arrangements for midwives working in the community, and occupational health nurses, to obtain
and administer medicines. Those relating to midwives are contained in the UKCC Midwife's Code of
Practice and those to occupational health nurses in the
Royal College of Nursing Society of Occupational
Health Nursing Information Leaflet No. 11 dated
November 1983. Also in pursuance of Regulation
10(3) of the Misuse of Drugs Regulations 1973 specific
"Group Authority" is given to certain registered
nurses employed at places of work.

5   Receiving (the patient's role)

The patient's role is as participant. The point of receiving provides the opportunity for:

(a) **Validation**

Ensuring that the patient understands the treatment, the need to complete the prescribed course and has consented to receiving it.

(b) **Education/Instruction**

Assessing and promoting the patient's knowledge and understanding regarding his/her medication, and reinforcing safety; this is essential before the patient can progress to independence. The role of the relatives and other informal carers is an important consideration in the rehabilitation of the patient.

(c) **Self-Administration**

Monitoring the patient's self-administration of prescribed medicines (where the practice is established) or preparing the patient for self-administration at home or in hospital as part of a planned programme towards independence. At home and at work account must be taken of the possibility of self-medication with non-prescribed medicines.

6   The legislative aspect

Medicinal products are subject to legislative controls relating to their manufacture, prescription, sale, handling, storage and custody. The nurse therefore operates within a legal framework in respect of:

(a) **Supplies.** Proper procedures should be employed for ordering. Checking deliveries and maintaining records are key factors. Orders should not be such that stocks will be excessive and wastage likely.

(b) **Storage.** As well as being kept in a secure place as required by legislation, drugs should be stored in the appropriate environment as instructed by the respective manufacturers.

(c) **Stocktaking.** This involves recording, checking stocks and disposing of unwanted medicines according to legislation. Discrepancies in stocks must be reported and investigated.

Collaborative working with the Pharmacist will ensure that appropriate systems are developed in respect of these three important aspects of the process aimed at safe administration of medicines.

SUPPLEMENT SUGGESTING VARIATIONS WHICH SHOULD APPLY WHERE THE SPECIFIC FRAMEWORK IS NOT APPROPRIATE

(a) **There are certain situations in which practitioners are involved in the administration of medicines where specific factors within the preceding framework are difficult to apply or could not be applied without introducing dangerous delay and its consequent risk to patients.**

(b) These will include occupational nursing settings in industry, small hospitals with no resident medical staff and possibly some specialist units within larger hospitals and a variety of community settings.

(c) **In any situations in which practitioners may be expected or required to administer 'prescription only' medicines to patients which have not been directly prescribed for those patients by a medical practitioner who has examined and made a diagnosis, it is essential that a clear policy be determined which enables action to be taken in the patients' interests and to protect the practitioners from risk of complaint which might jeopardise their employment or professional status.**

(d) It is therefore recommended that, in any situation where practitioners might be called upon or expected to administer 'prescription only' medicines which have not been directly prescribed as a result of examination, the following principles should be agreed and set down in a local policy which is known to all practitioners likely to be involved.

(i) It should first be agreed and then set down in writing by all the doctors working within a particular setting that there are circumstances in which particular 'prescription only' medicines may be administered in advance of examination by a doctor. Where frequent staff changes make this impractical one senior doctor should be appointed by his/her colleagues to establish such policies on their behalf, with them undertaking to honour his/her decision. A review of such policies must take place annually.

(ii) The particular circumstances in which a particular 'prescription only' medicine (and its form, route, etc.) could be administered must then be the subject of specific and well documented agreement, which must have similar support.

Wherever possible agreements should, in the particular organisation to which they apply, satisfy the needs likely to emerge in paragraph 2(g) on page 318.

(iii) Except where there is an appropriate senior nurse to provide this instruction it must be the responsibility of one of the doctors working in the setting (acting on behalf of all the doctors) or, where appropriate, a pharmacist to undertake instruction of any practitioner who will be expected to administer any 'prescription only' medicine which has not been specifically prescribed, this instruction to encompass information concerning the medicine, the indications for its use, its effects and side-effects, and any contra-indications. Where an appropriate senior nurse is available for this purpose he/she must not hesitate to call upon the services of the doctor, especially in relation to aspects of diagnosis, pharmacology and prescribing.

(iv) The above instruction should conclude with an assessment of knowledge and competence which is a necessary prelude to the preparation of the written document authorising a particular practitioner to administer a particular 'prescription only' medicine without a specific prescription in a particular set of circumstances.

(v) No practitioner should be expected to accept the responsibility for administering such medicines against his/her will, and those who do accept the responsibility must remember the requirements of the UKCC Code of Professional Conduct that they acknowledge any limitations in their competence and seek appropriate instruction.

(e) **Practitioners who engage in the administration of 'prescription only' medicines which have not been specifically prescribed for a particular patient following medical examination and diagnosis in any situation where the above 5 criteria have not been fully met are rendering themselves extremely vulnerable. However, where these criteria are fully satisfied the nurse would normally be protected from the consequences of his or her actions even if made the subject of a complaint to the Statutory Regulating Bodies.**

Index